D1740042

AGEING AND INVISIBILITY

Ambient Intelligence and Smart Environments

The Ambient Intelligence and Smart Environments (AISE) book series presents the latest research results in the theory and practice, analysis and design, implementation, application and experience of *Ambient Intelligence* (AmI) and *Smart Environments* (SmE).

Coordinating Series Editor:
Juan Carlos Augusto

Series Editors:
Emile Aarts, Hamid Aghajan, Michael Berger, Vic Callaghan, Diane Cook, Sajal Das,
Anind Dey, Sylvain Giroux, Pertti Huuskonen, Jadwiga Indulska, Achilles Kameas,
Peter Mikulecký, Daniel Shapiro, Toshiyo Tamura, Michael Weber

Volume 7

Recently published in this series

ISSN 1875-4163 (print)
ISSN 1875-4171 (online)

Ageing and Invisibility

Edited by

Emilio Mordini

and

Paul de Hert

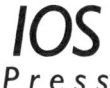

IOS Press

Amsterdam • Berlin • Tokyo • Washington, DC

© 2010 The authors and IOS Press.

All rights reserved. No part of this book may be reproduced, stored in a retrieval system, or transmitted, in any form or by any means, without prior written permission from the publisher.

ISBN 978-1-60750-614-0 (print)
ISBN 978-1-60750-615-7 (online)
Library of Congress Control Number: 2010933423

Publisher
IOS Press BV
Nieuwe Hemweg 6B
1013 BG Amsterdam
Netherlands
fax: +31 20 687 0019
e-mail: order@iospress.nl

Distributor in the USA and Canada
IOS Press, Inc.
4502 Rachael Manor Drive
Fairfax, VA 22032
USA
fax: +1 703 323 3668
e-mail: iosbooks@iospress.com

LEGAL NOTICE
The publisher is not responsible for the use which might be made of the following information.

PRINTED IN THE NETHERLANDS

Ageing and Invisibility
E. Mordini and P. de Hert (Eds.)
IOS Press, 2010
© *2010 The authors and IOS Press. All rights reserved.*

v

FOREWORD BY LAMBERT VAN NISTELROOIJ MEP

ICT and ageing: building the Silver Economy

Ageing and ICT

The direction of the demographic change societies all over the world are experiencing is clear: the population is ageing at a breathtaking pace. The number of people over 50 will increase by 35% in 2050, the number of people over 80 by 300%. This puts our social health- and social security systems under pressure.

ICT can assist the elderly in carrying out their daily work, keeping intact their social network, monitoring their health condition and improve their security. It can play an important role in enabling the elderly to stay at home longer and in good health while increasing their quality of living by supplying ways of keeping in touch with their loved ones. It can enable them to order their food and medicines online and participate in systems for monitoring and diagnosis.

These hardware and software applications should be integrated, easy to operate, economical and reliable. You can think of everything from consumer electronics, smart textiles, smart homes, telematics services to wellness and medical equipment.

In addition, products and services aimed at the ageing population can boost our economy. This is what I call the 'Silver Economy'.

The Ambient Assisted Living initiative

In Parliament, I was the speaker for the European Peoples Party (EPP) on the EU Ambient Assisted Living (AAL) Programme.

The AAL Programme consists of four parts: research, development, legislation and co-operation (with industry). Between now and 2013, the EU, the Member States and the private sector are investing more than 1 billion euros in research and innovation for ageing well, stimulating employment, innovation, competitiveness and the quality of life of the elderly.

Local and regional 'smart care' initiatives

Next to (inter)national programmes like AAL, there is an increasing role for regional cooperation in this field as they know best about local wishes and possibilities. The province of Noord-Brabant, where I was a regional minister for 12 years, recently took the initiative to launch a €9 million programme named 'Smart Care'. The programme is designed to provide tailor-made solutions in the region in the field of ICT solutions and services for the elderly. Such initiatives are important to scale up our research and development to the markets, all over Europe.

Ethical issues

The use of ICT involves serious ethical questions. It is encouraging to see that a recent SENIOR survey shows that 51% of surveyed IT companies in Europe have ethical codes. Another 31% will adopt one in the near future. Social aspects of ICT for ageing societies are very important: the discussion should not only be about techniques and research. The solutions should be people-centred, and supported by the networks people use.

Thank you, SENIOR!

The SENIOR project shows how the ethical aspects can be integrated into the evolution of new technologies. The European Parliament and the new European Commission will soon start with the mid-term evaluation of the 7th Framework Programme for research. Your approach should be safeguarded and funded in the years to come.

Thank you for the excellent research work and the debate on the underlying values for our Silver Economy.

Lambert van Nistelrooij
Member of the European Parliament for the EPP group
Vice president of the Intergroup on Ageing and Intergenerational Solidarity
February 2010

ABOUT THE AUTHORS

Emilio Mordini is a clinical psychoanalyst and founding director of the Centre for Science, Society and Citizenship.
emilio.mordini@cssc.eu

Paul De Hert is a core member of LSTS. He currently holds the chair of Human Rights, Legal theory, (European and Constitutional) Criminal Law of the VUB, where he also leads the Research Group on Human Rights (HUMR). Paul De Hert is a core member of LSTS the interdisciplinary Research Group on Law Science Technology & Society at VUB.
paul.de.hert@vub.ac.be

Eugenio Mantovani is a doctoral researcher at LSTS.
emantova@vub.ac.be

David Wright is the Managing Partner of Trilateral Research & Consulting LLP, which is based in London and which he co-founded in 2004.
david.wright@trilateralresearch.com

Kush Wadhwa is the Founder and Managing Director of Global Security Intelligence Limited, a London-based research consultancy.
kwadhwa@globalseci.com

Jesper Thestrup is the Managing Director and principal shareholder in In-JeT ApS. He has been involved in IST programme activities for more than 10 years.
jth@in-jet.dk

Guido Van Steendam is professor in ethics of science and philosophy of health care at the KULeuven, university Leuven. He teaches in the Faculties of Medical and natural Sciences, as well as in the Higher Institute of Philosophy.
guido.vansteendam@cs.kuleuven.be

Ira Vater is a partner of EBA where she is mainly responsible for project management of EU funded projects.
ira.vater@ebanet.eu

Antonio D'Amico has 15 years professional experience in the sectors of telecommunications, multimedia and information market.
antonio.damico@iaegeie.eu

GENERAL INTRODUCTION

The book *Ageing and Invisibility* flows from the research work carried out during 24 months within the EU FP7 project SENIOR, which is the acronym for 'Social ethical and privacy needs in ICT for older people'. SENIOR was asked to provide 'a systematic assessment of the social, ethical, and privacy issues involved in ICT and Ageing, to understand what lessons should be learned from current technological trends, and to plan strategies for governing future trends.'[1] While new technologies hold great promise, they also pose risks to privacy and ethical principles. The SENIOR consortium undertook to investigating how new ICT can meet the needs of senior citizens without compromising privacy and ethics. The project was based on three main principles which determined its main phases – inclusion as goal, dialogue as instrument, and technology design as target. As an FP7 support action, SENIOR was part of the wider EU strategy established by the Lisbon Treaty aimed at eradicating poverty and social exclusion by 2010. The Riga Ministerial Declaration on e-inclusion of June 2006 identified six themes for social inclusion. One of these themes was e-Ageing, whose goal is to empower older people to fully participate in the economy and society.[2] The SENIOR contribution to policy implementation has been twofold. First, SENIOR described the ethical and privacy impacts of ICT for inclusion. This objective was achieved through a series of thematic expert meetings organised throughout the year 2008. Such meetings (i) defined ICT systemic solutions and technology trends, (ii) discussed relevant ethical and privacy issues and (iii) weighed the trade-offs between privacy, ethics and technological innovation. Second, the project identified ICT services and solutions that avoid exclusion and promote inclusion of senior citizens. During the year 2009, SENIOR collected a series of best practices showing how ethics and privacy principles can be incorporated in technology design. The inclusion target was pursued by setting out key actions, highlighting risks and grounding milestones.

During two years of activity, the team of SENIOR reached out to a great number of stakeholders including policy-makers, industry, academia, civil society organisations and regional and local authorities, among others. The SENIOR team investigated and reported on the relevant legal, social and ethical dimensions of ageing and ICT. This work was turned into deliverables, papers, articles in peer-reviewed journals and a book of interviews with experts from around the world.[3] This is the second and last book produced by SENIOR. SENIOR's last effort aims to provide researchers, civil society organisations, policy-makers and companies with a resource to know more about some ethical, social and legal aspects involved in the inclusion of older persons

---

[1] From the project's Description of Work. SENIOR ran from January 2008 to December 2009. Partners are: Centre for Science, Society and Citizenship, Italy; European Business Associates Srl, Italy; Global Security Intelligence Limited, United Kingdom; Inclusion Alliance for Europe, Romania; IN-JET, Denmark; International Forum for Biophilosophy, Belgium; Trilateral Research & Consulting LLP, United Kingdom; Vrije Universiteit Brussel, Belgium. EU funding amounts to € 950.000. Website: http://www.seniorproject.eu.

[2] The Riga Ministerial Declaration on e-inclusion of June 2006 identified six themes which the European Commission uses to foster social inclusion: e-Accessibility (make ICT accessible to all), e-Ageing (empower older people to fully participate in the economy and society), e-Competences (equip citizens with the knowledge and skills for lifelong learning), Socio-Cultural e-Inclusion (enable minorities, migrants and marginalised young people), Geographical e-Inclusion (increase the social and economic well-being of people in economically disadvantaged areas with the help of ICT), and Inclusive e-Government (encouraging increased public participation in democracy). Further policy documents that constitute SENIOR background are COM (2005) 425/F of 13/09/2005; COM (2007) 332/F of 14/06/2007 and the COMMISSION STAFF WORKING PAPER [COM(2007)332] – Brussels, 14 June 2007 SEC (2007) 811

[3] Available at www. seniorproject.eu

in the Information Society. Readers with an interest in ageing societies will find here an overview on the process of e-inclusion of older persons in the EU's Information Society. Highlights are put on the EU policy background for e-inclusion (chapter one); chapter two considers critically the active ageing spirit of e-inclusion; the legal framework for e-inclusion of senior citizens is described in chapter three; given their importance, the rights to privacy and data protection and the notion of consent are given space in chapters four and five. Chapter six explains why the convergence of technologies is significant in terms of support to the elderly, what are the risks and barriers to take-up of ICT amongst senior citizens. An important element in the e-inclusion strategies has been the identification and promotion of good practices. Chapter seven discusses the merits of good practices exercise. Chapter eight takes *congedo* and suggests a few recommendations.

As chapter one explains, the relation between e-inclusion and the broader socio-economic objectives of the Union interrogates a period of time that goes from the origins of the Information Society in 1993 to the present. Since its definition at the beginning of the nineties, the Union's social and economic policies – gathered today under the formula of the 'Lisbon process' – have pursued, along macroeconomic deflationary objectives (the Maastricht criteria), an expansion of the number of people who stay active, employed or independent in society. Since the year 2000, the EU's policies on the information society have been integrated into the broader European Union social and economic policies. Within this framework, e-inclusion is meant to assist – as far as this is possible, necessary or desirable – (active) ageing. Demographic ageing announces hard times for the welfare state as we know it; politics press on the Information Society to devise solutions which can help organise risks and opportunities, social needs and economic priorities, of an increasing ageing population. As the reader will see, both the 1993 White Paper as well as the Lisbon strategy (2000–2010, and, later, the Commission's EU 2020 policy) bring together economic growth goals, technological development and the social needs of an ageing population. Since Lisbon 2000, public policy engages different stakeholders within the internal market, including social partners, end-user organisations, governments, technology developers, service providers and so on. In the future EU 2020, to assure stronger governance the Lisbon method is expected to deliver Information Society indicators which may include ethical, privacy and social needs of 'e-ageing'.

Drawing from literary sources, chapter two elaborates a series of reflections that emerged during the debates, conferences, meetings and talks held during the SENIOR project (2008–2009). In particular, chapter two discusses active ageing and e-inclusion policies. It acknowledges that ageing actively and living independently are of great value to elderly persons; it also acknowledges that technologies can play an important role in this. However, this chapter also suggests that social polices such as those on active ageing can bring with them practices that oddly counter their goal, the well being or protection of the aged. The lives of elderly people, we argue, today as well as a hundred years ago, are affected by the attitude or mentality of a given society towards what is 'old'. Modern technological societies woo the idea of decelerating, arresting or postponing ageing. Such an idea finds fertile ground in the prevailing cultural, social and market-led representations of ageing, which involve a great deal of falsification and removal. The removal and falsification of ageing appear rather awkward though. Soon the old will outnumber the young: is such a society of the elderly building an image where being old means little good? We suggest that this apparent paradox be viewed in the context of demographic change and active ageing. Being old is fine on the condition that one is...not old. From an ethical point of view it is questionable whether the ostracism of ageing is 'good' or 'bad' for elderly people and/or for society as a whole. We limit ourselves to conclude that the rescuing of active ageing as the mainstream narrative on old age is problematic for a society which commends pluralism of life-styles.

The law which, in our view, is most relevant for the e-inclusion of older persons in the EU, is discussed in chapter three. At the level of European Union, the sources of law include human rights law, treaty provisions on equality and anti-discrimination directives and, as a part of the internal market, the Information Society. Human rights law is arguably the most important body of law for inclusion: the European Convention of Human Rights (1950), the Revised European Social Charter (1996) and the 2000 EU Charter of Fundamental Rights of the European Union are analysed and their relevance for older persons highlighted. In addition, international human rights law provides for an ample body of 'soft law' provisions, the so called international framework on ageing. In 2002, for instance, the UN Madrid summit invited states to mainstream soft law principles on ageing throughout their national policies. Concerning discrimination, the Treaty of Lisbon in article 9 recognises as one of the policies and activities of the Union 'adequate social protection, the fight against social exclusion, and a high level of education, training and protection of human health[4].' In the European Union *acquis*, discrimination on grounds of age is forbidden in the context of employment. Old age discrimination, however, is increasingly treated as a horizontal public policy matter, for instance, in the area of services. A growing body of regulations is adopted in the Information Society. We follow the SWAMI[5] method to enlist and illustrate some relevant areas such as interoperability, e-health, consumer protection, product safety which we deem important for ICT and the aged.

The fundamental right to private life and data protection are the object of a separate analysis in chapter four. Privacy needs in e-inclusion of elderly people, we suggest, include a protective dimension shielding the individual from undue external pressures, and an emancipatory dimension, more difficult to conceptualise, which relates to the individual need and interest in sharing life with others. Often, in concrete situations, older persons will have both interests and needs at the same time. In the Information Society, the protective function of privacy boils down to shielding older citizens from unnecessary or excessive categorisation including techniques such as spam, targeted advertisements, commercial profiling, in general when it is not clear why and for which purpose one person's preferences, tastes, etc. need to be opened up. The emancipatory function of privacy recognises the right to establish relations with others. Here the task of privacy protection is to ensure that sharing personal experiences or information takes place without the individual having to care, or to stay alert, or anxious about the fact that there is a '(data) arms race' going on behind his or her back. In this sense, the crucial function of privacy is to protect networks, such as situations of dependency, so sharing can remain a trusted interpersonal exercise.

Concerning data protection, the realisation of ubiquitous environments, in particular in the field of health care and surveillance, draws the attention to the tension between data protection and the requirements of the new ICT environment, which needs extensive data collection and profiling in order to make the user's environment act in-

---

[4] Consolidated versions of the Treaty on European Union and the Treaty on the Functioning of the European Union Official Journal C 115 of 9 May 2008.

[5] D. Wright et al., *Safeguards in a World of Ambient Intelligence,* Springer, Dordrecht, 2008.

telligently. From the European data protection regime, we identify three areas that ought to be given consideration, at least from an elderly perspective. They concern the definition and implementation of privacy by design settings and regulations; rules on the transparency and accountability of processors and controllers; and consent requirements.

The latter, consent requirements, is dealt with in a separate chapter, chapter five. Starting from an analysis of consent in human rights law, where consent is a key notion in the field of medical law, we discuss the data processing context, where consent is an increasingly formalised notion. We surmise that sociological changes in the IT society, unbalanced relations between users and client organisations, complexity of data processing and increasing situations of incapacity affecting consent in large sectors of the ageing population pose challenges to the notion of consent. The snag, from an elderly perspective, is to find solutions that, while not frustrating individual self-determination and liberty, assist, where appropriate, the individual declaration of consent so as to avoid putting excessive responsibility on him or her.

Chapter six includes a review of the state of the art of technology for inclusion of elderly people. After discussing inclusion in the context of the Internet and computer technologies, the chapter focuses on ambient technologies. The aim is to explain why the convergence of technologies is significant in terms of support of the elderly. Cases are discussed which involve applications for cognitive support, support for ADLs, communications, health and mobility. The final pages focus on the barriers inhibiting the development or adoption of these technologies and on the risks that might arise from failure of such technologies to take proper root.

An important element in the e-inclusion strategies has been the identification and promotion of good practices. Noting increased emphasis on good practices as a matter of e-inclusion strategy, chapter seven considers what good practices are, what their perceived value is and what are the criteria used for selecting them. The success in using good practices as a matter of strategy and policy is critically dependent on how they are selected and by whom and how well they are promoted or disseminated. The chapter includes four examples of good practices.

As the title of the book suggests, the benefits associated with the use of modern technologies will not come automatically. Information Society technologies do not stand apart and develop autonomously from social life; not inevitable, nor neutral, technologies are the product of the human project and the result of the work of networks of people, scientists, research leaders, companies, sponsors, politicians, investors, experts, committees, etc. which take decisions and make choices. Similarly, technological developments are given direction by narratives which emphasise contrasting views of ageing. The point the book makes is a warning: society should question itself about the use of technology to deal with ageing, whether this is ultimately ethically good, to what extent and within which limits. The risk we run is that ageing and the role of old age go in disguise and disappear from societal sight.

Finally, the authors would like to thank everyone who contributed to the SENIOR project. Special thanks go to participants to the numerous SENIOR meetings who graciously shared their insights with us and brought their experienced perspectives into the project. We gratefully acknowledge support of the European Commission services at the DG Information Society and Media, and in particular to the ICT for Inclusion unit, its head Mr. Paul Timmers and project officers Silvia Bojinova and Giorgio Zoia.

A note of special thanks goes to Valeria Balestrieri from CSSC (Rome). Without her dedication and patience this book would not have been possible.

The authors

Emilio Mordini, Paul de Hert, Eugenio Mantovani, David Wright, Kush Wadhwa, Jesper Thestrup, Guido Van Steendam, Ira Vater, Antonio D'Amico.

CONTENTS

Ageing and Invisibility
E. Mordini and P. de Hert (Eds.)
IOS Press, 2010
© 2010 The authors and IOS Press. All rights reserved.
doi:10.3233/978-1-60750-615-7-1

CHAPTER ONE. THE EU AND THE E-INCLUSION OF OLDER PERSONS

By Paul De Hert and Eugenio Mantovani

INTRODUCTION

Since its definition at the beginning of the nineties, the Union's policies on economy and occupation – gathered today under the formula of the 'Lisbon process' – have pursued, along macroeconomic deflationary objectives (the Maastricht criteria), an expansion of the number of people who stay active, employed or independent in society. The policy objective of expanding active citizenry targets, for reasons which are both of economic sustainability (efficiency) and of social justice (equity), groups of persons who are excluded, disadvantaged or more vulnerable than those living within the boundaries of active life. In the wake of demographic change, such a group is, in the view espoused by the EU, elderly people.

The expansion of active citizenry to the aged elicits multi-disciplinary policy initiatives in spheres as diverse as social policy, transport, environment, family relations, health care, urban planning. One of such domains gaining momentum is Information Society. Rapidly developed since the beginning of the nineties – in the same years of the development of the European Union and European employment strategy – information society is today an integral part of the Lisbon agenda. Indeed, ageing and information and communication technologies (ICT) represents one the six thematic themes of the i2010 European Union policy initiative on e-inclusion. Within this framework, e-inclusion is meant to assist – as far as this is possible, necessary or desirable – active ageing.

This chapter seeks to illustrate how the policy of e-inclusion for elderly people came about and describes its relationship with European Union (EU) social and economic policies. We will review the main stages that have accompanied the emergence and organisation of an information society (IS) in Europe from the beginning of the 1990s to present. We endeavour to show how the development of the information society relates to the framework of EU growth and employment strategies drawing from a number of EU policy documents, communications, directives and action plans that have been issued in this period of time.

Contextual conditions at the beginning of the 1990s. The end of bipolarism; TEU and GATT.

The concept and the idea of an information society emerged in the 1970s in the United States (US), Canada, Europe and Japan.[1] In the EU, the information society

---

[1] For the USA, M.U. Porat, *The information economy: Definition and Measurement*, Washington, DC, Government Printing Office, 1977; for France, P. Nora, A. Minc, *L'informatisation de la societe*, La Documentation Francaise, Paris, 1978 (transl. *The computerisation of society,* intro by D. Bell., MIT

first appeared on the political agenda after the publication of the US National Information Infrastructure Initiative in 1993.[2] Europe's information society moved its first steps in times of important political, social and economic changes.[3] Suffice is to remember that in 1992 the Maastricht Treaty was signed. The European Union came about in the aftermath of the fall of the Berlin wall, the collapse of the USSR, the reunification of Germany, the break up of Yugoslavia and the first Gulf War. By 1992, the European Union achieved the completion of the internal market, started in 1986-87 with the Single European Act. When the Treaty of Maastricht came into force in 1993 the Community's competence had been extended to the growing sector of telecommunication and ICT. In those years a truly global electronic market was emerging in the field of telephony and GSM mobile communications. Various public bodies (such as ITU, ISO, ETSI, CEPT etc.) already supervise agreements in the telecommunications sector, give advices of on technical issues and promote the interconnection and interoperability of networks, standards and national frequencies. At international level, Europe is engaged in a number of agreements concluded under the auspices of the WTO, and the GATT, GATS and TRIPS agreements, which concern also the information society.[4] From an economic perspective, at the beginning of the nineties Europe was lagging behind[5] featuring high rates of unemployment over several years and across large sectors of society.[6] Furthermore, Europe began to feel the effects of the progressive ageing of its population on welfare systems and intergenerational relationships.[7]

Press, Cambridge (MA), 1980). For Japan, J. Masuda, 'The Information Society as Post-Industrial Society,' Institute for the Information Society, Tokyo, 1980 (US edition, Washington, DC: World Future Society, 1981).

[2] US House of Representatives, 'National Information Infrastructure Act. Report To Accompany H.R. 1757', 103d Congress, 1st Session, 1993. H.R. 1757 is the 1993 National Information Infrastructure Act of 1993. Full text available at http://www.eric.ed.gov/ERICDocs/data/ericdocs2sql/content_storage_01/0000019b/80/15/3d/9a.pdf (accessed on February 2010).

[3] There is ample literature on the origins of the information society. See, e.g, J. L. Selvaggio (ed.), *Information society. Economic Social & Structural issues*, Lawrence Erlbaum Associates Publishers, Hove and London, 1989; C. May, *The Information Society. A sceptical view*, Polity Press, Cambridge (UK), 2002. K. Ducatel, J. Webster, and W. Herrmann, *The Information Society in Europe. Work and Life in an Age of Globalisation*, Rowman & Little field Publishers, Inc., Lanham-Boulder-New York-Oxford, 2000.

[4] See GATS commitments and obligations, including Articles VI (Domestic regulation), XVI (Market access), and XVII (National Treatment), and the GATS Annex on Telecommunications ('measures affecting access to and use of Public Telecommunications Transport Networks and Services' (PTTN&S), including Sections 4 and 5. See also WTO, Dispute Settlement Body, *Mexico - Measures Affecting Telecommunications Services,* complaint by the United States, 1 May 2004, DS204. http://www.wto.org/english/tratop_e/dispu_e/cases_e/ds204_e.htm . See also B. Cammaerts, J-C. Burgelman (eds), *Beyond competition: broadening the scope of telecommunications policy*, VUB University Press, Brussels, 2000.

[5] International Monetary Fund (IMF), *World Economic Outlook*, Washington, October 1993.

[6] OECD, *JOBS strategy. Pushing ahead with the strategy,* Paris, 1996. http://www.oecd.org/dataoecd/57/7/1868601.pdf

[7] Intergenerational equity or generation divide refers to conflicts that arise in the allocation of scarce public resources and in terms of sharing the financial implications of population ageing. Consider, e.g., social security, education or health, gaps in the aspirations of the young generation, the threat of limited opportunities, terms of pay, job security, access to housing. See European Commission, 'Opportunities, access and solidarity: towards a new social vision for 21st century Europe', Communication from the Commission to the European Parliament, the Council, the European Economic and Social Committee and the Committee of the Regions, COM(2007) 726 final, Brussels, 20 Nov 2007, p.8. See below.

The 1993 Delors' White Paper. Active labour policies and integration of employment policies

In 1994, a study conducted by the Paris-based Organization for Economic Cooperation and Development (OECD) identified the causes of Europe's setback in the structure of its labour market. The OECD 'Jobs Study' lamented that employment policies were delaying adaptation of the workforce to the changing conditions and demands of the market.[8] On a similar string, within the European Union, the 1993 'White Paper on growth, competition and employment' suggested the Community's low employment creation could be traced back to the 1970s 'when it proved unable to increase its rate of job creation to match the increase in the number of people seeking employment'.[9] To reverse this trend, the White Paper advocated proactive labour market policies and the use of all regulatory instruments - from taxation, education, health care, to social security -- to spur higher employability (White Paper, p.135). Goetschy[10], who describes the White Paper as Jacques Delors' 'last major contribution before his departure, a sort of legacy', explains: 'The White Paper attempted to combine contradictory elements. The ambition was to meet the convergence criteria for EMU [the European Monetary Union], the implications of which were deflationary, and yet to achieve higher levels of employment. To meet such a challenge, one of the means was to broaden the debate beyond negative flexibility to more active labour market policies. The objective was also to integrate employment policy with other policy issues (fiscal, social protection, environment, equality of opportunities for men and women, new family patterns, demographic changes), linking Keynesian and supply-side measures.' In other words, it was suggested to promote higher, though not full, employability through structural reforms of the labour market while limiting public spending within the perimeters imposed on public debt by the economic and monetary union (EMU) (White Paper, p.31). In line with the conclusions reached by the OECD's Jobs strategy mentioned above, public employment policies would have to stimulate entry and promote longer stay in active productive life. The targets of 'active policies' would be primarily those groups who, being outside the labour market, live on and spend the resources of the welfare state. 'It is no longer possible to leave masses of unemployed people in Europe unoccupied', presses on the White Paper. 'Such is, however, the structure of

---

[8] OECD, *JOBS STUDY. Facts, Analysis, Strategies*, Paris, 1994, in particular part three, available at http://www.oecd.org/dataoecd/42/51/1941679.pdf. See also *Jobs Strategy. Pushing ahead with the strategy*, Paris, 1996, p. 19 where the OECD suggests that '…Although competition thereby increases efficiency and raises incomes, it means that companies and workers must be able to adapt in order to prosper.'
[9] European Commission, 'White Paper on Growth, Competitiveness, Employment: The Challenges and Ways Forward into the 21st Century', Brussels, 5 December 1993, COM (93) 700 final/A and B. Bulletin of the European Communities, Supplement 6/93, p.41-42. The architect of the White Paper was the head of the European Commission and former French Finance Minister M. Jacques Delors. Hereinafter (White Paper, p. 41-42) in the text.
[10] J. Goetschy, 'The European Employment Strategy: Genesis and Development', in *European Journal of Industrial Relations*, vol.5, n.2, p.117-137. The text is available free of charge at http://ec.europa.eu/governance/areas/group8/contribution_strategy-genesis_en.pdf . See also S. Klosse, 'The European Employment Strategy: Which Way Forward?, in *The International Journal of Comparative Labour Law and Industrial Relations*, 2005, vol.21, n.1, p. 5-36. A. Sapir, 'Globalisation and the Reform of European Social Models', Background document for the presentation at ECOFIN Informal Meeting, Manchester, 9 September 2005. B.H. Casey, 'The OECD Jobs Strategy and the Employment Strategy: two views of the labour market and the welfare state?' in *European Journal of Industrial Relations*, 2004, vol.10, n.3, p. 329-352.

government spending on unemployment: roughly two thirds of public expenditure on the unemployed goes on assistance and the remainder on active measures' (White Paper, p.18). By targeting groups excluded from employment Europe would a) reduce public expenditure on social security and b) be able to allocate more resources to active citizenry measures instead, such as education, training and long life learning (White Paper, p.12). More employment would then provide the fiscal base necessary to support the cost of pensions and welfare services, particularly in a context of demographic change.[11]

One of the most important consequences of the White Paper was to focus efforts, rather on the demand side, on the supply side, that is, to "activate" the reserves of work and the consumption capacities latent in the population, in particular women and also persons with disabilities, immigrants, and older adults.[12] Older persons, however, together with their work and consumption capacities, do not feature prominently in the White Paper, more concerned and focussed on enhancing participation of women and youth. The aged come under the spotlight in the mid-1990s when it becomes clear that Europe's working population - and consumption capacities - is affected by changes in Europe's demographic structure.[13]

Demographic change and Population Ageing

According to demographers we live in a demographic transition period which occupies a one hundred year time period, from 1950 to 2050.[14] This demographic transition is the result of the combined effect of two factors, 1) decline in mortality rate (higher number of people reaching old ages) and 2) decline in fertility rate (less children are born). Demographers foresee that by 2050 life expectancy in European countries will have risen to 82 years for men, and 87.4 for women.[15] As a

---

[11] P. Villa, 'La Strategia Europea per l'Occupazione e le Pari Opportunità tra uomini e donne', in M. Rossilli, *I diritti delle donne nell'Unione Europea. Cittadine, migranti, schiave*, Ediesse, Roma, 2009, p.163-199.

[12] Villa, Ibid., 169-172.

[13] Martijn Van der steen, 'Ageing or silvering? Political debate about ageing in the Netherlands', in *Science and Public Policy*, 35(8), October 2008, pages 575-583, where the author demonstrates that narratives on demographic ageing influence policy making. See below.

[14] UN DESA, Population Division, *Population Ageing 2006 Wall Chart*, August 2007, http://www.un.org/esa/population/publications/ageing/ageing2006.htm. Between 2005 and 2050, half of the increase in the world population will be accounted for by a rise in the population aged 60 years or over, whereas the number of children (persons under age 15) will decline slightly. Furthermore, in the more developed regions, the population aged 60 or over is expected to nearly double (from 245 million in 2005 to 406 million in 2050), whereas that of persons under age 60 will likely decline (from 971 million in 2005 to 839 million in 2050). See also Antonio Golini, demographer at Rome's La Sapienza University, in Paola Pilati, 'In pensione si andrà a settant'anni', *L'Espresso* (Italy) 6 agosto 2009.

[15] This point is repeatedly mentioned in various documents from the European Commission, the OECD and many other organisations. See, for example, Council Directive 2000/78/EC of 27 November 2000 establishing a general framework for equal treatment in employment and occupation ('the European Employment Directive'); 'Increasing labour-force participation and promoting active ageing', Joint Report released on 24 Jan 2002 and adopted by the Council (Employment and Social Policy) at its session on 7 March 2002; 'Increasing the employment of older workers and delaying the exit from the labour market', Communication from the Commission to the Council, the European Parliament, the European Economic and Social Committee ad the Committee of the Regions, of the European Communities, Brussels, 3 March 2004, COM(2004) 146 final; 'Working together for growth and jobs: A new start for the Lisbon Strategy, Communication to the Spring European Council from President Barroso in agreement with Vice-President Verheugen', Brussels, 2 February 2005, COM (2005) 24; Communication from the Commission on the Social Agenda, Brussels, 9 February 2005, COM(2005)

consequence, it is foreseen that there will be more old people than young people. More precisely, anticipatory knowledge indicates that by the year 2050 the number of people aged 60 and above will be three times what it was in 1950. By 2050, twenty five per cent of the EU's population will be over 60.[16] In the UK the number of people aged 65 (not 60 as below) and over is expected to exceed the number of people under 16 by 2021.[17]

From a socio-economic perspective, the relationship between number of people in retirement age (65 years and over) and the working age population (from 15 to 64 years) represents what is called 'old age dependency ratio'. The contraction of the working age population is expected to decrease by 48 million between 2005 and 2050.[18] For Eurostat, this means that if current trends prevail until 2050 'anyone in his working age then might have to provide for twice as many retired people as is usual today.'[19] Among the retirement age population, the fraction of people which is going to increase the most is, expectedly, that of older persons reaching very old age, 80 years old or more.[20] As a consequence, also the 'care dependency rate' may increase, i.e. the relationship between persons affected by a form of age-related cognitive of physical disability and the persons who care for them.[21] Currently, more is spent privately on aids, adaptations and assistive technologies than is spent by public authorities. States in the EU though spend between 30 and 40% of total health expenditures on elderly persons aged above 65. For health care, demographic changes may lead to increased public spending in the range of 0.7 to 2.3 percentage points of GDP over the next fifty years, with some Member States projecting increases above 2 percentage points. For long-term care, ageing would lead to increases in expenditure

---

33 final; European Commission, 'i2010 – A European Information Society for growth and employment', Communication from the Commission to the Council, the European Parliament, the European Economic and Social Committee and the Committee of the Regions, Brussels, 1 June 2005, COM(2005) 229 final. See also OECD, *Live Longer, Work Longer: A synthesis report*, Paris, 2006; N. Eberstadt and G. Hans, 'Healthy Old Europe', in *Foreign Affairs*, May/June 2007.

[16] European Commission, 'Accompanying document to the Communication from the Commission to the European Parliament, the Council, the European Economic and Social Committee and the Committee of the Regions, Ageing well in the Information Society', Staff Working Document, SEC(2007) 811, Brussels, 14 June 2007, p.6.

[17] United Kingdom, Office for National Statistics (ONS), Social Trends survey, Population ageing, 27 August 2009, http://www.statistics.gov.uk/cci/nugget.asp?ID=949

[18] European Commission, 'The Demographic Future of Europe – from Challenge to Opportunity', Communication from the Commission, COM (2006) 571 final, Brussels, 12 October 2006, pp.4-5. For an overview see also *The Economist*, 'Special report on ageing population', 27 June – 3 July, 2009.

[19] Eurostat, *Living conditions in Europe. Data 2002-2005*, Brussels, 2007, p.15.

[20] Eurostat, *The Social Situation in the European Union 2005-2006. The Balance between generation in an Ageing Europe*, Brussels, 2006. See also Eurostat, *The Life of Men and Women in Europe: A Statistical Portrait*, Brussels, 2008. According to this document, the proportion of very old people (aged 80 and more) is expected to almost triple in the EU-27, from 4% in 2005 to 11% in 2050, with the highest proportions expected in Italy, Germany and Spain. It is worth noting that the population aged 55 to 64 will also grow considerably over the next fifteen years.

[21] Dependency implies a disability which requires the provision of a care service. ADL dependency refers to difficulties in performing at least one Activity of Daily Living (ADL). These activities are listed in the Katz ADL scale and include bathing, dressing, feeding etc. See Katz S., Ford A.B., Moskowitz R.W., Jackson B.A., Jaffer M.W., *'Studies of illness in the aged. The Index of ADL: A standardized measure of biological and psychosocial function'*, in JAMA, 1963; 21: 94 – 919. Quoted from Sanna Räty, Arpo Aromaa, and Päivikki Koponen (National Public Health Institute, KTL Department of health and functional capacity), *Measurement of physical functioning in comprehensive national health surveys - ICF as a framework*, August 2003, especially pages 29-30. Available at http://ec.europa.eu/health/ph_projects/2000/monitoring/fp_monitoring_2000_annexe15_04_en.pdf

ranging from 0.2 to 2.5 percentage points of GDP – most notably in Member States having strong traditions of formally provided long-term care.[22]

A certain narrative develops based on anticipatory knowledge

It is against this background that Europe's Information Society unfolds. Keywords of this period are economic growth, social cohesion, employment strategies, and demographic ageing. In support to European policy making and, later, to the inclusion of older persons in the information society, a certain EU policy narrative outlines challenges and opportunities that lay ahead when the demographic mosaic of Europe predictably changes. Before proceeding to illustrate the policy factors that have accompanied the development of the EU policy architecture for the inclusion of older persons in the Information society, which is the goal of this chapter, it is important to bear in mind, as a caveat, the limits of any policy narrative or policy making discourse 'based on the future', such as population ageing. Indeed, the knowledge on which policy strategies to meet the challenges and opportunities of demographic ageing is, however well documented and accurate, necessarily 'anticipatory' or 'predictive' knowledge. It is, as Marteen Van der Steen nicely illustrated focussing on the case of The Netherlands, knowledge foundered on a blend of facts about the present and then on assumptions, aspirations, or predictions about what the future will be.[23] Skimming through reports and studies one stumbles across titles such as 'grey ageing', indicating a general worsening of conditions for all, including the youth; 'silver ageing', indicating ageing related new life chances and, mostly, a growth market sector, or 'intergenerational crisis', signifying feuds between social groups, the youth and the old, and suggesting changing circumstances for social justice. These narratives, contends Van der Steen, are based on facts available *today*, but give shape to visions of the post-demographic change society of *tomorrow*. Critically, by insisting on what the shift in demographic balance will do to society, grey, silver intergenerational crisis narratives give direction to rules-setting institutions, research planning, local governments projects, etc. 'Just as a researcher who anticipates that ageing will be one of the most important problems for the coming decades not only predicts a possible future, but also makes the case for further investments in research on that important topic', Van der Steen states, so governments drive investments, cut or increase taxes or social services or take any other decisions pleading on that anticipatory knowledge. Future narratives can be powerful frames for change. What is more, when evidence-based reasoning is associated with predictive 'what if' knowledge, the decision taking process tends to forget or ignore the 'ambiguous nature of anticipatory knowledge'. Anticipatory knowledge speaks the language plurality, as no one can foresee with certainty what the future is going to be.[24]

---

[22] Economic Policy Committee and DG ECFIN, Budgetary challenges posed by ageing populations: the impact on public spending on pensions, health and long-term care for the elderly and possible indicators of the long-term sustainability of public finances, Brussels, 24 October, 2001, EPC/ECFIN/630-EN final. See also by the EPC 'The impact of ageing on public expenditure, 2006 and the 2009 Ageing Report: Economic and budgetary projections for the EU-27 Member States (2008-2060)', Brussels, 2009. European Social Network, *Long-term care for older people. Statistical background 2. Present and projected expenditures by types of care*, Brussels, 2006, p. 7-8.
[23] Martijn Van der Steen, 'Ageing or silvering? Political debate about ageing in the Netherlands', op.cit.
[24] Ibid., p.582.

Having said that, in this chapter, we revise a list of policy documents that, in our view, have given shape to the EU's vision of the Information Society in times population ageing.

I. BUILDING THE INFORMATION SOCIETY (1993-1997)

One of the objectives of the 1993 White Paper was to activate the dormant production and consumption capacities of society. This required the activation of all policy resources, from social policies to transport, environment, family relations health care and so on. One domain rapidly gaining momentum was that of Information Society technologies. The birth of the information society is related to the White Paper's strategy for growth and occupation, mentioned above. In effect, the first response to the 1993 US National Information Infrastructure Initiative came with the influential 1993 Delors' White paper.[25] Further to the White paper, in December 1993, the European Council appointed a committee to detail 'specific measures to be taken into consideration […] for the infrastructures in the sphere of information.'[26] The committee requested the European Commission to draft a report to be presented for possible adoption at the European Council of the 24 and 25 June 1994 in Corfu, Greece. In response, the European Commission's DG VIII (Industry) set up a group of nineteen industry experts chaired by the then Commissioner Martin Bangemann from Germany.[27] The group's task was to spell out 'challenges' and suggest 'pathways' to the information highways of the 21st century and wrap them up in a report which became known as the 'Bangemann report'. The report paper consisted of a six-chaptered document reflecting the issues dealt with by the US National Information Infrastructure initiative.[28]

Set up clear competitive rules, the market will drive

In their message to the EU Council, experts from the industrial sector point out that 'information and communications technologies are generating a new industrial revolution already as significant and far-reaching as those of the past' (Bangemann Report, p. 5). The experts call on Europe to create an information society and encourage a coordinated European approach. The report seeks regulatory reforms without which, it is warned, 'our companies will lack the commercial muscle to win a share of the enormous global opportunities which lie ahead. Our companies will migrate to more attractive locations to do business. Our export markets will evaporate' (Bangemann Report, p. 8). To avoid this scenario, the group recommends

---

[25] European Commission, White Paper, op.cit., Theme I: Information Networks, p. 22-27. See also A. Henten, K.E. Skouby, M. Falch, 'European Planning for an Information Society', in *Telematics and Informatics*, 1996, Vol. 13. No. 213, p. 177-190.
[26] European Council, Brussels, 10-11 December 1993, EC Bulletin, n.12, p.10.
[27] Members of the High Level Group on the Information Society were: Martin Bangemann, Enrico Cabral da Fonseca, Peter Davis, Carlo de Benedetti, Pehr Gyllenhammar, Lothar Hunsel, Pierre Lescure, Pascual Maragall, Gaston Thorn, Candido Velazquez-Gastelu, Peter Bonfield, Etienne Davignon, Jean-Marie Descarpentries, Brian Ennis, Hans-Olaf Henkel, Anders Knutsen, Constantin Makropoulos, Romano Prodi, Jan Timmer, and Heinrich von Pierer.
[28] The text of the report is available at http://www.cyber-rights.org/documents/bangemann.htm#chap1, or http://www.epractice.eu/en/library/281360, last accessed on November 2009. In what follows we draw and quote from the version provided by the e-practice library. Hereinaftre, the Bangemann report in the text.

three major regulatory initiatives: 1) dismantling telecommunications monopolies, 2) reducing the cost of electronic communications by 'removing non-commercial political burdens and budgetary constraints imposed on telecommunications operators', and 3) ensuring uniform technical and legal standards coordinated with developments outside the European Union by setting 'clear rules, within a single, fair and competitive framework' (Bangemann Report, p. 12). Once regulation is in place, the infrastructures of the nascent information society should be entrusted to market and free competition. The formula proposed is catchy and straightforward: 'the market will drive ... the prime task of government is to safeguard competitive forces' (Bangemann Report, p. 9).

Though necessary pre-conditions, technical and regulatory measures may not be sufficient to guide the transition of Europe towards the Information Society.[29] The high level group seems to be aware of the risk of a digital divide between 'haves and have-nots', 'a society in which only a part of the population has access to new technology, is comfortable using it and can fully enjoy its benefits.' The group also warns against the risk that individuals will reject the new information culture and its instruments' (Bangemann Report, p. 7). Concerning the risk of digital divide, it is recommended that 'fair access to the infrastructure be guaranteed to all, as will provision of universal service, the definition of which must evolve in line with the technology' (Bangemann Report, p. 7). Education, training and promotion of ICT should be 'a priority task' of the Community's life-long education and vocational training competence. In order to stem the risk that individuals will reject the 'new information culture and instruments,' it is important to convince people that 'new technologies hold out the prospect of a major step forward towards a European society less subject to such constraints as rigidity, inertia and compartmentalization', and that they unleash 'unlimited potential for acquiring knowledge, innovation and creativity' (Bangemann Report, p. 5-9).

The Bangemann report was adopted without any reservation during the 1994 European Council meeting in Corfu and it became the Action Plan on Europe's Way to the Information Society (APEWIS).[30] In 1995, the Action Plan formed the backbone of European negotiations at the G7 Ministerial conference on the Information society in Brussels.[31] On that occasion, the Brussels G7 summit, the

---

[29] The list is very long: Interconnection of networks and interoperability of services and applications are recommended as primary Union objective as well as a review of the European standardization process. As a matter of urgency, international, long distance and leased line tariffs should be brought down into line with rates practised in other advanced industrialised regions and by the fair sharing of public service obligations among operators. European markets should also able to find its counterpart in markets and networks of other regions of the world. It is therefore of paramount importance for Europe takes 'adequate steps to guarantee equal access.' Eventually, the group recommends the establishment at the European level of an authority that oversees the deregulation and liberalization of the ICT market. In addition, a common and agreed regulatory framework should be created for the protection of intellectual property rights, privacy and security of information. *Ibid.* p. 12-15.

[30] European Commission, 'Action Plan on the Europe's Way to the Information Society (APEWIS)', COM (94)347, Brussels, 19 July 1994. See also the comments of the European Parliament in 'Report on 'Europe and the global information society. Recommendations to the European Council - a communication from the Commission of the European Communities: 'Europe's way to the information society: an action plan', Committee on Economic and Monetary Affairs and Industrial Policy, Rapporteur: Mr. Fernand Herman (COM(94)0347 - C4-0093/94)', (PE 217.506/fin., A4-0244/96), Brussels and Strasbourg, 16 July 1996.

[31] G7 summit, Ministerial conference on the information society, Brussels, 25-26 February 1995. The Bangemann report was presented as Europe and the Global information Society report. European Commission, 'Europe and the Global Information Society. Bangemann report recommendations to the European Council', Official Report, Brussels, 26 May 1994.

critics of the report gave voice to their concerns and reserves. They disapproved of the fact that the report had completely omitted to include the views of stakeholders other than industries, such as labour unions, cultural and academic institutions and citizens' organisations.[32] Opposition to the Bangemann Report invited the European Commission to give more thorough consideration to the impact that the nascent information society would have on society. The first effort in this direction materialised in 1996 when a High Level Group of Experts established under the aegis of the European Commission, Directorate General 'Employment and Social Affairs', delivered a report called 'Building the information society for us all', to which we now turn.

II. BUILDING THE INFORMATION SOCIETY FOR US ALL (1996)

1. INTRODUCTION

Well before plans for an information society unfolded in 1993, the development of personal computer technologies had aroused the interest and concern of academia. Preoccupations mostly concentrated on the possible dire consequences that the 'computerization of society' or 'telematics' would have over civil liberties, transparency of power, security of communications, respect for private life and control over personal data.[33] In the 1990s, when the construction of the information highways proceeds rapidly towards an information society, concerns were also aired about social issues: how would a computerized society affect work, education, health and, in general, the way people live together?[34]

---

[32] For a critical view on the first steps of the European Information Society and social issues see A. Torres, 'Une nouvelle vassalisation', in *Internet l'extase et l'effroi. Maniere de Voir*, Le Monde Diplomatique, Paris, August 1996. See also Sophia Kaitatzi-Whitlock, 'A redundant information society for the European Union?' in *Telematics and Informatics,* 2000, vol. 17, n.1-2, p. 39-76. See also ``Societe de l'Information Pour qui et Pourquoi?, Actes du 'Contre-Sommet du G7' organised on 24-26 February 1995 by disagreeing Members of the European Parliament and other social forces. One of the arguments of the Contre-Sommet was that, unlike the EU and the USA, other countries, such as Canada, had brought together trade unions, civil society representatives and industry since the early planning of that country information highways. On this see also D. Johnston, 'The Challenge of the Information Highway. Final Information Highway Advisory Council', Canadian Government, Ottawa, 1995. Johnston speaks of the role of government as a 'catalyst.'

[33] In 1978, the Nora and Minc report, mentioned in the Introduction, led to the adoption of a law on computer data and freedom by the French Parliament. An ad hoc Commission, the CNIL, was created to monitor its enforcement. In 1980 the OECD issued the 'Guidelines governing the protection of privacy and trans-border flows of personal data (OECD, Recommendation of the Council concerning guidelines governing the protection of privacy and transborder flows of personal data, 23rd September, 1980. In 1981, the Council of Europe opened to signature Convention 108 for the Protection of Individuals with regard to Automatic Processing of Personal Data (see also Council of Europe 1987: Recommendation R (87) 15 regulating the use personal data in the police sector). In 1995, the European Union adopted Directive 95/46/EC on the protection of individuals with regard to the processing of personal data and on the free movement of such data. On the data protection EU legal framework see Chapter 3.

[34] Already the Nora and Minc report announced social, economic and also political changes upon the emergence of *telematique*. Telematics was seen by these authors as 'increasing productivity, but causing short term unemployment'; [...] 'fostering administrative decentralisation and promote competitiveness of small and medium sizes businesses'; [...] 're-creating an information agora that would call into question the elitist distribution of power, which ultimately means knowledge and

Telematics raise civil, political and also socio economic concerns

As seen in the previous section, the 'to do' spirit of the Bangemann group left little room for such thoughts. Rejecting or missing out on ICT - the argument went - would turn society in a worse place while engaging in information society would in time be rewarding. The group limited itself to suggest that '[c]hanges in labour legislation and the rise of new professions and new skills require dialogue between the social partners, if we are to anticipate and to manage the imminent transformation of the work place.' The paucity of social analysis by industry was to some extent understandable. Catching up with the US in the field of leading-edge technology and facing the increasing pressure coming from global markets were seen as urgent matters. However, as another group of experts held out, 'now the debate is entering a new phase, and the time has come to focus on the many neglected and sometimes unexpected social aspects of the IS.'[35]

The group of experts we are talking about was formed as a High Level Experts Group (HLEG) under the aegis of the European Commission DG Employment and Social Affairs. In their report 'Building the European Information society for us all', twelve experts[36] of different backgrounds collected contributions, comments and observations from stakeholders such as governmental organizations, NGOs, trade unions, private companies, business organizations, academic institutions and religious organizations. For its width and depth, the 'HLEG report' represents the first attempt to formulate a social discourse about the information society. As we will see in this and in the next chapter, many of the ideas and reflections developed therein are recurrent themes in today's e-inclusion policy. In addition, the HLEG report contains reflections which are of great interest to older persons.

What's special with the information society?

What is noteworthy, the group adopted an open-ended definition of the information society, described neutrally as 'the society currently being put into place where low-

---

memory'; [...] 'knowledge will end up being modelled on the stock of available information and building data banks will become indispensable for sovereignty.'

[35] European Commission, Directorate-General for employment, industrial relations and social affairs Unit V/B/4, 'Building the European Information Society for Us All', Manuscript completed in April 1997, Luxembourg: Office for Official Publications of the European Communities. Hereinafter 'High Level Expert Group report' or 'HLEG report'. Available at   http://www.epractice.eu/files/media/ media_688.pdf

[36] The members of the high-level expert group (HLEG) were: Hans Blankert, President, Confederation of Netherlands Industry and Employers (VNO-NCW), The Hague, Netherlands. Gerhard Bosch, Professor, Head of Labour Market Department, Institut Arbeit und Technik,Gelsenkirchen, Germany. Manuel Castells, Research Professor, Consejo Superior de Investigaciones Científicas, Barcelona, Spain. Liam Connellan, former Director General of the Confederation of Irish Industry, Dublin, Ireland. Birgitta Carlson, Senior Advisor, Telia AB, Farsa, Sweden. Ursula Engelen-Kefer, Deputy President, Deutscher Gewerkschaftsbund (DGB), Düsseldorf, Germany. Chris Freeman, Emeritus Professor, Science Policy Research Unit, University of Sussex, United Kingdom. Lisbeth Knudsen, Chief Editor, Det Fri Aktuelt, Copenhagen, Denmark. Yves Lasfargue, Director, Centre d'Etude et de Formation pour l'Accompagnement des Changements (CREFAC), Paris, France. Isabelle Pailliart, Professor, Institut de la Communication et des Médias, Université Stendhal, Grenoble, France. Armando Rocha Trindade, President, Universidade Aberta, Lisbon, Portugal. Jorma Rantanen, Director, Finnish Institute of Occupational Health, Helsinki, Finland. Luc Soete (chairman), Professor, Director, Maastricht Economic Research Unit on Innovation and Technology (MERIT), University of Maastricht, Netherlands. Pier Verderio, Director, International Relations and Training, Federazione Informazione e Spettacolo - Confederazione Italiana Sindacati Lavoratori (FIS-CISL), Italy.

cost information and data storage and transmission technologies are in general use' (HLEG report, p. 16). According to the HLEG, the presence of automatic processing of information in 'general use' tells very little about how an information society could or should look like, 'just as we know different models of industrialised society.' In order to understand what use society can make of new technologies, the HLEG group considers it important to ponder upon and isolate its salient characteristics.

2. DATA, INFORMATION, AND KNOWLEDGE

What's so special about the information society which differentiates it from previous societal models and allows us to speak about an information society? According to the HLEG, one of its most significant features relates to the relationship between data, information and knowledge. The HLEG makes three points.

First, there is a substantial difference between data (in the information society) and raw materials (in modern industrialised societies), and their use. 'Use' of data or information is not comparable to 'use' of raw materials. The latter are in fact 'res extensa': they occupy space, it takes time to accumulate them, they are scarce by default. Data, by contrast, are by definition abundant: they accumulate in the space of few seconds, occupy limited or no space, they are so abundant that they require techniques to sort out and filter information and knowledge from noise. [37]

Second, while the Bangemann report discussed above was confident that ICT would *per se* energise every economic sector (Bangemann report, p.17), the HLEG cautions that data and information do not mobilise demand and supply of work or capital to an extent comparable to industrial societies.[38] The Fordist factory needs encumbering and demanding assets: the industry itself occupies hectares, space; lots of people work in it and share its fate, usually over a long period of time; common interests, including contrasts with management, and life personal experiences are shared. For sociologist Zygmunt Bauman the tight link between capital, raw materials (including infrastructures, such as the factory itself), labour and management – which live under a common roof – lead to the internalization by society of practices of collective mediation and compromise, which spill over from the roofs of the industry and become part of social life negotiations (the Fordist-industry based society).[39]

In the information society the so called 'Fordist compromise' looses the grip and is rapidly replaced by 'soft-ware' industry. A software industry does not mobilise as much work and capital nor does it engender practices of compromise and mediation. On the contrary, technology facilitates isolation of workers through means, such as multi-tasking, which reduce dependency between workers and between workers and management.

---

[37] HLEG Report, p.16. Algorithms, data mining, path dependency, profiling techniques are good examples of techniques and technologies used to separate noise from information. See M. Hildebrandt and S. Gutwirth, *Profiling the European Citizen,* Springer, 2009.

[38] Similarly, Y. Masuda, *The Information Society as Post-Industrial Society,* Institute for the Information Society, Tokyo 1980 (US edition, Washington, DC: World Future Society, 1981), p. 87, where the author claims that 'there will be a change from an industrial structure centering around goods, energy, and services to an information type of industrial structure.'

[39] Z. Bauman, 'Liquid Modernity', Polity Press, Cambridge, 2006, especially Chapter 3 on time and space.

Third, the HLEG group warns that 'the generation of unstructured data does not automatically lead to the creation of information, nor can all information be equated to knowledge. Still less to wisdom' (HLEG Report, p.17).[40] One can only hope, says the group, that the new technologies will be used to shape a 'wise' vision of society. But this will require investment in human resources and skills, not only ICT skills, but also education, training, study and 'tacit knowledge' (HLEG Report, p.18).

3. SOCIAL CONSTRUCTIVISM V. TECHNOLOGY DETERMINISM

The other important point to make about the Information society concerns, according to the HLEG group, the relationship between human factor and technological factor. For the report, such a relationship should be governed by a social integrationist approach to ICT and science, as opposed to a technological deterministic one. 'The social integrationist vision that the High Level Expert Group espouses explicitly rejects the notion of technology as an exogenous variable to which society and individuals, whether at work or in the home, must adapt. Instead it puts the emphasis on technology as a social process' (HLEG Report, p.19). Technologies are described as a 'process of change which is flexible and, as such, dependent on the particular conditions of application and use.'[41] From a regulatory point of view, the starting point should be the notion that 'social processes determine technology for social purposes'.[42] Concretely, this should boil down to the embedment, in all stages of technology development, of social or ethical decisions (concepts of social and 'organisational 'embeddedness', HLEG Report, p.19-20). We will see in chapter IV and V (on privacy and data protection, and on consent) that the notion of social embeddedness is central for the ethics of ICT for older persons, suggesting, e.g., that the use of assistive technology be accepted also by the networks of actors, families and informal carers who surround the end-user.

4. POLICY CHALLENGES: SOCIAL EXCLUSION, LITERACY, VIRTUALITY, AND FLEXIBLE ORGANISATION

Based on these two preliminary reflections, the HLEG group pauses on a series of policy challenges, some of which are particularly relevant for us.

Inspired by the social integrationist ethics, the information society should, first of all avoid fomenting social exclusion, and, secondly, create new opportunities for the least-advantaged. To explain this point, the 1997 HLEG report makes an interesting reference to the renowned 1993 White Paper 'Growth, Competitiveness, Employment' and to the Commission's opinion of 28 February 1996 'Reinforcing political union and preparing for enlargement.'[43] Both put emphasis on social cohesion as a core European value. The reference to the 1996 Commission opinion is

---

[40] For the HLEG group wisdom is ''distilled' knowledge derived from experience of life, as well as from the natural and social sciences, from ethics and philosophy.' Pages 17, ft. 12. On knowledge see Chapter II and Chapter VIII.

[41] On social determinism and technological determinism see, amongst others, J. Ellul, *The Technological Society*, Vintage Books, New York, 1964; L. Green, *Technoculture*, Allen and Unwin, Crows Nest, 2001; A. Murphie and J. Potts, *Culture and Technology*, Palgrave, London 2003.

[42] L.Green, *Technoculture*, op.cit., p. 21.

[43] European Commission, 'Reinforcing political union and preparing for enlargement', Opinion from the Commission, COM (96) 90 final, Brussels, 28 February 1996.

particularly relevant: 'Europe', the opinion reads, 'is built on a set of values shared by all its societies and combines the characteristics of democracy - human rights and institutions based on the rule of law - with those of an open economy underpinned by market forces, internal solidarity and cohesion. These values include access for all members of society to universal services or to services of general benefit, thus contributing to solidarity and equal treatment.' The *Building the European Information society for us all* report draws from the Commission's opinion to affirm the urgency of a 'clearly agreed common minimum social framework' for the information society. 'In the future', the report explains, 'there could be different models of information society. They are likely to differ in the degree to which they avoid social exclusion and create new opportunities for the disadvantaged' (The HLEG Report, p. 16).[44] Lacking a robust vision of social cohesion, the group fears that, under the drive of market globalisation, the Information Society may engender a 'harmonisation by erosion of Europe's social standards' (The HLEG Report, p. 52). The concern voiced by the group is that the information society will be for the less-favoured such as the disabled and elderly people, the unemployed and the immigrants, not a possibility of emancipation, but of increased exclusion (HLEG Report, p. 56); 'not a new social order, but more of the same.'[45] There certainly are, the HLEG concurs, opportunities where ICT can play an emancipatory role - for instance in the field of health, where technologies can help overcome physical or cognitive handicaps. But opportunities for the elderly, the unemployed, the immigrants or the disabled will not be there because "the technology exists" or through the market's invisible hand. The group takes a hearty view on this: 'What is not at issue in this debate, however, is that these opportunities will - with a few exceptions - not be forthcoming simply through the market. Excluded groups, as the term suggests, do not generally form 'consumer groups' of commercial interest' (HLEG Report, p. 56).

On these bases the High Level group puts forth its own definition of inclusion in the information society, ten years before the 2006 Riga Declaration launched its own e-inclusion definition. On the HLEG's account, '[w]e associate inclusion - what in Eurospeak is more commonly termed 'cohesion' - with the extent to which any individual is able to participate in society. Whether rich or poor, at a distance or at the centre, [young or old, we shall add], one would hope that in a future Information Society individuals will be able to play a full part in the social life of the community. Ideally, the IS should help to reduce exclusion, not increase it' (HLEG Report, p. 56).

Education, training, and life long learning practices. But ensure that information is available also in non e-format

One of the challenges comes from the rapid proliferation of ICT systems, new applications, and also new *modes d'emploi*. The pace of technological development,

---

[44] HLEG Report, p. 16. One may hear echoes of J. Rawls, (J.Rawls, *A theory of justice*, Harvard University Press, Cambridge (Mass), 1971) and in particular of the theory of 'primary goods' (p.127). For Rawls, the 'Difference Principle' is that social and economic inequalities are to be arranged so that 'they are to be of the greatest benefit to the least-advantaged members of society' (p.303). Accordingly, departures from equality of a list of what he calls primary goods – 'things which a rational man wants whatever else he wants' – are justified only to the extent that they improve the lot of those who are worst-off under that distribution in comparison with the previous, equal, distribution. (p. 92)'
[45] S. Cohen, *Visions of Social Control: Crime Punishment and Classification*, Cambridge: Polity/Basil Blackwell, 1985. For the HLEG, the main concern is that current exclusion problems will remain by and large the same in the future IS.

epitomised in the so called Moore law[46], contrasts sharply with the obsolescence of knowledge in human beings. Men and women usually have waning capacities to accumulate information, let alone assimilate it; people forget how to do things. Technology instead changes continuously and rapidly; it is only because we are constantly using it that we know how to deal with it, and yet difficulties arise at all times. Yet occasional use and/or passing of time engender rapid obsolescence of practical knowledge, for instance when he or she who retires and stops using pc applications and may have to re-learn how to deal with and cope with ICT.[47] The rapid obsolescence of knowledge places great importance on training, education and life long learning practices. 'There is nothing automatic about the way various individuals of different capabilities or different educational qualifications will access or are likely to respond to new ICT opportunities' the expert group holds (The HLEG Report, p.56). It is recommended to advance understanding about how individuals with different backgrounds or of different ages learn how to deal with technology. A good way to begin would be to make high quality and low cost learning materials as well as opportunities to learn available to all members of society. Exclusion linked to cost or access to study material should be avoided and be the joint responsibility of both the private sector and public institutions. On the HLEG's mind, 'to limit the involvement of the public sector to an economic enabling function is to grossly underestimating the role and importance of public agencies and services as information providers and processors in a multitude of economic, social and policy areas' (The HLEG report, p.28).

In particular, the role of the public is seen as that of *content* provider setting clear guidelines on the development, distribution and maintenance of ICT. It is too important to have friendly, universally accessible information and communication technologies. At the same time, it is key task of public policy to maintain the possibility of direct access to non-electronic information or through human contact (The HLEG report, p.30[48]).

---

[46] The so-called Moore law, named after Gerard Moore, one of the founders of INTEL, a leading company in microprocessors and semiconductors, describes a long-term trend in the history of computing hardware. It holds that the number of transistors that can be placed inexpensively on an integrated circuit has doubled approximately every two years. Rather than being a naturally-occurring 'law' that cannot be controlled, however, Moore's Law is effectively a business practice in which the advancement of transistor counts occurs at a fixed rate. (source: wikipedia)

[47] Birgit Jæger, 'The Inclusion of Senior Citizens in the Information Society', Discussion on Ethical, privacy and legal issues related to ageing at work, SENIOR Project, Expert meeting on Ubiquitous communication', 22 September 2008, Brussels. See also Chapter III on consent and the right to access information in non electronic format. Research conducted under SENIOR suggested that 'feeling too old to learn' is often a perception molded by dominant social perception about ageing, than by seniors themselves. Compare Øyvind Nøhr, Lillehammer University College, 'The competent Seniors: Aging and use of digital media – conflict or happiness?' , SENIOR project, Socio-Anthropological Workshop, Brussels, 2-3 June 2008. See also SENIOR project, Work Package 1 final, prepared by D. Wright, p. 105 and SENIOR project, D.2.3, 'Intelligent User Interface' final, prepared by P. De Hert & E. Mantovani, p. 5.

[48] The HLEG report, p.30. '3c. Public services as a model of service provision: The public service sector should be a model of service provision for the general public, particularly in combining remote access by means of communication technologies with the option of human contact for those citizens who so desire. Information access systems must be developed to be geared to the needs of the entire population. In other words, remote-access information systems must be user-friendly, guarantee universal access, including to public records, and enable individual enquiries, etc. In addition, maintaining the possibility of direct access through human contact is vital to ensure that no one is excluded.' On accessibility and interface see SENIOR project, D2.3, 'Intelligent User Interface', prepared by P. De Hert and E. Mantovani, 2008.

What are the implications of being constantly 'on call'?

Our quality of life in the Information Society may be affected by whether or not we will be able to 'master the impact of virtuality.' Virtuality is used to describe situations in which human activities are increasingly based on representations of reality, for instance online social networks, rather than on reality itself. For the drafters of the report, it is essential that we understand how technologies are used. One of the implications of being constantly on call, for instance, may be to limit opportunities for conviviality and increase social isolation (The HLEG Report, p. 36).[49] The group suggests that ICT solutions stay tuned and sensitive to the social context in which they are used – isolated areas, rural or urban environments, care of frail elderly people may involve different actors such as family, formal caregivers and small communities. The use of ICT should thus be assessed not only with and by the user, patient, or worker but also against the larger context of, e.g., family members, care takers, work places.[50]

Collective dimension of ICT: decisions should be taken with others

One of the domains of social life which is expected to be transformed by technological development is work. If we are 'all' to benefit from the advantages of ICT in this area, the report holds, technology alone will be 'insufficient.' Technological developments should be introduced in the structure of firms, production and work processes, labour and skill requirements, and be accompanied by organisational discussions about, *e.g.*, staff versatility, training, flexible hours, new pay systems, teamwork and flatter hierarchies (The HLEG Report, p. 37). The path to follow is, according to the experts, collective agreements.[51] The trust of the group is that the emerging information society will need reinforced organisational mechanisms. Collective participation in the area of technology in the workplace could, following Baumann's hint seen above, be adopted outside the domain of work too - for instance in living institutions or situations of dependency. We will encounter the collective dimension below when we discuss consent (Chapter V) and ethical recommendations (chapter VIII).

---

[49] See E.Mordini & S. Massari, *Including Seniors in the Information Society. 28 World Leaders talks on Privacy, Ethics, Technology and Ageing*, CIC Edizioni internazionali, Roma, 2008, in particular p.181-185 (Final remarks).
[50] This point was made by M. Starr, 'The Perspective of caregivers', SENIOR project, Final Conference, 27 November 2009. See also SENIOR, D.1.5, WP 1 Report Final, prepared by D. Wright, 2008, p. 97
[51] A similar point is made by P. De Hert in the field of workplace privacy. P. De Hert, 'The Use of Labour Law To Regulate Employer Profiling: Making Data Protection Relevant Again', in M. Hildebrandt and S. Gutwirth (eds), *Profiling the European citizen. Cross Disciplinary Perspectives*, Springer, 2008.

III. TOWARDS LISBON (1997-2000)

1. THE ROLLING ACTION PLAN FOR THE INFORMATION SOCIETY (1997)

EU economic goals, Information Society and early signs of demographic change

While the HLEG report was being drafted, the 1996 'Living and Working in the Information Society: People First' Green Paper made an attempt to stimulate new thinking in three areas, i) organisation of work, ii) employment, and iii) social cohesion in the information society.[52] With respect to iii) (social cohesion), the Community drew attention to the relationship between information society and demographic change. The Green Paper acknowledges (paragraph 109) that 'changing demographic and social welfare trends means that an increased number of people will require some form of care.' It thus encourages better understanding of the potential of ICT to a) improve the quality of life of older people and people with disabilities, b) facilitate independent living in the community, and c) open up new possibilities for participation and socio-economic integration.[53]

Delivered during the European Year of Lifelong Learning, 'Living and Working in the Information Society: People First' also calls for investments 'in the architecture of life long training and education of those [...] who are often perceived as being less geared to the use of ICTs and unable to take part in the IS, such as older people and people with disabilities' (paragraph 110-111).

The reflection developed by the 1996 Green Paper fed in a Commission communication titled 'The Information Society: From Corfu to Dublin: The New Emerging Priorities', published in the same year. The communication establishes four priorities, two of them related to the development of an internal and global Information society market. The other two concern 1) the development of the information society in a knowledge-based society, and 2) the reduction of digital divide, protection of consumers, public services and cultural diversity.[54] The 'New emerging priorities' paper was, for its part, slotted in the revised version of the Action Plan to Europe's Way to the Information Society, 'Europe at the Forefront of the Global Information Society: Rolling Action Plan'[55], issued in 1997. The aim of the

---

[52] European Commission, 'Living and Working in the Information Society: People First', Green Paper, COM (96) 389 final, Brussels, 24 July 1996.

[53] For example, the Green Paper states that ICT applications can provide alternative modes of communication and information presentation, such as multimedia services for people with sensory impairments. Equally, they can offer the opportunity to carry out activities from home (telework or distance learning for people who have difficulties accessing employment and educational opportunities). They can also facilitate remote access to medical and social care and other support services. COM (96) 389 final, para. 111.

[54] European Commission, 'The Information Society: From Corfu to Dublin: The New Emerging Priorities', Communication from the Commission to the Council, the European Parliament, the Economic and Social Committee and the Committee of the Regions, COM(96) 395 final, Brussels, 24 July 1996. Four priorities are listed, namely: complete the liberalisation of the Telecommunication market by January 1998; make the information society a 'knowledge-based society' (four years ahead Lisbon); closer cooperation between structural funds and Information Society policies to avoid a two tier IS Europe, protect consumers interests, improve public sector services, and ensure cultural diversity; bring the market of Information society's goods and services in line with the WTO framework.

[55] European Commission, 'Europe and the Forefront of the Global Information Society: Rolling Action Plan', Communication from the European Commission to the Council, the European Parliament, the

Plan was to 'present a list of all important actions [...] required to further implement the Information Society in Europe' (Rolling Action Plan, paragraph III).

The Rolling Action Plan recommends advancing penetration of technology

The Rolling Action Plan delves into the market aspects of the Information society and, only marginally, on social cohesion or inclusion. As far as the market aspects are concerned, the Plan emphasises the need to buttress the business environment by putting in place a legal framework for electronic commerce including rules on copyright, data protection, digital signature and global WTO rules. In the area of social inclusion, 'People at the centre', the Plan insists on the need to stem inertia and resistance to technology penetration. The Commission draws the attention to employment opportunities in the Information Society economy, notably in e-commerce, services and content providers, and multimedia sectors. It also stresses the importance of ICT training at school and of life long learning. The role of the public policy is limited to the, though surely important task, of providing 'opportunities to develop the employability of workers, support change in the organisation of enterprises, reinforce social cohesion and cultural diversity and enhance people's ability to participate in the Information Society' (Rolling Action Plan, paragraph III). The Plan also contains a reference to the 'protection of fundamental rights and freedoms, in particular the right to privacy' (Rolling Action Plan, paragraph II) in the Information Society, but it does not give any guidance about how to do this and put 'people at the centre'.

Avoid technologies which raise barriers and exclude people

Unlike the Rolling Action Plan, the communication 'Social and Labour Market Dimension of the Information Society People First - The Next Steps,' issued in 1997[56], is noteworthy because it suggests one way to use information society to pursue social inclusion goals. The communication stresses the need to attain equal access to ICT specifying that 'IT hardware and services should be designed in such a way that they do not discriminate against certain groups, raising barriers and excluding them *from their use* (italics face added)'(paragraph XIII). In order to avoid discrimination in the access to technology the Commission suggests the adoption of 'universal design' guidelines and recommends that software and hardware stay user friendly. Human-computer interfaces should be responsive to the needs of users 'who may face problems in accessing the new technological environment' (paragraph XIII).

2. THE EUROPEAN EMPLOYMENT STRATEGY AND ELDERLY PEOPLE

As was pointed out in the introduction, the construction of Europe's Information Society evolves in parallel with the European strategy for growth, competitiveness and jobs initiated by the 1993 Delors' White Paper. It is now time to put on hold the

---

Economic and Social Committee and the Committee of the Regions, COM (97) 106 final, Brussels, 27 November 1996, updated and revised on 31 July 1997.
[56] European Commission, 'The Social and Labour Market Dimension of the Information Society: People First - The Next Steps', Communication from the Commission, COM (97) 390 final, Brussels, 23 July 1997.

Information society and look at the making up of Europe's employment strategy between 1997 and 2000.

In 1997, the 1993 White Paper achieves momentum. One of the White Paper's aims was to 'activate' the work capacities of European societies starting from those sectors or groups deemed to be most 'inactive' and therefore disadvantaged. By targeting groups excluded from employment, the argument went, Europe would increase occupation while reducing public expenditure, and augment the fiscal basis needed to finance appropriate 'active life' social security schemes.[57] The 1997 European Employment Strategy (EES) is the instrument through which the European Union and Member States set to achieve this end, *viz.* the expansion of employed and/or active citizenry. As we will see, one of the groups targeted is older persons.

The 1997 European Employment Strategy rested on four pillars: employability, entrepreneurship, adaptability and equal opportunities.[58] The four pillars were branched out into nineteen guidelines, later expanded to twenty-two by the 1998 Vienna European Council.[59] Guidelines on 'equal opportunities' did not address elderly people, being more directed at combating gender discrimination in employment, career breaks, parental leave, part-time work, and care for children. Older persons are mentioned under the 'employability' pillar. 'It is important', guideline number four states, 'to develop, in the context of a policy for active ageing, measures such as maintaining working capacity, lifelong learning and other flexible working arrangements, so that older workers are also able to participate actively in working life' (EU Council, 1999/C 69/02, Annex, para. 4). The development of a policy context conducive to active ageing requires increased employability of older adults. 'In order to reinforce the development of a skilled and adaptable workforce,' guideline six calls on Member States and social partners 'to develop possibilities for lifelong learning, particularly in the fields of information and communication technologies, and […] define lifelong learning in order to set a target according to national circumstances for participants benefiting from such measures' (EU Council, 1999/C 69/02, Annex, para. 6). In the same place, it is specified that 'easy access [to lifelong learning] for older workers will be particularly important.'

The European Employment strategy gained impetus in the year 2000 when the Lisbon agenda was adopted. Crucially, it is with Lisbon 2000 that the burgeoning information society gets fully associated in the pursuit of the Europe's broader socio-economic policy and objectives. ICT could be one way to help older persons staying active longer.

---

[57] The White Paper, 1993, *above*. This vision returns in *The Economist,* 'Special Report on Ageing', 'Work till you drop', 27 June – 3 July 2009: 'By carrying on, older persons will not only save the public purse money by not drawing a pension but will also continue to pay taxes and social-security contributions.'

[58] European Council, Presidency Conclusions, Luxembourg, 12-13 December 1997. Recall that the 1997 Amsterdam Treaty includes a title (Title IX) on employment and equal opportunities.

[59] EU Council, Resolution on the 1999 Employment Guidelines, 1999/C 69/02, Brussels, 22 February 1999 which incorporates the conclusions of the Vienna European Council of 11 and 12 December 1998.

IV. THE LISBON AGENDA (2000)

1. THE LISBON STRATEGY, AGEING POPULATION, AND ICT

The 2002 Kok report: Delaying the average age at which people leave the labour force and promotion of active ageing

In March 2000 the Lisbon European Council famously set the (overly)-ambitious objective of attaining an overall employment rate of 70% by 2010.[60] In 2001, in Stockholm, the European Council took note of 'an ageing population of which people of working age constitute an ever smaller part' and added an additional objective to the already-crowded Lisbon agenda, *viz.* an employment rate objective of at least 50% of the population aged between 55 and 64.[61] Already in 2002, however, the Lisbon objectives for growth and jobs seemed out of reach. A European Employment *taskforce*[62] guided by former Dutch Prime Minister Mr. Wim Kok said it was necessary to energise flexibility in work, to provide incentives active life, and to invest on human capital, if the Lisbon objectives wanted to be achieved. One of the areas to be energised was the ageing population. The report could not be clearer: it states that '[…] for years the so-called "Demographic Timebomb" has been debated as if it were a distant problem on the far horizon. This attitude is no longer sustainable' and concludes that 'delaying the average age at which people leave the labour forces is crucial.'[63] The taskforce suggested comprehensive active ageing strategies and a radical policy and culture shift. Three key recommendations are set forth: (a) providing the right legal and financial incentives for workers to work longer and for employers to hire and keep older workers; (b) increasing participation in training for all ages, especially for the low-skilled and for older workers; and (c) improving working conditions and quality in work.[64]

Promotion of active ageing

After the 2002 Kok review, the EES' four-pillared structure (based on employability, entrepreneurship, adaptability, and equal opportunities) was disbanded. It was

---

[60] The March 2000 Lisbon European Council famously aimed to make Europe 'the most competitive and the most dynamic knowledge-based economy in the world' by 2010. The Lisbon strategy built on three pillars, *an economic*, a *social and an environmental pillar*. The objectives were not achieved. *European Voice*, '2020 vision', by Jim Brunsden, 14 January 2010.

[61] Stockholm European Council, Presidency conclusions, 23 and 24 March 2001. 'The challenge to create more and better jobs, accelerate economic reform, modernise the European social model and harness new technologies and the reality.' Available at http://www.consilium.europa.eu/ueDocs/cms_Data/docs/pressData/en/ec/00100-r1.%20ann-r1.en1.html

[62] W. Kok et al., 'Jobs, Jobs, Jobs. Creating more employment in Europe', Report of the European Commission Employment Taskforce, November 2003, p.8.

[63] 'The labour market situation for workers aged 50 and over is a major cause for concern, all the more so in the light of demographic ageing. Urgent action is needed not only to ensure that a higher share of those currently aged 55-64 stay in work, but also to keep a much larger share of those currently in their 40s and 50s in employment.' Ibid., p.9

[64] *Ibid.*, page 9 and 10. See also Barcelona European Council, Presidency conclusions, 15-16 March 2002, para.9, where the Presidency takes not of the need to increase response to the challenge of ageing, stressing that early retirement should cease to be the immediate response to the problems of restructuring enterprises. Opportunities must be given to older workers to keep their jobs, since flexible work organisation formulas (part time and teleworking among others) and the guarantee of lifelong learning tools that can help make those opportunities a reality.' http://www.consilium.europa.eu/ueDocs/cms_Data/docs/pressData/en/ec/71025.pdf

replaced by ten priorities, one of which is the 'promotion of active ageing'.[65] *'Promotion of active ageing'* can be attained thanks to improvement of working conditions, notably health and safety at work, access to vocational training, flexibility of work organisation, elimination of incentives for early exit from the labour market and early retirement. It is conceded, however, that active ageing requires that jobs are available, attractive, and reasonable for all age groups, including older persons.[66]

The IS and the Lisbon agenda: Access to ICT is relevant for economic growth and social justice. Focus on accessibility and user requirements

Let us now return to the Information Society and see what place and role the 2000 Lisbon agenda gave to it. In sum, with the launch of the Lisbon strategy or agenda the information society becomes instrumental to the attainment of the socio-economic polices of the European Union. By the year 2000, the European Union had rapidly progressed in the construction of the IS highways. The telecommunication sector is opened up to private competitors; a legal framework on the cross border flow of personal data is established; R&TD efforts are spearheaded by the EU through heavily funded multiannual programmes; ICT research has gone from pc technologies to Ambient Intelligence technologies; ICT applications growingly converge with nanotechnologies, cognitive sciences, biology.

In the knowledge-based society that Lisbon had envisaged technology penetrates all sectors of society both for the sake of social justice and for the sake of economic growth. Technology should basically enable both dimensions and all citizens. According to Paul Timmers, head of the 'ICT for Inclusion' Unit at the European Commission DG Information Society and Media, 'new technologies represent an instrument which can enable social, economic and also political relations by linking the individual to the community-network.'[67] Timmers makes a reference to Castells, who explains how within social, economic, leisure, health care, etc. networks the individual moulds his or her identity. The Information Society requires 'acting on information'.[68] Access to networks alimented by ICT therefore becomes part of the repertoire of capabilities of today's and tomorrow's European citizen. Promoting the use of ICT for all, including the least advantaged, and to empower them through, *e.g.*, access to broadband networks, friendly interfaces, mobile communication and so on is responsibility of the modern state.

Therefore, the burgeoning information society can not be entrusted solely to market forces. Led by the market, ICT has targeted services, applications, content,

---

[65] EU Council, 'Guidelines for the employment policies of the Member States', Council Decision, Brussels, 22 July 2003, published in OJ L 197 of 5 August 2003. The ten priorities are:
1) active and preventative measures for the unemployed and inactive; (italics face added); 2) job creation and entrepreneurship; 3) promotion of adaptability and mobility, social dialogue and corporate social responsibility; 4) promotion of the development of human capital, education and lifelong learning; 5) promotion of active ageing; 6) promotion of gender equality; 7) integration of and combating discrimination against people at a disadvantage on the labour market, notably early school leavers, low-skilled workers, people with disabilities, immigrants and ethnic minorities; 8) tax and financial incentives to enhance work attractiveness; 9) transformation of undeclared work into regular employment; 10) addressing regional employment disparities.
[66] Member States will aim to achieve an increase by five years of the effective average exit age from the labour market (estimated at 59,9 in 2001).
[67] Paul Timmers, 'EU e-inclusion policy in context', VOL. 10 NO. 5/6 2008, pp. 12-19, Q Emerald Group Publishing Limited. At the time of writing Paul Timmers is Head of Unit of ICT for inclusion at the European Commission
[68] M. Castells, *The Rise of the Network Society*, Blackwell Publishers, London, 1996. .

and also consumers deemed to be the most profitable.[69] As a result, some geographical areas have been left out; some places, institutes, schools, libraries, universities have been neglected and not equipped with the appropriate ICT means. Also, the special needs and requirements of some groups of persons have been overlooked. This model is no longer sustainable.

2. E-EUROPE AND THE CHOICE FOR ACCESS AS PIVOTAL PRINCIPLE

In the relationship between information society and Lisbon agenda one may hear echoes of the technological determinism and social constructivism approaches adopted by the Bangemann and HLEG reports.[70] Rather than relying on one approach, the Lisbon strategy seems to be a blend of both.

The March 2000 European Council paves the way to the integration of ICT in fields of public interest such as health, education, work, services, and active citizenry policies.[71] The objectives of the Lisbon agenda are translated in the Information Society book with the key word of 'usage.' For its part, usage invites questions of affordability, accessibility, and usability of systems, including for people with functional limitations or for those who lack digital literacy and competences.[72] Accessibility in all its features occupies a central position in 'An information society for all[73]' *e*Europe initiative. Presented as a complementary initiative to the 23 and 24 March 2000 Lisbon European Council, *e*Europe set three main objectives:

1) Bringing *every citizen*, home and school, every business and administration, into the digital age and online;
2) Creating a *digitally literate* Europe, supported by an entrepreneurial culture ready to finance and develop new ideas; and

---

[69] Gerard Cronet, 'The perspective of gerontology', SENIOR Final Conference, 27 November 2009, Brussels. 'Market competition and short term profit business logic result with selecting the most profitable targets for products and services.'

[70] The Bangemann report insisted on the energising contribution of ICT to economy and society in general. By contrast, the HLEG report considered technology as social process. See above Paragraph III.3 'Social constructivism v. technology determinism'

[71] European Commission, DG INFSO, 'The Lisbon strategy and the Information Society' presentation delivered on March 2007.
http://ec.europa.eu/information_society/eeurope/i2010/ict_and_lisbon/index_en.htm

[72] *Availability* acquires particular relevance for the e-inclusion of citizens who live in remote or rural areas and do not have access, for instance, to broadband networks; *affordability* hints at economic issues, such as cost of buying a computer or subscription fee to be paid to internet service provider. *Ability and ICT accessibility* are related more closely to human computer interaction. *Ability* points at (lack of) digital competence: many citizens do not know how to use a computer or experience difficulties in understanding computer language. Senior citizens, for instance, experience hearing and vision impairments as a natural part of the ageing process; some develop arthritis making it difficult to use mainstream interfaces (the mobile phone, e.g.); others suffer from reduced mobility; impaired manual dexterity, physical impairments and so on. *ICT accessibility* is concerned with design, interface, and usability requirements to meet those needs. See, SENIOR project, D2.3, 'Intelligent User Interface', prepared by P. De Hert and E. Mantovani, November 2008, available at www.seniorproject.eu

[73] European Commission, 'eEurope - An information society for all', Communication on a Commission initiative for the special European Council of Lisbon of 23 and 24 March 2000, COM(1999) 687 final, Brussels, 8 December 1999.

3) Ensuring the whole process is *socially inclusive*, builds consumer trust and strengthens social cohesion. (italics face added)

The *e*Europe initiative brings to the spotlight the issue of the so called digital divide. The digital divide manifests itself in various ways. According to the analysis of David Wright[74], there is a social digital divide, which concerns, e.g., persons who do not know how to use a computer, users who do not see any benefits in ICT, and users who may have some disability that hampers their ability to gain access to the information society. There is also an economic social divide, where the use of ICT is hampered by the cost, *e.g.*, to buy a computer or to pay the subscription fees demanded by an Internet service provider. There is a geographical digital divide which concerns mostly communities living in areas without access to, e.g., broadband networks. There is eventually a technological digital divide which is created by the lack of interoperability, common standards or hard to understand human-computer interfaces. It seems there is also an age-related digital divide. In Europe, surveys indicate that only 10 per cent of senior citizens over the age of 65 use the Internet, compared to 68 per cent of those aged 16-24.[75] According to Eurostat 2006, the digital divide in Europe is mainly a matter of age and education.[76] But there also other reasons such lack of infrastructure or access, lack of incentives to use ICT, unfriendly interfaces, lack of training which contribute to widen the gap. For the European Commission age-related and other forms of digital divides cumulate over time and generations, instead of disappearing. The accumulation of divides may become a stable phenomenon and be translated into social stratification.[77]

To fill in the gap, the EU does not dispose of a unitary strategy. The 2005 'i2010 initiative', discussed below, emphasises the need to teach Europeans basic digital skills and to mobilise structural funds and rural development funds in this direction.[78] In its Ageing Well in the Information Society Action Plan[79], the Commission criticises the lack of common standards which hampers the take up of existing and new services such as smart homes, integrated health and social care ICT systems, and assistive technologies. For its part, *e*Europe envisages policy actions in different areas: e-youth; Internet access; e-Commerce; fast Internet for researchers and students; smart cards for secure electronic access; risk capital for high-tech SMEs; eParticipation for the disabled; Healthcare online; Intelligent transport; Government online, etc.

The age related digital divide and e-ageing are not included as a priority in *e*Europe although there are areas, *viz. e*participation for the disabled, health care online, government online, that clearly affect older persons' interests.

[74] See SENIOR project, Work Package 1 Report, prepared by D. Wright, 2008, p.32. www.seniorproject.eu

[75] Riga Ministerial Declaration made by EU Ministers on eInclusion concerning 'Inclusive eGovernment', 11 June 2006. See also, for the UK, Ofcom, Older people and communications technology: An attitudinal study into older people and their engagement with communications technology, London, July 2006.

[76] See C. Demunter, 'The digital divide in Europe', Statistics in focus, 38/2005, Eurostat, 12 Oct 2005.

[77] European Commission, 'Commission Staff Working Document, Accompanying document to the Communication from the Commission to the European Parliament, the Council, the European Economic and Social Committee and the Committee of the Regions, Ageing well in the Information Society, COM(2007) 332 final', SEC (2007) 0811 final, Brussels, 14 June 2007.

[78] COM(2005) 229 final, p. 10.

[79] COM(2007) 332 final, Brussels, 14 June 2007, p. 7. See below.

3. DEMOGRAPHIC AGEING DRIVES THE EU 'TOWARDS A EUROPE FOR ALL AGES'

As was pointed out above, the Lisbon strategy and the development of the information society are accompanied by increased attention to Europe's ageing population and on the impact of this demographic trend on European societies and economies. Demographic ageing also takes to the the the EU social, economic and information society agendas a rather new group of citizens, the elderly.

Demographic ageing at international level

Demographic ageing and its impact on quality of life of older persons elicited the interest and concern of United Nations organs since the beginning of the eighties.[80] In effect, the General Assembly first debated the issue of old age in 1948 during its third session, when it received a draft declaration of old age rights submitted by Argentina.[81] Argentina's initiative stayed unheeded until 1971, when the twenty-sixth session of the GA adopted a resolution on the question of the elderly and the aged.[82] In 1973, a study on the changing social, economic and cultural roles of the aged prepared and presented to the GA by the UN Secretary General Kurt Waldheim illustrated the absolute and relative increase of ageing populations in the world and suggested that population ageing might have far-reaching and unpredictable consequences on the social and economic structures of societies.[83] In 1978, the General Assembly resolved to organise a World Assembly on ageing for the purpose of 'launch[ing] and international program of action aimed at guaranteeing economic and social security to older persons, as well as opportunities for them to contribute to national development.'[84] Four years later, in Vienna, the World Assembly on Ageing adopted the 1982 Vienna International Plan of Action on Ageing.[85] This document, discussed in chapter III, later endorsed by the General Assembly[86], detailed in sixty-two recommendations the measures that Member States should adopt in order to safeguard the rights of older persons in their national legislations. In 1991, the UN General Assembly promulgated the United Nations principles on older persons, which consists of eighteen points divided into five sections, rubricated under the principles of independence, participation, care, self-fulfillment, and dignity.[87] In 2002, the United Nations hosted its Second World Assembly on Aging in Madrid. The Madrid summit drew up the Madrid International Plan of Action on Ageing (MIPAA)[88] with

---

[80] The recommendations of the World Assembly on Ageing were endorsed by the General Assembly in its resolution 37/51 of 3 December 1982. The framework of international human rights for elderly people is discussed in Chapter 3, Human Rights.
[81] UNGA resolution 213 (III) of 4 December 1948
[82] UNGA resolution 2842 (CXXVI) of 18 December 1971.
[83] Report presented to the General Assembly, UN Doc. A/9126
[84] UNGA resolution 33/52 of 14 December 1978.
[85] Report of the World Assembly on Ageing, Vienna, 26 July-6 August 1982, United Nations publication,. Sales No. E.82.I.16.
[86] A/RES/37/51 of 3 December 1982. The Vienna summit was the first major international initiative in response to the 'question of aging'. http://www.un.org/documents/ga/res/37/a37r051.htm (last visited 15 February 2009). See chapter III, Human Rights of older persons.
[87] The UN Principles on older persons were adopted by the General Assembly with resolution 46/91 of 16 December 1991. http://www2.ohchr.org/english/law/pdf/olderpersons.pdf . See chapter III, Human Rights of older persons.
[88] Second World Assembly on Ageing Madrid, 8-12 April 2002, Report A/CONF.197/9 of 23 May 2002. Available at http://www.un.org/swaa2002/documents.htm (last visited 15 October 2009). The

the goal of 'ensur[ing] that older persons are mainstreamed into overall policy, not treated as a separate group in need of remedial care.' By mainstreaming, the MIPAA intends assessing the implications of any planned action, including legislation, policies or programmes, in all areas and at all levels, in relation to the concerns, needs as well as experiences of the elderly.[89]

For the growing importance on social and economic matters, it is worth mentioning the initiative taken by the G8 summit in the year 2000. Meeting in Turin (Italy), the G8 adopted the document 'Towards Active Ageing.'[90] The Turin Charter encouraged states to facilitate and support the participation of old people in economic and social life so 'older persons [to] contribute to the goals of economic growth, prosperity and social cohesion in all countries' (paragraph I). Active labour market policy measures should also be reviewed in order to fit the needs of older workers. These measures – it is suggested - should include *inter alia* improvements in ICT skills with the aim of bridging the 'digital divide' (paragraph VIII).

In their studies on demographic change, the Organisation for Economic cooperation and Development (OECD) repeatedly encouraged its members to reform public pension schemes, taxation systems, and social transfers to incentive late retirement.[91] In general, from the OECD viewpoint, ageing is a horizontal matter that decision makers ought to consider when they deal with occupation, transport, housing and urban developments policies.[92] In particular, the OECD invites the rationalisation of ageing policies in the health care sector.[93] The suggestion is to strike a sustainable balance between investments in 'health care' and investments in 'long term health care,' the latter being about adopting better life styles and exploitation of new technologies.

---

text of the International Plan of Action on Ageing is available at http://www.un.org/esa/socdev/ageing/documents/building_natl_capacity/guiding.pdf (last visited 15 February 2010)

[89] *Ibid.,*p.12. For a commentary see Sidorenko, Alexandre, & Alan Walker, 'The Madrid International Plan of Action on Ageing: From conceptualization to implementation' in *Ageing & Society,* 2004, 24 (2): 147-165.

[90] G8, Labor Ministers Conference, Turin Italy, November 10-11, 2000. the G8 produced the 'Turin Charter: Towards Active Aging', available at http://www.g7.utoronto.ca/employment/labour2000_ageing.htm. See V. Marshall, 'ICT and the Social Inclusion of Older Adults: Can the Social Sciences Contribute to New Solutions to Old Problems?' Opening lecture for the Socio-Anthropological Workshop, Project, 'The Social, Ethical and Privacy Needs in ICT for Older People: Dialogue for a Roadmap', Brussels, Belgium, June 2-3, 2008. Available at http://seniorproject.eu/index.php?module=CMpro&func=listpages&subid=4 (last visited 15 October 2009)

[91] OECD, *Maintaining prosperity in an ageing society*, Paris, 1998. Available at http://www.oecd.org/dataoecd/21/10/2430300.pdf ; See also OECD, *Ageing and Income: Financial Resources & Retirement in 9 OECD Countries*, Paris, 2000; OECD, *Policy Brief: Maintaining the Economic Well-Being of Older People - challenges for retirement income policies,* Paris, December 2001; OECD, *Age of Withdrawal from the Labour Force in OECD Countries: Labour Market & Social Policy. Occasional Papers no. 49*, Paris, January 2002. See also David Carey, *Coping with Population Ageing in the Netherlands*, OECD Economics Department Working Papers 325, OECD, Economics Department, 2002.

[92] See, e.g., OECD, *Getting older, getting poorer?*, Paris, February 2002; OECD, *Ageing, Housing & Urban Development*, Paris, January 2003. OECD, *Governments Must Rethink Transport Safety for Elderly*, Paris, 2001; *Ageing and Transport: Mobility Needs and Safety Issues*, April 2002; *Public Support for Governmental Benefits for the Elderly Across Countries and Time*, 2000

[93] In a study titled 'The Health of Older Persons in OECD Countries: Is it improving fast enough to compensate for population ageing?,' the OECD suggests that 'decisions taken now in terms of the balance of care, support for informal care and choices offered to older populations will also largely determine the future', OECD, Series OECD Labour Market and Social Policy Occasional Papers with number 37, Paris, 2000.

Within the European Union, in the year 1999, demographic ageing was the object of a comprehensive communication from the European Commission entitled 'Towards a Europe for all ages - Promoting prosperity and intergenerational security.'[94] Conceived of as Europe's contribution to the UN-sponsored International Year of Older Persons, celebrated in 1999, 'Towards a Europe of all ages' is a rather detailed document. At the beginning of its communication, the Commission heartily points out that in the next twenty years the number of older Europeans will outpace the number of younger generations. The report reads as follows:

'The European population will soon stop growing in size [...] It will then gradually start decreasing, though at different times and speeds in different countries and regions. In almost one quarter of European regions the population will already have stopped growing before the end of the century. Soon our societies will have a much larger proportion of older persons and a smaller working age population (see graph 2). The youngest generation, the 0-14 age group, representing 17.6% of the population in 1995, will fall to 15.7% in 2015, a decline of almost 5 millions. The generation 15-29, from which entrants into the labour market are drawn, will decrease even more rapidly (- 16%, equivalent to a decline of 13 million). Among older age cohorts, the exact opposite will occur. The generation 50- 64 will increase by more than 16 million (26%) while the growth of people of retirement age (65+) and the very old (80+) will approach 30% and 40% respectively. The changes in the 80+ group will be larger and happen faster than changes in any other age group.'[95]

In the first part, the communication illustrates the challenges that demographic ageing poses to European societies, while in the second part it elaborates a series of policy recommendations. The main challenges are clustered under four headings dealing, respectively, with 1) decline of the working age population and the ageing of the workforce, 2) pressure on pension systems and public finances, 3) the growing need for old age care and health care, and 4) the growing diversity among older people in terms of resources and needs (in particular the gender issue).

Who will support the cost of social protection for the large pool of inactive old people? Flexible employment policies are in demand.

According to the Commission, the growing number of retired people and the decline of the working age population will put pressure on pension systems and public finances. This will raise a problem of equity between generations. Who will support the cost of social protection for the large pool of inactive old people? The Commission suggests that a broader base for social protection systems must be secured through a higher employment rate for those of working age. As it was agreed in Lisbon – our reader will recall that the Lisbon agenda of March 2000 and, in particular, the 2002 'Kok report' set out 'to bring about a significant increase in the employment rate of Europe on a lasting basis' - Europe needs to retain workers' capacities. To achieve this, it is necessary to create life-long learning opportunities,

---

[94] European Commission, 'Towards a Europe for all ages - Promoting prosperity and intergenerational security', Communication from the Commission, COM(1999) 221 final, Brussels, 21 May 1999.
[95] COM(1999) 221 final, p.7.

support flexible working arrangements, plan tax and benefit schemes which can give incentive to taking up job offers and training opportunities, and induce employers to reconsider the age dimension in human resource management.[96] In addition, exploring new forms of gradual retirement could help reform pension systems, a sensitive issue in many EU member states, and make them 'more sustainable and flexible' (Towards a Europe for all ages, COM (1999) 221 final, p.5. See also below, on flexicurity).

Long term care, healthy ageing, prevention and rehabilitation

The growing need for old age care and health care is likely to augment dependency on health care systems. This situation will arguably induce a rethinking of formal health care systems as well as new thinking on 'healthy ageing, accident prevention and post-illness rehabilitation.' (Towards a Europe for all ages, COM (1999) 221 final, p.5-9) In order to support health care in old age, research programmes of the EU are encouraged to deepen medical, technological and social research on 'new public health instruments.'[97] The Commission indicates that informal care, that is, care which is not remunerated as service, will need to be integrated by formal care, which is likely to increase in size. This could result in 'possible moves towards a combination of public, voluntary and private for-profit providers in the supply of care.'[98] The Commission also points out that 'a greater use of assistive technologies may significantly improve the capacity for self-reliance and the quality of life of older people, even for the severely disabled.'

Diversity in old age

Meeting the needs of elderly people must also consider the growing diversity among older people in terms of resources and needs. The group of elderly people is a heterogeneous one.[99] The Commission acknowledges 'differences in family and housing situation, educational and health status and in income and wealth crucially determine the quality of life of older people.' (Towards a Europe for all ages, COM (1999) 221 final, p.19) The Commission also acknowledges that, as a consequence of population ageing, 'living conditions of elderly people may worsen as a result of heightening social exclusion and increased risk of poverty in later age. Women, who account for almost two-thirds of the population above 65, are particularly vulnerable due 'to historically weak labour market participation of women, social protection systems based on the model of the male breadwinner, and gender differences in longevity.' (Towards a Europe for all ages, COM (1999) 221 final, p.5)

---

[96] COM(1999) 221 final., p.4. Research conducted under the SENIOR project shows that many private companies, whose organisation of work relies almost exclusively on information and communication technologies, are wary of hiring older adults also because they fear old age is a barrier to pick up ICT skills. Experience shows that when properly trained or assisted, seniors can learn to use the few applications that usually run in an enterprise. SENIOR project, D1.5 'Work Package 1', prepared by D. Wright, p. 5.

[97] Ibid. p.5

[98] Ibid. p.19.

[99] Mordini E. et al., 'Senior citizens and the ethics of e-inclusion', in *Ethics and Information Technology*, (2009) 11: 203-220.

4. DEMOGRAPHIC AGEING, INFORMATION SOCIETY AND ELDERLY PEOPLE

Starting from the year 2000, the European Union strategy for the inclusion of elderly people in the information society takes shape. The strategy of Lisbon is to develop the information society so it includes the special needs and preferences of an ageing population. The market will be the driving force but, unlike in the past, all stakeholders, *viz.* social partners, end-users organisations, governments etc...shall be involved. The trust is that structured consultation between relevant stakeholders will deliver a reasonable compromise between economic goals, technological developments, and the personal and social needs of an ageing population. However, as the 1999 communication 'Towards a Europe of All Ages' demonstrates, e-including elderly citizens is a complex matter. As we will see in the next chapter, there are several life conditions and amongst senior citizens there is great heterogeneity, which makes it problematic devising one-fits-all solutions.

V. THE REVIEWED LISBON AGENDA AND THE EMERGENCE OF E-INCLUSION FOR ELDERLY PEOPLE (2005-TO DATE)

1. A MORE INTEGRATED APPROACH

In the year 2005, a second review of the Lisbon process is in order. The results of the 2005 review are included in the communication by the European Commission, 'Working together for growth and jobs: A new start for the Lisbon Strategy.' The 2005 mid-term review warns that 'current dynamics', including demographic ageing, cast a shadow over both long-term growth and social cohesion.' European societies must be ready to help more people to work, to work longer, and work in a way that uses their talents to best effect: 'Creating more and better jobs is not just a political ambition: it is an economic and social necessity.'[100]

Integration of low public spending and high employment rates

The Spring European Council of 22 and 23 March 2005[101] set forth a simplified system of coordination between EU macroeconomic politics (broad economic policy guidelines (BEPG))[102] and labour market policies. Formally, it produced a single framework of sixteen broad economic policy guidelines and eight guidelines on employment.[103] As far as broad economic guidelines are concerned, the first six detail

---

[100] The first review is based on the Kok report, seen above. The results of the 2005 review are included in European Commission, 'Working together for growth and jobs: A new start for the Lisbon Strategy', Communication to the Spring European Council from President Barroso in agreement with Vice-President Verheugen, COM(2005) 24, Brussels, 2 Feb 2005, p.24.

[101] Spring European Council, Brussels, 23 March 2005.

[102] The broad economic policy guidelines (BEPG) takes the form of a Council recommendation) based on article 99 of the Treaty. It is the central link in coordination of the Member States' economic policies. They ensure multilateral surveillance of economic trends in the Member States. Since 2003, the BEPG have been published for a period of three consecutive years.

[103] European Commission, 'Integrated guidelines for growth and jobs (2005-2008), COM(2005) 141 final, Brussels, 12 April 2005.

macroeconomic policies.[104] Guidelines 7 to 16 concern structural microeconomic guidelines including investments in research, ICT, competition, internal market, business environment, infrastructures and so on. Most important for our purposes are the eight guidelines on occupation,[105] which introduce, *inter alia,* two new notions, viz. 'flexicurity' and 'life cycle approach.'

THE EMPLOYMENT GUIDELINES (2005)[106]
Guideline No 17: Implement employment policies aiming at achieving full employment, improving quality and productivity at work, and strengthening social and territorial cohesion
Guideline No 18: Promote a lifecycle approach to work (italics face added)
Guideline No 19: Ensure inclusive labour markets, enhance work attractiveness, and make work pay for job-seekers, including disadvantaged people, and the inactive
Guideline No 20: Improve matching of labour market needs
Guideline No 21: Promote flexibility combined with employment security and reduce labour market segmentation, having due regard to the role of the social partners
Guideline No 22: Ensure employment-friendly labour cost developments and wage-setting mechanisms
Guideline No 23: Expand and improve investment in human capital
Guideline No 24: Adapt education and training systems in response to new competence requirements

Guideline number 18 - 'Promote a life cycle approach to work' – encourage states to adopt employment policies which help people find jobs at every stage of their working lives and remove barriers for those who wish to work. Active ageing policies, it is maintained, may include adaptation of working conditions, adequate incentives to work, and discouragement of early retirement. Social protection systems, *viz.* pensions and social security, should 'support participation and better retention in employment and longer working lives' through adapting welfare schemes to the principles of 'social adequacy', 'financial sustainability' and 'responsiveness' to changing needs.

These 'principles' are further elaborated in guideline 21, which introduces the concept of 'flexicurity.' In essence, flexicurity is a social welfare model which combines labour market flexibility with employment security[…].'[107] The idea at work behind it is that (job) flexibility, which gives a prerogative and an advantage to the employer, and (job) security, which grants financial support to the individual/employee, are not necessarily in tension but can be made mutually

---

[104] They are: 1) secure economic stability, 2) safeguard economic sustainability, 3) promote an efficient allocation of resources, 4) promote greater coherence between macroeconomic and structural policies, 5) ensure that wage developments contribute to macroeconomic stability and growth, 6) contribute to a dynamic and well-functioning EMU. Ibid. p.10.

[105] EU Council, 'Guidelines for the employment policies of the member states', Council Decision 2005/600/EC, Brussels, 12 July 2005.

[106] Ibid., In Annex.

[107] Compare European Commission, 'Towards Common Principles of Flexicurity: More and better jobs through flexibility and security', Communication from the Commission to the European Parliament, the Council, the European Economic and Social Committee and the Committee of the Regions, COM(2007) 359 final, Brussels, 27 June 2007.

supportive.[108] To be mutually supportive security and flexibility need to be planned on a common basis, which is provided by the continued contribution to economy by individuals throughout different periods of their work life. Guideline 18 on 'life cycle approach' here acquires significance. In order to 'support participation and better retention in employment and longer working lives' (guideline 18), social security should tap in the needs and the work capacities of a individual work-life trajectories. According to the report 'Jobs, Jobs, Jobs', flexibility could be advantageous for employers as well as for workers and their families: 'Flexibility is not just in the interest of employers; it also serves the interest of workers, helping them to combine work with care and education, for example, or to allow them to lead their preferred lifestyles.'[109]

The initiative 'Time to move up a gear: Partnership for Growth and Jobs'[110] applies the notions of 'flexicurity' and 'life cycle approach' to the opportunities and challenges posed by an ageing population. 'Active employment policies', listed in Part II, page 21 of the initiative, should 'provide incentives for elderly people to remain in work' and also 'appraise social protection systems that continue to offer the security needed to help people embrace change.' Employment policies should help older people find jobs while pension systems should be able to respond to individual social and also economic needs or changes. For example, older employees could, instead of stopping work, take up less demanding jobs, benefit from partial retirement and partial employment, enjoy continued training, or give training.[111] In line with guidelines 21 and 23, mentioned above, the EU and Member States are therefore encouraged to organise life long learning programmes for those who are over 45 years old, and to provide financial incentives for those who prolong their working lives or engage in part-time work.[112]

In conclusion, the 2005 'new impulse' or 'fresh impetus'[113] did not modify the structure of the 1997 European Employment and 2000 and 2002 Lisbon strategies, which remains the same, *viz.* attracting and retaining skilled people in the labour

---

[108] Wilthagen, T. and F. Tros (2004). 'The concept of 'flexicurity': a new approach to regulating employment and labour markets', in *Transfer: European Review of Labour and Research*, Vol. 10, No. 2, 2004, 166-186. Flexicurity is described as a policy strategy to enhance, at the same time and in a deliberate way, the flexibility of labour markets, work organisations and employment relations on the one hand, and security — employment security and social security — on the other. See R. Blanpain & M. Tiraboshi (eds.), *The Global Labour Market. From Globalization to Flexicurity*, Kluwer Law International, The Netherlands, 2008. Frank Hendrickx, Sonja Bekker, Roger Blanpain (eds.), *Flexicurity and the Lisbon Agenda. A Cross-Disciplinary Reflection*, Intersentia, 2008.

[109] W.Kok, 'Jobs Jobs Jobs', *op.cit.*, 2003, p. 27-32; W. Kok, *et al.*, 'Facing the Challenge: The Lisbon Startegy for Growth and Employment', Report from the High Level Group, Brussels, 2004, p. 33.

[110] European Commission, 'Time to move up a gear: The new partnership for growth and jobs', Communication from the Commission to the Spring European Council', COM(2006) 30, Brussels, 25 January 2006. The communication is supported by a Union Action Programme and National Action Programmes.

[111] T. Wilthagen, *Mapping out flexicurity pathways in the European Union*, Tilburg University - Flexicurity Research Programme, The Netherlands, March 2008. This paper was presented at the seminar 'Flexicurity: a new paradigm for employment and labour market regulation?', London 19 June 2008, Cabinet Office (UK).

[112] P. Villa, 'La Strategia Europea per l'Occupazione e le Pari Opportunità tra uomini e donne', op.cit., p.187-188.

[113] Council Decision, 'Guidelines for the employment policies of the Member States', 2005/600/EC, Brussels, 12 July 2005 on whereas n. 2 states 'The Lisbon European Council in March 2000 launched a strategy aimed at sustainable economic growth with more and better jobs and greater social cohesion, with long term employment targets, but five years later the objectives of the strategy remain far from being achieved.'

market. However, the introduction of flexicuirty and life cycle approach introduce new elements. Flexicurity arrangements for older persons in times of demographic ageing favour the integration of longer working lives and preferred life styles with appropriate social security arrangements. The question is how to plan state interventions in the field of labour and social security without running the risk of normalizing one's life cycle or life project.

2. THE SOCIO-ECONOMIC CHALLENGES OF AGEING SOCIETIES: A NEW APPRAISAL

Towards a new social vision for 21st century

The 2005 review of the Lisbon process was accompanied by a Social Agenda[114] designed to guide the European Union's action in the 'modernisation of the European social model and promote social cohesion.' The Agenda suggested a two-pronged strategy. The first segment, 'Building confidence', concerns the structure of the labour market[115]; the second segment purports to generate 'a more cohesive society', *viz.* to modernise social protection and intervention in heath care and long term health care, organise minimum income schemes, and include people excluded from the labour market (Social Agenda, COM(2005) 33 final, p.9-10). Announced in the Social Agenda these policy objectives were elaborated in more detail in the Commission's document 'Opportunities, access and solidarity: towards a new social vision for 21st century Europe.'[116]

'Opportunities, access and solidarity: towards a new social vision for 21st century Europe' consists of a detailed communication built on the reflections collected by the Commission Bureau of European Policy Advisers (BEPA)[117] and based on the results of Eurobarometer polls.[118] Its main merit lies in trying to unravel the complexities of European society showing how demographic ageing is both the result and it generates complex economic, social and cultural dynamics.

Demographic ageing itself is difficult to understand. While it is true that Europe's population enjoys – overall - greater life-expectancy than yesterday, the Commission policy advisers recall that healthy life expectancy and access to health still vary considerably between income groups and regions in Europe ('Opportunities, access and solidarity: towards a new social vision for 21st century Europe', p.4).

---

[114] European Commission, 'Social Agenda', Communication from the Commission, COM(2005) 33 final, Brussels, 9 February 2005.

[115] Namely: '1) Achieving full employment through greater involvement of social partners (revision of the Directive on European Works Councils (94/45/EC)); 2) A new dynamic for industrial relations based on development of a legal framework, especially on labour law, promotion of social dialogue, and promotion of social responsibility; 3) Removal of obstacles to workers' mobility, such as those arising from occupational pension schemes, and an optional European framework for transnational collective bargaining.' Ibid.

[116] European Commission, 'Opportunities, access and solidarity: towards a new social vision for 21st century Europe', Communication from the Commission to the European Parliament, the Council, the European Economic and Social Committee and the Committee of the Regions, COM(2007) 726 final, Brussels, 20 Nov 2007.

[117] The Bureau of European Policy Advisers is a department of the European Commission. It was established in order to provide professional and well-informed advice to the President and the European Commissioners.

[118] Eurobarometer, 'European Social Reality Report', Special Eurobarometer 273 / Wave 66.3 – TNS Opinion & Social – February 2007.

While there is evidence that birth rates are declining across Europe, the 'desire for children', says the Commission, 'often remains unfulfilled.' ('Opportunities, access and solidarity: towards a new social vision for 21st century Europe', p.4) Context and organisational factors do influence the decision of a couple to have or not to have children. This may also be the result of uneven sharing of parenting responsibilities, sub-optimal presence of childcare facilities, housing situations, and family-unfriendly work organizations.

Needs of care unmet

Demographic ageing may generate a high number of situations in which the caring needs of older persons are unmet.[119] Up to two-thirds of people over 75 are today dependent on informal care, which is mostly provided by the immediate family, especially women. Today, however, many elderly persons (28% of the population over 70) live alone. Financial means also vary. In Europe the risk of poverty is higher among older people[120], with elderly women particularly exposed to low pensions as a result of incomplete careers. Family structures are also changing. Marital break ups, single parenthood, weakening bonds of extended family, shifting work/life balance and care responsibilities, higher risk of unstable employment... These conditions affect millions of middle age Europeans today and may become source of social exclusion in few years time.

Risk of inter-generational divides

New risks of a generation divide are emerging between younger and older generations. Relations between generations are important given the number of generations (four or five) living together in society.[121] The 'gap', it is suggested, 'is between the aspirations of the young generation and the threat of limited opportunities [...]. Conflicts concern terms of pay, job security, access to housing, as well as in terms of sharing the financial implications of population ageing.' What is at stake is the solidarity between generations.

Concerning immigration flows, they may be more sustained in the coming years, but probably more varied than traditional immigration waves, with an increasing

---

[119] The growth of the population aged 80 or more will be even more pronounced in the future as more people are expected to survive to higher ages. The proportion of very old people (aged 80 and more) is expected to almost triple in the EU-27, from 4% in 2005 to 11% in 2050, with the highest proportions expected in Italy, Germany and Spain. It is worth noting that the population aged 55 to 64 will also grow considerably over the next fifteen years. European Commission, ' The Social situation in the European Union 2007', Directorate-General for Employment, Social Affairs and Equal Opportunities – Unit E.1 Eurostat – Unit F.3, April 2008

[120] 'Elderly people also face a higher risk of poverty than the total population. In 2008, the at-risk-of-poverty rate for those aged 65 years and over was 19% in the EU27. The highest rates were observed in Latvia (51%), Cyprus (49%), Estonia (39%) and Bulgaria (34%), and the lowest in Hungary (4%), Luxembourg (5%) and the Czech Republic (7%).' Eurostat, *Living conditions in 2008*, Brussels, 18 January 2010. It should be noted that the 'at-risk-of-poverty rate' is a relative measure of poverty, and that the poverty threshold varies greatly between Member States.

[121] Compare it with Roger Liddle and Frederic Lerais of the Bureau of European policy advisers (BEPA), *Europe's Social Reality*, Health & Consumer Protection DG, 2007. In particular questions asked at page 42: 'As life expectancy increases, how much will the burden of care for the elderly rise and who should meet it - in both financial cost and personal time? What are the social implications of the increasing numbers of elderly people living alone? Where should the balance of responsibility lie between family, community and state?' http://ec.europa.eu/health/ph_overview/health_forum/docs/ev_20070601_rd03_en.pdf

number of people leaving and then returning to their country of origin ('Opportunities, access and solidarity: towards a new social vision for 21st century Europe', p.8).

The employment landscape may be more complex than only 'shrinking.' The Eurobarometer poll[122] indicates that some 44.6 million people aged between 16 and 64 - 16% of the EU working-age population - consider themselves to have a longstanding health problem or disability. Many of them, though, are willing and able to take up work, provided appropriate conditions are in place.

'All of this', concludes the BEPA group 'means that European societies will have to become more open, diverse and complex', promote equality by accepting diversity and eradicating forms of discrimination. The implications of ageing may be obvious, notably in relation to health and social protection systems, yet they 'pose comprehensive challenges that would seem illusory to solve only through targeted actions.'[123] The new concept of flexicurity, it is pointed out, entails 'a radical policy and culture shift away from a 'job-for-life' ending with early retirement towards 'employment for life.' (The demographic future of Europe – from challenge to opportunity, p.7) Active ageing or active ageing employment strategies acquire meaning if social and organisational conditions are at the core of 'a life cycle perspective'[124] and of a 'substantial rethink of intergenerational responsibilities and the way the associated costs are shared between generations.' [125]

3. I2010 EUROPEAN INFORMATION SOCIETY: ENTERS E-INCLUSION

Our reader will recall the 2000 *e*Europe initiative 'An information society for all'[126], discussed above. *e*Europe supported the 2000 Lisbon agenda harnessing the growth

---

[122] Eurobarometer, op.cit., 2007.

[123] See European Commission, 'The demographic future of Europe – from challenge to opportunity', Commission Communication, COM(2006) 571 final, Brussels, 12 Oct 2006. where the Commission identifies five ways to address the 'Demographic Timebomb': helping to balance work-family-private life; improving work opportunities for older people; increasing productivity and competitiveness by valuing the contributions of older employees; harnessing the positive impact of migration for the job market; and ensuring sustainable public finances for social protection in the long-term.

[124] It is not clear what the Communication intends by 'life-cycle perspective'. Lights are provided by Steven Ney, 'Active ageing policy in Europe: between path dependency and path departure', in *Ageing International*, Fall 2005, Vol. 30, No. 4, pp. 325-342, especially p.10: 'The Life-cycle approach relates individual and collective wellbeing over time to the complex interaction of a wide variety of factors. These include family life, employment, education, socio-cultural participation, material security and health.' Ney holds that the life-cycle approach is alternative to an approach focussed on demographic aging and its financial consequences: 'Adopting a holistic life-cycle approach implies that successful aging policymaking embrace all generations. Aging policy is fundamentally about providing and safeguarding social, economic and political rights for citizens of all ages. In short, effective citizenship for older people presupposes real citizenship for everyone.' For reflection on active ageing see Chapter 2.

[125] European Commission, 'Opportunities, access and solidarity', *op.cit.*, p.8. In 2008, the Renewed Social Agenda continued the reflection on the priority areas identified in the European Commission's recent Communication Opportunities, access and solidarity: towards a new social vision for 21st century Europe. European Commission. (2008a). Renewed social agenda: Opportunities, access and solidarity in 21st century Europe. Brussels. COM(2008), 412 final. See below, Post i2010.

[126] COM(1999) 687 final, 8 December 1999.

and jobs strategy to the information society.[127] Five years later, the 'i2010: European Information Society for growth and employment' is presented to the 2005 Spring European Council with the goal, *inter alia*, of achieving an Inclusive European Information Society that promotes growth and jobs.[128]

Three priority areas are listed in the *i2010 Strategic Framework,* which implements the i2010 initiative. 'Fully in-line with the new governance cycle of the re-launched Lisbon Strategy' the three areas for action are:

(a) the completion of a Single European Information Space and open competitive internal market for information society and media;
(b) strengthening Innovation and Investment in ICT research to promote growth and more and better jobs; and
(c) achieving an Inclusive European Information Society that promotes growth and jobs in a manner that is consistent with sustainable development and that prioritises better public services and quality of life. [129]

In paragraph (c) of the i2010 strategic framework, the expression '[...] Inclusive European Information Society[...]' introduces the concept of e-inclusion as one of the key enablers of the economic and social progress of the i2010 initiative, and thus of the Lisbon agenda. E-inclusion is seen as an enabling tool for anyone - who so wishes - to participate in the advantages of the information society, thus helping to reduce individual or social exclusion. The i2010 initiative reaffirms the idea that the information society must satisfy social justice and for economic goals. A few years later, addressing the theme of ICT accessibility, Commissioner Vivian Reding would back the launch of a public consultation on e-accessibility calling ' [...] on the web publishing industry and public sector administrations to make a much more determined effort to ensure the web is accessible to everyone. Those responsible should remember that in a few years time, they will probably find themselves amongst those having trouble to read the screen.'[130]

4. THE RIGA DECLARATION (2006)

The 2006 Riga declaration marks an important phase in the architecture of Europe's Information Society. In the year 2006, the European Union is already well engaged in ICT. Actions and initiatives target penetration of ICT[131], e-government[132], e-health[133],

---

[127] *eEurope* aimed at creating a digitally literate Europe, bringing every citizen into the digital age and online, and ensuring *socially inclusive* information society.
[128] European Commission, 'i2010 – A European Information Society for growth and employment', Communication from the Commission to the Council, the European Parliament, the European Economic and Social Committee and the Committee of the Regions, COM(2005) 229 final, Brussels, 1 June 2005.
[129] COM (2005) 229 final, *i2010*, p. 12.
[130] Viviane Reding, EU Commissioner for the Information Society and Media, Brussels, European Commission Press Release (IP/08/1074), 2 July 2008. The Commission's public consultation document is available at http://ec.europa.eu/einclusion
[131] European Commission, 'eAccessibility', Communication from the Commission to the Council, the European Parliament and the European Economic and Social Committee and the Committee of the Regions, COM(2005) 425 final, Brussels, 13 September 2005.
[132] European Commission, 'i2010 eGovernment Action Plan: Accelerating eGovernment in Europe for the Benefit of All', Communication from the Commission to the Council, the European Parliament, the European Economic and Social Committee and the Committee of the Regions, COM(2006) 173 final,

and even 'e-democracy'[134]. Ubiquitous computing and the convergence of ICT with other technologies and disciplines hold out opportunities to assist or enable individuals to lead active and independent lives. Against this backdrop, one year after the review of the 2005 Lisbon strategy, EU member states agree to join efforts to upgrade the development of Europe's Information Society. On 11 June 2006, e-inclusion is officially launched in the town of Riga by the Ministers of European Union (EU) Member States and European Free Trade Area (EFTA) countries responsible for media and communication.[135] The Declaration's aim is to create an information society for all through targeted actions designed to include those who are, for different reasons, more vulnerable to be excluded from it. The Declaration defines e-inclusion as meaning both inclusive technologies and the use of technologies to achieve wider inclusion objectives.[136] In line with the 'i2010' communication and the broader renewed Lisbon agenda, e-inclusion sets out six thematic areas, also known as the six 'flagship' initiatives of e-inclusion. They are geographical digital divide, accessibility, digital literacy and competences, cultural diversity, inclusive eGovernment, and ative ageing.[137]

In the field of active ageing, ICT should empower older people so they can fully participate in the economy and in society, continue independent lifestyles and enhance their quality of life. In tune with the spirit of the renewed Lisbon strategy, the Riga approach to ICT for the elderly brings together social and economic needs and opportunities in four main ways.[138] First, it seeks to reduce market fragmentation by promoting interoperability, standards and common specifications. Second, the Declaration calls for exploiting the occupational possibilities offered by innovative ICT solutions in order to, e.g., improve working conditions or help reorganise the work-life balance of older workers. Third, ICT penetration among the elderly should afford better access to goods and services as well as promote personal interactions and social contacts. Last, the Ministerial summit encourages independent living initiatives, the promotion of assistive technologies, and ICT-enabled services for integrated social and healthcare, including personal emergency and location-based services[139].

Brussels, 25 April 2006. See also the *eGovernment Action Plan. A roadmap for Inclusive eGovernment: towards making all citizens, and especially disadvantaged groups major beneficiaries of eGovernment*, drafted by the eGovernment Unit of the DG Information Society of the European Commission and the Inclusive eGovernment ad hoc group, Brussels, 27 Nov 2006. http://www.umic.pt/images/stories/publicacoes/inclusive_egovernment_roadmap.pdf

[133] European Commission Information Society and Media, 'ICT for Health and i2010: Transforming the European healthcare landscape: Towards a strategy for ICT for Health', Office for Official Publications of the European Communities, Luxembourg, June 2006.

[134] OECD, *Promise and Problems of e-democracy*, Paris 2003. http://www.oecd.org/dataoecd/9/11/35176328.pdf

[135] Ministerial Declaration approved unanimously on 11 June 2006, Riga, Latvia. The text of the Riga declaration is available at http://ec.europa.eu/information_society/events/ict_riga_2006/doc/declaration_riga.pdf

[136] *Ibid.*: 'E-inclusion focuses on participation of all individuals and communities in all aspects of the information society.'

[137] In detail, concerning e-Competences: ICT skills should become a repertoire of citizens' capacities. Lifelong learning is necessary. Socio-Cultural e-Inclusion, to enable minorities, migrants and marginalised young people to fully integrate into communities and participate in society by using ICT. Geographical e-Inclusion, to increase the social and economic well being of people in rural, remote and economically disadvantaged areas with the help of ICT. Inclusive eGovernment, to deliver better, more diverse public services for all using ICT while encouraging increased public participation in democracy. Ageing in the text.

[138] See Riga Declaration, para. 9.

[139] *Ibid.*, para. 12.

The Riga Declaration, however, warns that technological solutions should always increase quality of life, autonomy and safety while respecting privacy and ethical requirements.

To be part of the information society: accessibility and personalization

The guidelines and objectives of Riga are elaborated upon and detailed in the 2007 European Commission initiative 'To be part of the information society.'[140] The communication clarifies what is meant by e-inclusion and why it is worth pursuing it. 'E-Inclusion', writes the Commission, 'refers to the actions to realise an inclusive information society, that is, an information society for all. The aim is to enable every person who so wishes to fully participate in the information society, despite individual or social disadvantages.' 'E-Inclusion is necessary', explains the communication, 'for social justice, ensuring equity in the knowledge society. It is also necessary on economic grounds, to fully realise the potential of the information society for productivity growth and reduce the cost of social and economic exclusion. Finally an inclusive information society brings large market opportunities for the ICT sector (Initial estimates indicate that benefits from e-Inclusion in the EU could be in the order of €35 to €85 billion over five years).'[141]

The communication acknowledges the objectives of the 'i2010 initiative' and of the Riga Declaration, such as bridging the digital divides. However, it warns that putting in place enabling conditions, such as broadband connection[142], may not be sufficient for groups such as elderly people, people with disabilities, and cultural minorities.[143] Innovative solutions should factor in users' special requirements and consider the contexts in which they are used. To this end, the 'To be part of the information society' communication calls for cooperation of stakeholders involved in ICT, industries, user organisations, trade unions, and governmental agencies. Concerted efforts and structured consultations should strive to deliver on the real needs of users. From a policy viewpoint, this means that 'policy makers should consider the potential of ICT within social and economic policies and, also, assess the impact of ICT on social inclusion, non discrimination and participation.'[144]

---

[140] European Commission, 'To be part of the Information Society', Communication from the Commission to the European Parliament, the Council, the European Economic and Social Committee and the Committee of the Regions COM (2007) 694 final, Brussels, 8 November 2007.

[141] COM (2007) 694 final. Compare it with the definition offered by the 1997 HLEG report, discussed above. The HLEG said 'We associate inclusion - what in Eurospeak is more commonly termed 'cohesion' - with the extent to which any individual is able to participate in society. Whether rich or poor, at a distance or at the centre, [young or old, we shall add], one would hope that in a future Information Society individuals will be able to play a full part in the social life of the community. Ideally, the Information Society should help to reduce exclusion, not increase it.'

[142] It is explained, e.g., that 'In a few years time a minimum speed of 20 Mbit/sec will be needed for services such as telemedicine that are of great importance for many people of risk of exclusion, in particular for the growing population of elderly persons.' COM (2007) 694 final, p. 7.

[143] COM (2007) 694 final, under paragraph 3.2 'Accelerating effective participation of target groups at risk of exclusion and improving quality of life', p.8. See also Riga Declaration, para. 20.

[144] COM (2007) 694 final, p.11.

Action Plan 'Ageing well in the information society':   Coordinate R&DT in ICT for the elderly while respecting privacy and ethical requirements (2007)

As far as older persons are concerned, the point of arrival of the 2005 'e-inclusion-after-Lisbon' strategy is the Action Plan 'Ageing well in the Information Society.'[145] The aim of the 2007 Action Plan 'Ageing well in the information Society' is to create industrial momentum for a significant effort in developing and deploying user-friendly ICT tools and services; mainstreaming older users' needs; and supporting other policy areas in addressing the challenges of ageing.[146] Concretely, the Action Plan launched a joint European research programme on ICT for improving the life of older people at home, in the workplace and in society in general. The Commission also set up a wholly new research initiative, 'Ageing well in the Information Society' which, leveraging on Article 169 of the Treaty[147], would coordinate Member State research programmes on ICT for ageing.

Most importantly, the Ageing Well in the Information Society Action Plan adhered to the recommendation made in Riga that technology for elderly must always 'increase quality of life, autonomy and safety, while respecting privacy and ethical requirements.'[148] The Action Plan goes further, arguing that recognising and protecting ethical, social and privacy needs involved in ICT for the elderly respond to market interests too. Lack of attention to privacy and ethical requirements can engender fear or distrust in users and prevent adoption of technology.

The Staff Working Document on Ageing well in the Information Society Action Plan (2007)

A comprehensive analysis and concrete proposals are included in the Commission's 'Staff Working Document' which supports the 'Ageing well in the Information Society action plan.'[149] The staff working document is a long paper which attempts to bring together an analysis of the general policy issues at stake - demographic ageing, information society, and Lisbon objectives - with proposals addressing different domain areas, such as health, work, standards, education, access, ethics, etc. relevant to ageing well in the information society. The analysis rehearses the line according to

---

[145] European Commission, 'Ageing well in the Information Society: Action Plan on Information and Communication Technologies and Ageing. An i2010 Initiative,' Communication from the Commission to the European Parliament, the Council, the European Economic and Social Committee and the Committee of the Regions, COM (2007) 332 final, Brussels, 14 June 2007.
[146] 'The action plan addresses market barriers and seeks to realise the opportunities for the older people of today and tomorrow, by raising awareness, building common strategies, removing technical and regulatory hurdles, and promoting take-up, joint research and innovation. It coordinates existing efforts, adds new actions to integrate, complement and reinforce existing work.' COM (2007) 332 final, p.4.
[147] Included under Title XVIII 'Research and Technological Development' (by the Single European Act 1986-87), article 169 provides as follows: 'In implementing the multiannual framework programme, the Community may make provision, in agreement with the Member States concerned, for participation in research and development programmes undertaken by several Member States, including participation in the structures created for the execution of those programmes.'
[148] Riga Declaration, op.cit., para 10.
[149] European Commission, 'Commission Staff Working Document, Accompanying document to the Communication from the Commission to the European Parliament, the Council, the European Economic and Social Committee and the Committee of the Regions, Ageing well in the Information Society, COM(2007) 332 final', SEC (2007) 0811 final, Brussels, 14 June 2007.

which 'ageing well in the information society' is both a social necessity and an economic opportunity and makes three points.

First, ageing societies should enable older people to continue 'participating in and contributing to economic and social life – where they wish to do so'. This would reduce social isolation and exclusion while allowing Europe's knowledge society to benefit from 'the knowledge and experience of elderly people.'

In the second instance, economy and society at large could contain 'the rising cost of care, while safeguarding the quality of social and health care and respect for human dignity.' The economic challenges also include keeping people productive in work when getting older, in view of the rising dependency ratio.[150] The Staff working document goes into great detail to illustrate the economic advantages of ageing well in the information society: the size of the growth sector in the market of ICT for the elderly[151], 'not only in Europe but increasingly globally'[152]; containment of the costs of care (SEC (2007) 0811 final, paragraph 2.2, p.9.); retaining older workers and increased occupation rates and employability for older workers. (SEC (2007) 0811 final, paragraph 3.3.2, p.31-33)

Third, it is suggested that the information society should 'enable older people – where they wish to do so - to be active and empowered citizens and consumers, thereby contributing to a positive perception of ageing in Europe' (SEC (2007) 0811 final, paragraph 1, p.5 and paragraph 3.4.2, p.35. On ethical conditioning, paragraph 3.2.7, p. 26).

The staff working paper recognises that companies failed to penetrate the area of ageing. 'Industry', it is argued, 'has limited understanding of comparative user requirements, such as socioeconomic factors, gender needs and income levels' that may impede access to ICT. Personal attitudes, sensitivities to ICT, and lifestyles need to be understood in order to offer what users actually need or want. (SEC (2007) 0811 final, paragraph 2.2[153]) Products and services, for the Commission, are often not adapted to meet the specific needs of frail older users or they are not adequately available.[154] The 'Staff Working Document' warns that the potential of ICT for elderly people cannot unfold if needs and contextual factors are not considered. It is key to take into account the cultural, economic, social, as well as psychological characteristics of the ageing group, before ICT is implemented. Diversity in needs and preferences may be due to many factors such as income, education, geographic location, health impairments, disabilities, or gender; it is important to know whether or not the ICT solution is mediated by professionals, doctors, rehabilitation experts, field experts, family members, informal care providers, and family members (SEC

---

[150] The relation between people in working age and retired people. See Eurostat, *Living conditions*, op.cit., 2007.

[151] SEC (2007) 0811 final, paragraph 3.2.1 on informational asymmetries'. 'User empowerment is a reality more than ever before with the help of new technologies, notably the Internet, and increasingly it is recognised that the ageing group represents significant buying power (over 3000 B€ in wealth and revenues for the over 65) and voting power.'

[152] SEC (2007) 0811 final, paragraph 2.2., p11-13. Concerning the health sector paragraph 2.3.5, p.14-15 and paragraph 3.3.1, p.29-30.

[153] SEC (2007) 0811 final, paragraph 2.2: 'the European mainstream industry has so far not exploited the full potential for products and services targeted at the mass-market of older people. While ageing is becoming a mainstream phenomenon, industry and providers do not yet sufficiently capture the needs of the ageing society in mainstream products and service.'

[154] SEC (2007) 0811 final, 'Older people, when faced with new technologies, can find themselves in a relatively weak position. If they fail at any point, the older person can feel utterly powerless.' E.Mordini *et al.,* 'Senior citizens and the ethics of e-inclusion', *Ethics and Information Technology* (2009) 11: 203-220.

(2007) 0811 final, paragraph 5.5.1); due consideration ought to be given to the organisation or reimbursement and insurance schemes as well as of liability issues (SEC (2007) 0811 final, paragraph 5.5.1.5)

In order to better accommodate research in ICT to the concrete situations in which elderly people live and age, the proposal of the Commission is to distinguish and focus on the three institutional contexts of 'Ageing well.' They are ageing at home, at work, and in the community.

1) Ageing well at work or staying longer active and productive in high-quality work. The Commission espouses the Lisbon strategy goal of increasing retirement age and keeping people working longer.[155] Unemployment often affects older workers more than others; jobs in traditional industries are made precarious by increasing competition. Furthermore, older workers need to adapt to knowledge-intensive jobs and learn how to cope with new technologies. 'ICT solutions', it is suggested, 'could help to keep older workers in the labour market productively, thus retaining their knowledge and skills.'[156] This, however, requires also 'new work patterns with better work-life balance and life long learning[157], and sustainable reconciliation of work and family life.

2) Ageing well in the community or 'being a member of the community: continuing to participate actively in society.' 'Acting on information' is becoming necessary to get access to public and commercial services; more generally, it is also getting increasingly important for social participation. However, the Internet[158], as well as other modern technologies, are more easily and quickly adopted, the Commission contends, 'by urban, skilled and financially well off communities and then spread to more peripheral, lower-skilled or lower-income social categories – and in this context, also tend to be taken up only later by the ageing population.' Interestingly, the Commission warns that the age-related and other forms of digital divides cumulate over time and generations, instead of disappearing. The accumulation of age related divides and other sources of social exclusion may, against the fast paced developments in ICTs, risk becoming a permanent phenomenon, 'thus translating into social stratification.' The risks of exclusion for those who those who stand in the dark side of the digital divide are real, and they should be lessened with enhanced access, accessibility, affordability, and usability requirements for ageing population. [159]

3) Ageing well at home or living a longer, independent and healthy daily life suggests the possibility of enjoying a healthier and higher quality of daily life for longer, assisted by technology, while maintaining a high degree of independence, autonomy and dignity. The aim of the 'living independently at home' plan is to provide social and health care to older people, while keeping these services financially sustainable and, possibly, reducing costs.[160] The challenges go together

---

[155] Employment and/or reduced productivity of 55 to 64 year old people creates substantial pressure on the long term sustainability of public finance, says the working paper, SEC (2007) 0811 final, paragraph 2.4

[156] SEC (2007) 0811 final, Ibid. at paragraph 2.4.

[157] SEC (2007) 0811 final, paragraph 3.2.1

[158] SEC (2007) 0811 final, Executive statement. 'Elderly people have a large buying power with persons over 65 representing some 20% of GDP. However, they also still have a low participation in the information society with only 10% of persons over 65 having Internet access.'

[159] On the digital divide between 'info-rich' and 'info-poor' see D. Zolo, *Glabalizzazione. Una mappa dei problemi*, Laterza, bari, p. 63-64.

[160] SEC (2007) 0811 final, paragraph 2.4. 'The increasing demand for social and health care services will generate additional costs that a lower growth cannot sustain. Projections suggest that age-related

with the opportunities. The delivery of efficient health care and independent living services is a social responsibility, on the one hand, and it is also an opportunity which can help raise productivity, on the other. Technological solutions can be integrated in formal and informal care, thus supporting the general need for health and social care. For instance, ICT can ensure sound, reliable health information for older adults and effective provision of continuity of care via telemedicine and social care in the home.[161] It is a long term investment, says the Commission, that is worth pursuing vigorously.[162]

Ethical concerns

Ethical concerns will emerge. The Action Plan Ageing well in the Information Society had warned that where solutions require a degree of monitoring and intervention, there is no specific reference point for ethics [...] in safeguarding human dignity and autonomy.'[163] The Staff Working paper implementing the Action Plan attempts to formulate some research questions which should be part of a high-level debate.[164] In order to preserve his or her autonomy, the user 'must have the right to overrule or switch off the technology' and 'to opt out completely from using the services, should they so wish.'[165] 'Such rights', it continues, 'must be built into the services.' In general, it is pointed out, '[b]ringing technology with monitoring functions into a person's home also raises important ethical questions with regard to possible conflicts with the principles of dignity, independence and privacy.'[166] More specifically, the paper identifies as a major barrier to the uptake of ICT the concern of older persons that they will spend the last years of their lives entangled in a technological fix. This leads to the formulation of an important principle, i.e., that ICT services should not aim to substitute existing care networks, but that they should be promoted and implemented as complementary solutions. Smart home devices, for example, should be seen as a means to enhancing social care rather than as a substitute for it.

ICT-based solutions should not increase isolation but contribute to maintaining or strengthening social networks.[167]

Finally, in the year 2009, the distinction among the areas of ageing, home, work and community is reviewed by the 'AAliance report.'[168] According to the drafters of the report the use and presence of ambient intelligence applications blurs the boundaries between different living contexts. As we shall see in chapter IV (the

---

spending on pensions, health and long-term care will increase by between 4 and 8 % of GDP in coming decades. Longer life expectancy poses challenges for health treatment, the effectiveness and financial viability of pension schemes, and the opportunity (sometimes formulated as a right) to pursue enhanced forms of healthy and independent living.'

[161] For instrance, personal health systems include implantable, wearable and portables systems for monitoring and diagnosis, therapy and repairing/substitution of functionality. SEC (2007) 0811 final, paragraph 3.3.1.

[162] SEC (2007) 0811 final, Ibid.. 'ICT can deliver the necessary improvement in efficiency and productivity of these services and help to assure their provision to future generations.'

[163] COM(2007) 332 final, p.7.

[164] The highly level debate was launched in Bled (Slovenie) on 12 May 2008. On Bled and its successor Vienna, see below.

[165] SEC (2007) 0811 final, paragraph 5.3.4.

[166] SEC (2007) 0811 final, Ibid.

[167] SEC (2007) 0811 final, paragraph 5.3.4.

[168] G. Van Den Broek, F. Cavallo and C. Wehrmann (eds.), *AALIANCE Ambient Assisted Living Roadmap,* IOS Press, Amsterdam, 2010.

technology context), during the day older individuals traverse multiple physical and virtual spaces (room, shop, garden, e-shopping, chatting, or planning an itinerary), whether they are at home, at work or 'on the move.' The distinction between home, community and work is still valid for research, but it does not provide practical guidance to the development of ambient assisted living technologies.

5. THE BLED AND VIENNA SUMMITS (2008)

In search of an ethics of digitalization for older persons in the Information Society

During the year 2008, the ethics of inclusion of older people were at the centre of two ministerial meetings organised by the European Commission with participation of Ministries from the Member States.

At the meeting of 12 May 2008 in Bled (Slovenia) it was agreed to promote study of an 'ethics of digitalisation which incorporates not only the need for assistance and protection, but also the need for empowering individuals with different capabilities (for instance, old and frail elderly), to forge relationships, to stay authentically active in society, to express and share their lives.[169] Few months later, the European Ministerial E-Inclusion (Vienna, 30 November 2008), undertook to describe in greater detail the age related divide in Europe. Europe faces a growing number of older people, including the very old (aged 85 or more) who are likely to suffer some form of disability in later age. Many older persons will live alone; there will be smaller households and more fragile family networks; demands for health and social care will increase at a time when public budgets are under strain. Meeting the real needs of older persons is complicated by the difficulty of forging a uniform narrative about 'the elderly' as a group. Older persons are not a homogeneous group and the diversity of that group ought to be preserved. ICT goods and services are usually produced on a large or mass scale basis which levels down differences. They should instead be flexible and able to adapt. Adaptation should consider not only the individual user's physical needs but also family and networks. To this end, based on the ethical imprint rounded off in Bled, the Vienna Ministerial proposes a set of actions aimed at giving practical weight to an ethics of digitalisation for elderly people. The suggestions laid forth concern i) the promotion and development of corporate statements of social responsibility and codes of ethics in e-Inclusion and implement EC Corporate Social Responsibility policies in this field; ii) the collection and comparison between best practices at local and regional level and to create more structured exchanges between stakeholders by creating regular consultative mechanisms, platforms, and forums; iii) the creation of a monitoring mechanism study the ethical and privacy implications of emerging technology for e-Inclusion. We will elaborate further on some of these recommendations in chapter III (Legal framework), chapter VII (Best practices), and chapter VIII (Ethical recommendations).

6. TOWARDS EU 2020

During the year 2009 the European Commission organised a series of workshops on good practices in ICT for elderly people, on which we report in chapter VII. The

---

[169] Mordini E, Wright D, et.al., SENIOR Discussion Paper, 'Ethics of e-inclusion of older people', 2008. http://ec.europa.eu/information_society/events/cf/ict2008/document.cfm?doc_id=5808.

European Union also started to reflect on the continuation of the Lisbon strategy, EU2020. The Commission anticipates that in the EU2020 agenda there will be tighter coordination of member states policies. The governance of 'Lisbon II' will work on categories, such as levels of innovation, discrimination, environment, or e-inclusion, and the EU will benchmark member states' performances in the selected areas.[170]

As in the previous experiences, *viz.* the 2000 Lisbon strategy and the 2005 reviewed agenda, a new initiative on information society and e-inclusion will, most likely, accompany EU2020. A consultation was launched on the post i2010 (opened on 4 August 2009 and closed on 9 October 2009).[171] In November 2009 the Swedish Presidency of the EU organized in Visby (Sweden) a panel, called the 'Visby Agenda', with the goal of 'creating impact for an e-Union 2015.' The Visby conference[172] gave the incoming presidency of the European Union, held by Spain, the opportunity to illustrate plans for the post-i2010. Spain foresees a new, post i2010 European Strategy (until 2015).[173] The future 'Granada Strategy' will be based on five points: ICT for the environment, the single digital market, next generation networks, overcoming the 'second' digital divide, and the drawing up of a Charter of Users' Rights. The formula 'second digital divide' means digital divide between the young and well-educated on one side and older generations and the less-educated on the other. This re-branding of the digital divide may lead to new initiatives on elderly people and ICT.[174] The second interesting point concerns the promotion of European Charter of ICT Users' Rights, which would ideally reinforce also older users. Eventually, in Visby, it was proposed to draw up a harmonised framework of Information Society indicators, based on easy and free to access statistical data.[175]

On its part, the European Commission's 'i2010 e-Inclusion Subgroup Committee' drew up a report titled 'Vision, priorities and actions for e-Inclusion Beyond i2010.'[176] It was agreed that the beneficial effects of e-inclusion still need to be proved. Presented in Limassol, Cyprus, on 6-8 April 2009, the paper identifies a number of areas and topics that e-inclusion policies may consider in the future. They can be conveniently grouped under four headings:

1) Improve ICT access and skills to stimulate greater use
2) Address the ageing trend by promoting ICT-enabled solutions

---

[170] *European Voice*, '2020 vision', by Jim Brunsden, 14 January 2010.

[171] European Commission, 'Consultation on the future 'EU 2020' strategy', Commission Working Document, COM(2009) 647 final, Brussels, 24 November 2009.

[172] http://www.se2009.eu/en/meetings_news/2009/11/10/webcast_visby_agenda_creating_impact_for_a n_eunion_2015_10_november

[173] Under the announced name of "For a digital Europe: the Granada Strategy. Information and Communication Technologies, Productivity and Quality of Life'.

[174] In its 2935th Meeting of 30 and 31 March 2009, the EU Council committee on telecommunications concurred that 'everyone should have the possibility of accessing services including users with disabilities and elderly users as well as all those who have particular difficulties in becoming part of the digital society.'

[175] See presentation by Professor H. Rosling (Karolinska University), Conference, Visby Agenda: 'Creating Impact for an eUnion 2015', 10 November. Professor Rosling calls for public solid and stable data bases compiled in machine readable unified format and available for free. http://www.se2009.eu/en/meetings_news/2009/11/10/webcast_visby_agenda_creating_impact_for_an_ eunion_2015_10_november

[176] Limassol e-Inclusion Report: Vision, priorities and actions for e-Inclusion Beyond i2010, prepared by the i2010 e-Inclusion Subgroup as a result of its meeting in Limassol, Cyprus, on 7-8 April, 2009 June 2009 (The report is provisional while it awaits endorsement by the i2010 High Level Group).

3) Enhance accessibility and personalisation to foster equality and inclusive ICT markets
4) Improve coordination and implementation of e-Inclusion measures for greater impact

Concerning the second point, viz., 'address the ageing trend by promoting ICT-enabled solutions', the group suggests targeted actions in the areas of work, active ageing, and care. Regarding work, the committee invites European states to actively support the 50-65 age group 'to prolong their work lives, as a means to increase their income and personal satisfaction, as well as ease and delay burden on pension systems.'[177] In the area of active ageing, the group advices better coordination in the area of ICT products and services in order to ensure that the latter are accessible and usable also by elderly people. In the field of care and independence, the group calls for 'enhanced interoperability between e-heath systems, innovative business and reimbursement models'. Technological developments in this area should, it is explained, be supported and directed social security and healthcare policies.[178]

At the level of member states, in the year 2009 Finland became the first country in Europe to make broadband internet access a legal right. Starting from July 2010, telecommunications companies operating in Finland will be under the legal obligation of providing all Finnish residents with broadband lines that can run at speeds of at least 1 megabit per second.[179] Other states may follow Finland's example.[180] Such initiatives are likely to give rise to new rights related to end-users' access, use, or suspension of services and applications through electronic communications networks.

A new directive to combat discrimination outside the field of employment may be approved in the next months or years. Together with the Treaty of Lisbon, which provides in Article 10 that new EU policies are to be examined on the basis of their effect on equality, the directive may have a positive impact on senior citizens. As suggested *infra* in Chapter III, fundamental rights may play an important role in the post-i2010 period. With the entry into force of the Lisbon Treaty, the 2000 EU Charter of Fundamental Rights has in effect gained full access to the EU legal framework.

VI. ACTIVE AGEING ON THE EU AGENDA

In this chapter we gave an account of the background against which Europe's Information Society unfolded.

---

[177] 'Measures should be adopted for ICT to be an enabler rather than a barrier for longer and balanced work lives, e.g. ad-hoc digital training, more friendly work environments and solutions such as telework, user-friendly tools for collaborative work environment, assistive technologies and services.'
[178] 'This should help', says the committee, 'to scale up the market for ICT supported independent living, mobility and personalised health monitoring, and improve quality of life while relieving the burden on social and health care.'
[179] See Chapter 1. Bobbie Johnson, 'Finland makes broadband access a legal right', The Guardian, 14 October 2009.
[180] For instance, in 2009 Belgium unveiled the Digital Belgium Action Plan 2010-2015. The Plan includes measures for driving internet penetration from 64% today to no less than 90% in 2015. The Belgian government will give incentives for PC ownership, as well as donate refurbished pc's to the poor and unemployed. For an overview on see also e-Government Factsheet, 'Belgium', September 2009, edition 12.0, prepared and available at www.epractice.eu

Europe's socio-economic vision, suggested in the 1993 White Paper, took shape in 1997 with the signing of the Amsterdam Treaty (and the introduction of Title IX), and the launch of the European Employment Strategy (EES), later reformulated in the language of Lisbon strategy. Keywords of the underlying socio-economic vision are economic growth, social cohesion, and employment strategies, and also demographic ageing. The main objective of the employment strategies, we underlined, is to activate the dormant production and consumption capacities of an ageing society.

Concerning the information society, we have paused on what can be considered the building blocks of Europe's Information society, the 1994 'Bangemann report' and the 1997 'Building the European Information society report.' The Bangemann report obtained the result that the nascent information society is steered by market forces.[181] Rejecting or missing out on ICT - the argument went - would turn society in a worse place to be, while engaging vigorously would in time be rewarding to society in general, not only to the market. The HLEG report or 'Building the information society for us all' report, by contrast, shunned the idea that the market leads and social questions come only 'after' the game is started. As the group of experts held out, the neglected and sometimes unexpected social aspects of the Information Society need to be addressed together with technology development plans, not overseen or postponed.[182]

Starting from the year 2000, the EU's policies on the information society are integrated in the broader European Union's social and economic strategy and vision. Pressing socio and economic policy issues directly affect information society strategies and give them direction. In particular, demographic ageing interrogates how technological developments can tame, limit or exploit the risks and opportunities, both social and economic ones, of an increasingly ageing population. What Lisbon proposes is structured consultation between relevant stakeholders to espouse economic goals, technological developments, to the social and ethical needs of an ageing population.

Eventually, the 2005 mid term review of the Lisbon strategy introduces the concept of active ageing, flexicurity and life cycle approach in work. Active employment policies should provide incentives for elderly people to remain in work and, at the same time, appraise social protection systems that continue to offer the security needed to help people embrace change.

On the escort of the mid-term review, in 2006 the Riga Declaration launched a policy of e-inclusion of older persons. E-inclusion promotes the development of technologies which can activate and increase participation of the elderly in social and economic life and allow them to live independently. Consequently, ICT for the elderly becomes part of complex web of the policy, social and also ethical issues: Active ageing.

---

[181] The ministers of the EU in Corfu took the group's recommendations 'lock stock and barrel' leaving one a member of the Bangemann group rather surprised himself: 'The Council of Ministers acted on all these recommendations without exception. Some of us wonder if they understood exactly what they did. It is not that they lack intellectual capacity, but decisions were taken fast.' Gyllenhammar, P., 'Let us liberalise cross-media ownership. Extract from the IIC Conference', Keynote speech, Intermediate, London, 1994, p.48. Retrieved from Sophia Kaitatzi-Whitlock, 'A redundant information society for the European Union?', in *Telematics and Informatics,* vol. 17, n.1-2, p. 39-76, 2000, p. 70

[182] European Commission, Directorate-General for employment, industrial relations and social affairs Unit V/B/4, 'Building the European Information Society for Us All', Manuscript completed in April 1997, Luxembourg: Office for Official Publications of the European Communities. Hereinafter 'High Level Expert Group report' or 'HLEG report'. Available at http://www.epractice.eu/files/media/media_688.pdf

REFERENCES

Alexandre, S., and Walker, A., 'The Madrid International Plan of Action on ageing: From conceptualization to implementation' in *Ageing & Society*, 2004, 24 (2): 147-165.

Bauman, Z., *Liquid Modernity*, Polity Press, Cambridge, 2006.

Blanpain R., Tiraboshi M., (eds.), *The Global Labour Market. From Globalization to Flexicurity*, Kluwer Law International, The Netherlands, 2008.

Broek van den, G., et al. (eds), '*Ambient Assisted Living Roadmap*', ALLIANCE report, August 2009.

Burgelman, J-C., Servaes, J., 'European approaches to the information society: a gold rush over bumpy roads?' in *Telematics and Informatics*, vol.134, n.2/3, p.63-66, 1996.

Cammaerts, B., Burgelman, J-C. (eds), *Beyond competition: broadening the scope of telecommunications policy*, VUB University Press, Brussels, 2000.

Casey, B.H., 'The OECD Jobs Strategy and the Employment Strategy: two views of the labour market and the welfare state?' in *European Journal of Industrial Relations*, 2004, vol.10, n.3, p. 329-352.

Castells, M., *The Rise of the Network Society*, Blackwell Publishers, London, 1996.

Cohen, S., *Visions of Social Control: Crime Punishment and Classification*, Cambridge: Polity/Basil Blackwell, 1985.

Collective, 'Overcoming the Barriers and Seizing the Opportunities for Active Ageing Policies in Europe', in *International Social Science Journal*, Vol. 58, No. 190, December 2006, pp. 617-631.

De Hert, P., "The Use of Labour Law To Regulate Employer Profiling: Making Data Protection Relevant Again", in M. Hildebrandt and S. Gutwirth (eds), *Profiling the European citizen. Cross Disciplinary Perspectives*, Springer, 2008, p. 226-237.

Di Gennaro & Dutton, 'Reconfiguring Friendships: Social relationships and the Internet', in *Information, Communication & Society*, Volume 10, Issue 5, 2007, p. 591.

Ducatel, K., Webster, J., and Herrmann, W., *The Information Society in Europe. Work and Life in an Age of Globalisation*, Rowman & Little field Publishers, Inc., Lanham-Boulder-New York-Oxford, 2000.

Eberstadt, N. and G. Hans, 'Healthy Old Europe', in Foreign Affairs, May/June 2007.

Ellul, J., *The Technological Society*, Vintage Books, New York, 1964.

Frissen, P., *De Staat*, Uitgeverij de Balie, Amsterdam, 2002.

Gavigan, Ottitsch, Greaves et al., *Demographic and Social Trends*, European Commission, Joint Research Centre Institute for Prospective Technological Studies, 1998.

Goetschy, J., 'The European Employment Strategy: Genesis and Development', in *European Journal of Industrial Relations*, vol.5, n.2, p.117-137. The text is available free of charge at http://ec.europa.eu/governance/areas/group8/contribution_strategy-genesis_en.pdf

Green, L., *Technoculture*, Allen and Unwin, Crows Nest, 2001.

Gyllenhammar, P., *Let us liberalise cross-media ownership. Extract from the IIC Conference*, Keynote speech, Intermediate, London, 1994.

Hendrickx, F., Bekker, S., Blanpain, R. (eds.), *Flexicurity and the Lisbon Agenda. A Cross-Disciplinary Reflection*, Intersentia, 2008.

Henten, A., Skouby, K.E. , Falch, M. 'European Planning for an Information Society', in *Telematics and Informatics*, 1996, Vol. 13. No. 213, p. 177-190.

Hildebrandt, M. and Gutwirth, S., *Profiling the European Citizen*, Springer, 2009.

Iakovidis I., Maglavera, S., Trakatellis, A., *User acceptance of Health Telematics Applications. Looking for convincing cases*, IOS Press, Amsterdam, The Netherlands, 1998.

Kaitatzi-Whitlock, S. "A redundant information society for the European Union?" in *Telematics and Informatics*, 2000, vol. 17, n.1-2, p. 39-76.

Katz S., Ford A.B., Moskowitz R.W., Jackson B.A., Jaffer M.W., *Studies of illness in the aged. The Index of ADL: A standardized measure of biological and psychosocial function*, in JAMA, 1963; 21: 94 – 919.

Klosse, S., 'The European Employment Strategy: Which Way Forward?, in *The International Journal of Comparative Labour Law and Industrial Relations*, 2005, vol.21, n.1, p. 5-36.

Kok W. et al., "Jobs, Jobs, Jobs. Creating more employment in Europe", Report of the European Commission Employment Taskforce, November 2003.

Martijn Van der steen, 'Ageing or silvering? Political debate about ageing in the Netherlands', in *Science and Public Policy*, 35(8), October 2008, pages 575-583.

Masuda, J., *The Information Society as Post-Industrial Society*, Institute for the Information Society, Tokyo, 1980 (US edition, Washington, DC: World Future Society, 1981).

May, C., *The Information Society. A sceptical view*, Polity Press, Cambridge (UK), 2002.

Mesch & Talmud, 'e-Relationships – the blurring and reconfiguration of offline and online social boundaries', in *Information, Communication & Society*, Volume 10, Issue 5, 2007, p. 585-590;

Mordini E, Wright D, et.al., SENIOR Discussion Paper 'Ethics of e-inclusion of older people', 2008. Avialable at http://ec.europa.eu/information_society/events/cf/ict2008/document.cfm?doc_id=5808.

Mordini E., et al., 'Senior citizens and the ethics of e-inclusion', in *Ethics and Information Technology* (2009) 11: 203-220.

Mordini, E., Massari, S., *Including Seniors in the Information Society. 28 World Leaders talks on Privacy, Ethics, Technology and Ageing*, CIC Edizioni internazionali, Roma, 2008

Murphie A., Potts, J., *Culture and Technology*, Palgrave, London 2003.

Ney, S. 'Active ageing policy in Europe: between path dependency and path departure', in *Ageing International*, Fall 2005, Vol. 30, No. 4, pp. 325-342.

Nora P., Minc, A., *L'informatisation de la société*, La Documentation Française, Paris, 1978.

Porat M.U, *The information economy: Definition and Measurement*, Washington, DC, Government Printing Office, 1977.

Rawls, J., *A theory of justice*, Harvard University Press, Cambridge (Mass), 1971

Sapir, A., 'Globalisation and the Reform of European Social Models', Background document for the presentation at ECOFIN Informal Meeting, Manchester, 9 September 2005.

Selvaggio, J. L.(ed.), *Information society. Economic Social & Structural issues*, Lawrence Erlbaum Associates Publishers, Hove and London, 1989.

Timmers, P., 'EU e-inclusion policy in context', in *Emeraldinsight*, Vol. 10 No. 5/6 2008, pp. 12-19, Emerald Group Publishing Limited. Available http://www.emeraldinsight.com/Insight/ViewContentServlet?Filename=/published/emeraldfulltextarticle/pdf/2720100502.pdf

Vedder, A., Custers, B., Leenes, R., Koops, B-J., Vudisa, J., *Impact of Converging Technologies on Future Security Applications,* TILT and Telematica Institute and Mesa+, Enschede,2008. http://www.tilburguniversity.nl/faculties/law/research/tilt/research/completed/converging/

Van Den Broek, G., F. Cavallo and C. Wehrmann (eds.), *AALIANCE Ambient Assisted Living Roadmap,* IOS Press, Amsterdam, 2010

Villa, P. , 'La Strategia Europea per l'Occupazione e le Pari Opportunità tra uomini e donne', in M. Rossilli, *I diritti delle donne nell'Unione Europea. Cittadine, migranti, schiave*, Ediesse, Roma, 2009, p.163-199.

Wilthagen, T. and F. Tros,'The concept of 'flexicurity': a new approach to regulating employment and labour markets', in *Transfer: European Review of Labour and Research*, Vol. 10, No. 2, 2004, 166-186.

Zolo, D., *Globalizzazione. Una mappa dei problemi*, Laterza, Bari, 2004.

EUROPEAN UNION

European Commission, *White Paper on Growth, Competitiveness, Employment: The Challenges and Ways Forward into the 21st Century*, Brussels, 5 December 1993, COM (93) 700 final.

European Commission, *Europe and the Global Information Society (The Bangemann report)*, Brussels, 26 May 1994.

European Commission, *Action Plan on the Europe's Way to the Information Society (APEWIS)*, Communication from the Commission to the Council, the European Parliament, the Economic and Social Committee and the Committee of the Regions, Brussels, 19 July 1994, COM (94) 347.

European Parliament, *Report on 'Europe and the global information society. Recommendations to the European Council - a communication from the Commission of the European Communities: 'Europe's way to the information society: an action plan*, Committee on Economic and Monetary Affairs and Industrial Policy, Rapporteur: Mr. Fernand Herman (COM(94)0347 - C4-0093/94)', (PE 217.506/fin., A4-0244/96), Brussels and Strasbourg, 16 July 1996.

European Commission, *The Information Society: From Corfu to Dublin: The New Emerging Priorities*, Communication from the Commission to the Council, the European Parliament, the Economic and Social Committee and the Committee of the Regions, Brussels, 24 July 1996, COM(96) 395 final.

European Commission, *Europe and the Forefront of the Global Information Society: Rolling Action Plan*, Communication from the European Commission to the Council, the European Parliament, the Economic and Social Committee and the Committee of the Regions, Brussels, 27 November 1996, COM (97) 106 final, updated and revised on 31 July 1997.

European Commission, *Living and Working in the Information Society: People First*, Green Paper, Brussels, 24 July 1996, COM (96) 389 final.

European Commission, *Reinforcing political union and preparing for enlargement*, Opinion from the Commission, Brussels, 28 February 1996, COM (96) 90 final.

European Commission, Directorate-General for employment, industrial relations and social affairs Unit V/B/4, *Building the European Information Society for Us All*, April 1997, Luxembourg: Office for Official Publications of the European Communities. Available at http://www.epractice.eu/files/media/media_688.pdf

European Commission, *The Social and Labour Market Dimension of the Information Society: People First - The Next Steps*, Communication from the Commission, Brussels, 23 July 1997, COM (97) 390 final.

European Commission, *eEurope - An information society for all*, Communication on a Commission initiative for the special European Council of Lisbon of 23 and 24 March 2000, Brussels, 8 December 1999, COM(1999) 687 final.

European Commission, *Towards a Europe for all ages - Promoting prosperity and intergenerational security*, Communication from the Commission, Brussels, 21 May 1999, COM (1999) 221 final.

European Commission, *eEurope - An information society for all*, Communication on a Commission initiative for the special European Council of Lisbon of 23 and 24 March 2000, Brussels, 8 December 1999, COM(1999) 687 final.

"Jobs, Jobs, Jobs. Creating more employment in Europe", Report of the European Commission Employment Taskforce, November 2003

European Commission, *Increasing the employment of older workers and delaying the exit from the labour market*, Communication from the Commission to the Council, the European Parliament, the European Economic and Social Committee and the Committee of the Regions, of the European Communities, Brussels, 3 March 2004, COM(2004) 146 final.

European Commission, *Working together for growth and jobs: A new start for the Lisbon Strategy*, Communication to the Spring European Council from President Barroso in agreement with Vice-President Verheugen', Brussels, 2 February 2005, COM (2005) 24.

European Commission, *eAccessibility*, Communication from the Commission to the Council, the European Parliament and the European Economic and Social Committee and the Committee of the Regions, Brussels, 13 September 2005, COM(2005) 425 final.

European Commission, *i2010 – A European Information Society for growth and employment*, Communication from the Commission to the Council, the European Parliament, the European Economic and Social Committee and the Committee of the Regions, Brussels, 1 June 2005, COM(2005) 229 final.

European Commission, *Integrated guidelines for growth and jobs (2005-2008)*, Brussels, 12 April 2005, COM(2005) 141 final.

European Commission, *Social Agenda*, Communication from the Commission, Brussels, 9 February 2005, COM(2005) 33 final.

European Commission, *ICT for Health and i2010: Transforming the European healthcare landscape: Towards a strategy for ICT for Health*, Office for Official Publications of the European Communities, Luxembourg, June 2006.

European Commission, *The Demographic Future of Europe – from Challenge to Opportunity*, Communication from the Commission, Brussels, 12 October 2006, COM (2006) 571 final.

European Commission, *Time to move up a gear: The new partnership for growth and jobs*, Communication from the Commission to the Spring European Council, Brussels, 25 January 2006, COM (2006) 30.

European Commission, *i2010 eGovernment Action Plan: Accelerating eGovernment in Europe for the Benefit of All*, Communication from the Commission to the Council, the European Parliament, the European Economic and Social Committee and the Committee of the Regions, Brussels, 25 April 2006, COM(2006) 173 final.

European Economic and Social Committee and the Committee of the Regions, COM (2007) 332 final, Brussels, 14 June 2007.

European Commission, *Ageing well in the Information Society,* Communication from the Commission to the European Parliament, the Council, the European Economic and Social Committee and the Committee of the Regions, Brussels, 14 June 2007, COM(2007) 332 final

European Commission, *Ageing well in the Information Society*, Staff Working Document, Accompanying document to the Communication from the Commission to the European Parliament, the Council, the European Economic and Social Committee and the Committee of the Regions, Brussels, 14 June 2007, SEC(2007) 811.

European Commission, *Towards Common Principles of Flexicurity: More and better jobs through flexibility and security*, Communication from the Commission to the European Parliament, the Council, the European Economic and Social Committee and the Committee of the Regions, Brussels, 27 June 2007, COM(2007) 359 final.

European Commission, *Opportunities, access and solidarity: towards a new social vision for 21st century Europe*, Communication from the Commission to the European Parliament, the Council, the European Economic and Social Committee and the Committee of the Regions, COM(2007) 726 final, Brussels, 20 Nov 2007.

European Commission, *Limassol e-Inclusion Report: Vision, priorities and actions for e-Inclusion Beyond i2010*, prepared by the i2010 e-Inclusion Subgroup as a result of its meeting in Limassol, Cyprus, on 7-8 April, 2009

European Commission, *Consultation on the future 'EU 2020' strategy*, Commission Working Document, Brussels, 24 November 2009, COM(2009) 647 final.

Council of the EU, *Resolution on the 1999 Employment Guidelines*, Brussels, 22 February 1999, *OJ C 69, 12.3.1999.*

Council Directive 2000/78/EC of 27 November 2000 establishing a general framework for equal treatment in employment and occupation ('the European Employment Directive'), Official Journal L 303 , 02/12/2000 P. 0016 – 0022.

Economic Policy Committee and DG ECFIN, *Budgetary challenges posed by ageing populations: the impact on public spending on pensions, health and long-term care for the elderly and possible indicators of the long-term sustainability of public finances*, Brussels, 24 October, 2001, EPC/ECFIN/630-EN final.

Council of the EU, *Increasing Labour Force Participation and Promoting Active Ageing*, 6707/02, Council of the European Union, Brussels, Joint Report from the Commission and the Council: Report requested by Stockholm European Council, 2002.

Council Decision, Brussels, 22 July 2003, OJ L 197, 05.08.2003.

Council of the EU, *Guidelines for the employment policies of the member states*, Council Decision, Brussels, 12 July 2005, 2005/600/EC, OJ L 205/21.

European Council, Presidency conlusions, Brussels, 10-11 December 1993, EC Bulletin, n.12.

European Council, Presidency conclusions, Barcelona, 15-16 March 2002.

European Council, Presidency Conclusions, Luxembourg, 12-13 December 1997.

European Council, Presidency conclusions, Stockholm , 23 and 24 March 2001.

Presidency of the EU, Sweden, *Visby Agenda: Creating Impact for an eUnion 2015*, November 2009.

Ministerial Declaration approved unanimously on 11 June 2006, Riga, Latvia. (*The Riga Declaration*), The text of the Riga declaration is available at http://ec.europa.eu/ information_society/events/ict_riga_2006/doc/declaration_riga.pdf

European Social Network, *Long-term care for older people. Statistical background 2. Present and projected expenditures by types of care*, Brussels, 2006.

Eurostat, *Living conditions in Europe. Data 2002-2005*, Brussels, 2007.

Eurostat, *The Life of Men and Women in Europe: A Statistical Portrait*, Brussels, 2008.

Eurostat, *The Social Situation in the European Union 2005-2006. The Balance between generation in an Ageing Europe*, Brussels, 2006.

http://www.se2009.eu/en/meetings_news/2009/11/10/webcast_visby_agenda_creating_im pact_for_an_eunion_2015_10_november

EuroBarometer, *European Social Reality Report*, Special Eurobarometer 273, February 2007.

SENIOR project, "The Inclusion of Senior Citizens in the Information Society", by Birgit Jæger, in Discussion on Ethical, privacy and legal issues related to ageing at work, SENIOR Project, Expert meeting on Ubiquitous communication", 22 September 2008, Brussels.

SENIOR project, 'The competent Seniors: Aging and use of digital media – conflict or happiness?', by Øyvind Nøhr, Lillehammer University College, Socio-Anthropological Workshop, Brussels, 2-3 June 2008.

SENIOR project, Work Package 1 final, prepared by D. Wright, 2008.

SENIOR project, "Intelligent User Interface", D2.3 final, prepared by P. De Hert & E. Mantovani.

SENIOR project, 'The perspective of gerontology', by G., Cronet, SENIOR Final Conference, 27 November 2009, Brussels.

SENIOR project, "The Perspective of caregivers", by M. Starr, Final Conference of the SENIOR project, 27 November 2009.

SENIOR project, , 'ICT and the Social Inclusion of Older Adults: Can the Social Sciences Contribute to New Solutions to Old Problems?', by

Marshall, V., Opening lecture for the Socio-Anthropological Workshop, SENIOR Project, Brussels, Belgium, June 2-3, 2008.

Non EU entities

G7 summit, Ministerial conference on the information society, Brussels, 25-26 February, 1995.

G8, Labor Ministers Conference, Turin (Italy), 10-11 November, 2000.

International Monetary Fund (IMF), *World Economic Outlook*, Washington, October 1993.

OECD, *Age of Withdrawal from the Labour Force in OECD Countries: Labour Market & Social Policy*. Occasional Papers no. 49, Paris, January 2002.

OECD, *Ageing and Income: Financial Resources & Retirement in 9 OECD Countries*, Paris, 2000;

OECD, *Ageing, Housing & Urban Development*, Paris, January 2003.

OECD, *Coping with Population Ageing in the Netherlands*, Economics Department Working Papers 325, Paris, 2002.

OECD, *Getting older, getting poorer?*, Paris, February 2002;

OECD, *Governments Must Rethink Transport Safety for Elderly*, Paris, 2001;

OECD, *JOBS strategy. Pushing ahead with the strategy*, Paris, 1996. http://www.oecd.org/dataoecd/57/7/1868601.pdf

OECD, *JOBS STUDY. Facts, Analysis, Strategies*, Paris, 1994, available at http://www.oecd.org/dataoecd/42/51/1941679.pdf.

OECD, *Live Longer, Work Longer: A synthesis report*, Paris, 2006;

OECD, *Maintaining prosperity in an ageing society*, Paris, 1998. Available at http://www.oecd.org/dataoecd/21/10/2430300.pdf ;

OECD, *Policy Brief: Maintaining the Economic Well-Being of Older People - challenges for retirement income policies*, Paris, December 2001;

OECD, *Promise and Problems of e-democracy*, Paris 2003. http://www.oecd.org/dataoecd/9/11/35176328.pdf

UN General Assembly, Resolution 213 (III) of 4 December 1948.

UN General Assembly, Resolution 2842 (CXXVI) of 18 December 1971.

UN General Assembly, Resolution 33/52 of 14 December 1978.

UN General Assembly, Resolution 37/51 of 3 December 1982.

United Kingdom, Office for National Statistics (ONS), Social Trends survey, Population ageing, 27 August 2009, http://www.statistics.gov.uk/cci/nugget.asp?ID=949

US House of Representatives, *'National Information Infrastructure Act. Report To Accompany H.R. 1757'*, 103d Congress, 1st Session, 1993. Full text available at http://www.eric.ed.gov/ERICDocs/data/ericdocs2sql/content_storage_01/0000019b/80/15/3d/9a.pdf (accessed on February 2010).

World Trade organisation (WTO), Dispute Settlement Body, *Mexico - Measures Affecting Telecommunications Services*, complaint by the United States, 1 May 2004, DS204. http://www.wto.org/english/tratop_e/dispu_e/cases_e/ds204_e.htm .

European Voice, '2020 vision', by Jim Brunsden, 14 January 2010.

Le Monde Diplomatique, 'Une nouvelle vassalisation', by Torres, A., in Internet: l'extase et l'effroi. Manicre de Voir, Le Monde Diplomatique, Paris, August 1996.

L'Espresso, In pensione si andrà a settant'anni', by Pilati, P., 6 August 2009.

The Economist, 'Special report on ageing population', 27 June – 3 July, 2009.

CHAPTER TWO. AGEING IN THE INFORMATION SOCIETY

By Emilio Mordini and Eugenio Mantovani

INTRODUCTION. E-INCLUSION, VULNERABILITY, AND ACTIVE AGEING

The lives of elderly people, today as well as a hundred years ago, are affected by the attitude or mentality of a given society towards what is 'old', because it belongs to the past, or because it is deteriorating towards death. Modern technological societies woo the idea of decelerating, arresting or postponing ageing. Such an idea finds fertile ground in the prevailing cultural, social and market-led representations of ageing, which involve a great deal of falsification and removal. The removal and falsification of ageing appear rather awkward though. Soon the 'old' will out number the young, and what is more, such a society of elderly is building an image where being old means little good. We suggest that this apparent paradox be viewed in the context of demographic change around the image of active ageing. Being old is fine on the condition that one is...not old. From an ethical point of view it is questionable whether the ostracism of ageing is 'good' or 'bad' for elderly people and/or for society as a whole. We limit ourselves to conclude that the rescuing of active ageing is problematic for a society which commends pluralism of life-styles.

We have learned from Chapter I that the policy e-inclusion of older persons is intertwined with complex cultural, social and economic realities. The 2005 'i2010 initiative' and the 2006 Riga declaration on e-inclusion are strictly related to the governance of social and economic objectives of the consolidated Lisbon agenda. In the Lisbon book, demographic ageing poses a number of challenges to European societies. As citizens age, they tend to fall out from the boundaries of work, or they become more frail. Predictive knowledge based on the incumbent demographic trend suggests the number of seniors who, because they retire, because they are very old, or because they are not able to live independently, fall out from active life, will increase.

As *The Economist* puts it, 'by carrying on, older persons will not only save the public purse money by not drawing a pension but will also continue to pay taxes and social-security contributions.'[1] The information society is a key instrument to this.

Information society technologies, however, are not a product of single policy decision. They do not stand apart and develop autonomously from social life; neither inevitable, nor neutral, technologies are the product of human projects and networks of people, scientists, research leaders, companies, sponsors, politicians, investors, experts committees, etc...which take decisions and make choices.[2] For instance, the day Philips pet robot will be toddling elderly nursing houses it will have gone through a list of small and major decisions that will have moulded the product and led to its final use and commercialisation.[3] Technological developments are part of such a fabric of 'micropolitical decision making' which is at work also after technological

---

[1] *The Economist*, 'Special Report and Ageing', 'Work till you drop', 27 June – 3 July, 2009.
[2] S. Gutwirth, *Privacy and the Information Age*, Lanham: Rowman & Littlefield, 2002, p.65-68
[3] The iCat. http://www.hitech-projects.com/icat/index.php

artefacts have become part of our daily life.[4] The use of technology may in effect change to fit purposes or operate functions different than the original ones.[5] Also in this case, politics and human beings are involved. They take decisions and give technology direction.[6]

The rationale lying behind the e-inclusion of older persons rests on the risk that elderly people remain excluded from the information society and, therefore, from the socio-economic objectives of the Lisbon process, of which the Information Society (IS) is an integral part. In the e-inclusion narrative, the risk of exclusion of elderly people (as well as migrants, disable people, marginalised youngsters, rural communities and so on) is expressed in terms of vulnerability. What makes older persons vulnerable in the information society, however, may be more biased than what EU documents suppose. The term 'vulnerable' indicates the 'easiness of being hurt.'[7] A person can be hurt either by an offender who is more powerful than him or her, or when he or she is unable to deal with contextual conditions and he or she succumbs to them. In both cases it is a matter of power relations, but the former condition speaks of inter-human, social, relations; the latter speaks of human-ambient relations. No doubt that power is also based on body functions: the altered or impaired body functions that come as a consequence of the natural process of ageing do have an impact on personal power. Yet, everybody would agree that considering e.g., the Pope, who is often an old person, but who is also one of the few absolute monarchs in the world, to be more vulnerable than a young priest would be exorbitant. Likewise, an old professor aged 80 is hardly more vulnerable than a young migrant sheltered in the university campus, who is penny-less and paper-less. At the same time, however, there is little doubt that the prostate of the professor makes him more impaired or disable than the young migrant. Thus, while the condition of frailty in old age is a rather natural condition, the link between old-age frailty and vulnerability speaks of cultural, political and economic 'individual-ambient' power relations. Vulnerability in old age is thus the result of mix of personal conditions of frailty and power relations. The development and use of technological developments, as enabling inter-human and individual-ambient relations, should consider also the 'ageing and power' dynamics.

From a public policy perspective, the relation between old-age frailty and power relations invites prudence. In the 1977 lessons at the College de France, Michel Foucault explained how enlightened welfare polices bring with them practices that naturally counter them.[8] For Foucault, modern social sciences produce categories or models which can, when run together or appropriated by welfare policies, erode legal freedoms. The erosion of legal freedoms, unlike blunt intrusion or deprivation of liberty, works through subtle and quiet processes of differentiation and normalisation. Social disciplines or sciences, such as psychiatrics, psychology, and sociology are active throughout the social field and contribute, through structured observation, to the disciplinarisation of patterns of behaviour. The erosion of legal freedoms takes place to the extent that the social constructions resulting from social sciences or

---

[4] S. Gutwirth, *op.cit.*, p.67.

[5] They can be re-invented, converted; they can be used (or abused) for different purposes. For instance, ten years ago a supermarket fidelity card offered some advantages to the consumer. Today, data about the consumer's purchasing habits can be used for personalised marketing. *L'Echo*, 'Colruyt se lance dans le marketing personnalisé', 27 January 2010.

[6] S. Gutwith, Ibid., p.65.

[7] For the New Collins Dictionary (1982) vulnerability means 'capable of being physically or mentally wounded or assailable.'

[8] M. Foucault, *Dits et écrits,* Paris 1994, vol. III, p. 719.

disciplines are associated with relations of power. Their combined effect is to give relief to what is the norm, and separate it from that which is not norm(al behaviour). But, as Gutwirth observes, this 'happens within a framework of a norm which is sheer balance and comparison, without any reference as such to the individual', and her or his legal freedoms.[9]

Active ageing is an example of a norm of sheer balance and comparison that does not consider individual traits. In short, such a norm singles out old age frailty or old age dependency and promotes physical fitness and independency as the norm of old age, which it calls inclusion. We have already seen that staying active longer, in particular postponing the age of retirement, may soon become necessary from an economic viewpoint, rather than choice.[10] When welfare systems come under strain and demographic changes mounts, the EU policy response suggests longer working lives[11] and welfare systems adjustments.[12] The narrative of 'active ageing', or productive ageing, emphasises that productivity and ageing are not contradictory. Also living independently is considered productive in the sense that it relieves family and/or society from providing care and from giving support.[13]

The active ageing narrative crowds popular media. TV programs and advertisements offer an ample set of stories about old age, which often reflect vested interests. Comforted by statistics about extraordinary longevity of human life, the market feeds an image of young and happy seniors. Women keep their charms, men re-gain their strengths; together they travel, go to university, animate clubs, nurse gardens, engage in politics; they can work, they can make plans for the future. And they are solvable. 'Being old is beautiful,' - says a recent ad. Few years ago, 72 years old Sofia Loren, after being voted 'world's most naturally beautiful person' posed for the 2007 Pirelli calendar. Summer 2009, to arrive on the sex-book shelf is 'Obsession,' an erotic tale written by an 85 years old lady 'in juicy details', writes the New York Times on its 27 July 2009. November 2009, Playboy magazine hires a 60-year-old Dutch reality star and model to strip off for a nude shoot. The Olympic games of older persons are being organised in several countries, as the 'Olympage Games' in Wales (UK). Commercials advertise anti-ageing cosmetics, rejuvenating medicaments, nano-cosmetics, liposuctions, plastic surgery, whitening or blackening of the skin, viagra and other performance enhancing drugs. Senior citizens feature in fairly good shape on the TV screen and on the silver screen, in magazines, on the Internet, and also in novels. Constance Rook coined the term 'Vollendungsroman' ('novel of completion') to define a new fiction paradigm which concentrates on the last stages of life.[14] Older seniors usually have a role as source of memories and old

---

[9] S. Gutwirth, op.cit., p. 68.

[10] *The Economist*, 'Special Report and Ageing', 'The end of retirement?', op.cit..

[11] See the OECD Jobs Strategy and for the EU, the 2002 Kok report and the 2005 revised Lisbon agenda, discussed in Chapter 1.

[12] ACTIVEAGE, *Overcoming the Barriers and Seizing the Opportunities for Active Ageing Policies in Europe*, 30 December 2005, p.18. See Chapter 1. The ACTIVAGE project was funded by the European Community under the HPSE programme 'Improving the Socio-Economic Knowledge Base' (1998-2002).

[13] Robert N. Butler is credited with the paternity of the expression 'productive ageing.' See Robert N. Butler, *The Longevity Revolution: The Benefits and Challenges of Living a Long Life*, Public Affairs Press, New York, 2008.

[14] SENIOR project, *Text analysis report*, D.1.2, prepared by Guido Van Steendam, 30 September 2008. At p.11: 'The 'novel of completion' follows the complex trajectory of the hero from maturity to death is conceived as the opposite of the more traditional 'Bildungsroman' ('novel of growth'), which follows the hero from infancy to maturity.' See also C. Rooke, 'Oh What a Paradise It Seems: John

stories. Younger seniors play more active, important roles, though they seldom take the role of main character.

Against this backdrop, the prevailing social representation of old age is marked by the birth of an 'extended middle age' category applying roughly to the post-65 age group, also known as 'third age', and the creation of a 'fourth age' group or older senior citizens. Third age includes senior people who enjoy physical and mental conditions which put them closer to the middle-aged than to the older senior citizens. The expression 'extended middle age' hints at a grey area between adulthood (40 years old) and seniority ('middle age') corresponding roughly to the age of retirement. The term 'extended' indicates continuity in life-style, but a change in circumstances: 'continuation,' because during extended middle age the main physical and mental abilities remain unaltered; likewise life-style, activity patterns, medical needs, social needs remain similar to the life-habits of adult citizens. 'Change,' because the person though gradually enters the role of senior citizen: retirement, in particular, drives, sometimes abruptly, individuals outside the boundaries of active life towards the role of the senior citizen. The other category, 'fourth age,' applies to older senior citizens aged eighty or above. These older senior citizens comfort the image of the wise, slow, frail elderly, affected by mild forms of dementia or physical impairments. Here again, more than age, the distinctive character of this category is life style. Older senior citizens live outside the boundaries of active life. They are more affected by losses in physical mobility and cognitive functioning and are in need of care and assistance.

Media, market, and society tend to stylize ageing across the boundaries of active life. On the one hand, these narratives contain a great deal or removal and falsification, as they simply neglect the realities of the frail older persons. On the other hand, however, active ageing images message the idea that old age is not only about being physically fit. Sitting idle watching TV, feeling useless, merely surviving makes little sense. The admittedly invasive consumerist brunt of active or productive ageing may well contain opportunities for older persons well being. Active or productive ageing comes as an empty shell stuffed with benevolent intentions which needs to be filled in with meaning and content.

In this chapter, we put forward our vision on ageing in highly technological societies. We ask ourselves what the characteristics of ageing are and how the fixtures of the information society affect the experience of getting old. To reflect upon the meaning of ageing in the information era we endeavor using as sources novels, poems, and plays. Admittedly, writings on ageing very often offer very personal thoughts; as readers, too, we tend to read them selectively, taking what we like about an author's ideas on ageing. We should therefore acknowledge that the representations of old age contained in this chapter are biased by our own, partial, and personal review and text analysis. Having said that, we do think there is a good point in using literary texts as sources. Most novels, poems, plays we have looked at were not written with the 'question of ageing' in mind; which makes them somehow sharper. Most importantly, literary sources offer the possibility, through their language of metaphor and simile, to learn about significant dimensions of human ageing which have, across societies and time, acquired meaning today.

Advancing understanding on ageing, we surmise, is necessary to bring to surface the real source of vulnerability for elderly people in highly technological societies and conceive of an ethical approach to their inclusion in the EU Information Society.

Cheever's Swan Song', in Anne M. Wyatt-Brown and Janice Rossen (eds), *Aging and Gender, Studies in Creativity*, University Press of Virginia, Charlottesville and London, 1993, pp. 204-225.

I. DIVERSITY AND COMMONALITIES

1. DIVERSITY

Reflections on ageing can be found in almost every single piece of literature, well before Constance Rook made a literary genre of it.[15] Between Cicero's famous *De Senectude,* written in 45 B.C, and Norberto Bobbio's homonymous book written in 1996 A.D.[16], we find Shakespeare's *King Lear*, Ionesco's *Le roi se meurt*, Lev Tolstoj *Ivan Ilich*, Hemingway's *The old man and the sea* just to name but really a few, as well as a wealth of poems.[17] Cicero recalls the figure of Cato 'the elder', whom he presents as a model of meaningful ageing.[18] Cato, Cicero writes in admiration, when he was 80 started learning Greek. 'What need of more?' the roman orator asks. Contemporary poet Kelly Cherry's 'Lines Written on the eve of a birthday' smack, by contrast, a gloom and sad note on the perspective of getting old. Ageing, she says, is the 'loss of possibility that claims you bit a bit'; 'it takes down brown hair and gives you gray instead'; 'it is the loss of possibility that murders us.'[19] Contrasting views often emerge in the writings of a same author. Plato, who lived until 83 (428 BC-348 BC), seems to think about old age as a bay of moderation and wisdom: 'Old age', he writes in the first book of the Republic, 'has a great sense of calm and freedom. When the passions have relaxed and diminish their hold, as Sophocles said, we are freed not from one mad master, but from many.' Less known is the observation Plato gives immediately after; where he suggests that one may bear old age 'not because of happy disposition, but because he is rich'. 'Wealth, they say, brings many consolations.'[20]

Richard A. Posner, the famous law scholar[21], turns to Aristotle and his contradictory, or apparently so, accounts of old age. In the Nichomachea Ethics, for Aristotle 'a wise man of young age cannot be found.' The reason is that the young man, unlike the old, has no experience. 'For it is length of time that gives experience'.[22] Elsewhere, in the Rethoric[23], the Stagirite is taking notes on how to persuade an audience of elderly men ('So people think well of speeches adapted to, and reflecting, their own character.'[24]). Elders are portrayed as 'men who are past their prime' in both body and spirit. Pessimism is their tune: 'They have lived many years; they have often been taken in, and often made mistakes; and life on the whole is a bad business. The result is that they are sure about nothing and under-do everything. They 'think', but they never 'know'; and because of their hesitation they always add a 'possibly' or a 'perhaps', putting everything this way and nothing

---

[15] Constance Rook coined the term 'Vollendungsroman' ('novel of completion'), mentioned in the introduction.

[16] N. Bobbio, *De Senectude*, Einaudi, Torino, 1996.

[17] Wayne C. Booth, *The art of growing older: writers on living and aging*, Poseidon, New York, 1992.

[18] Marcus Tullius Cicero (45 BC), *Cato Major De Senectude*, with introduction and notes by James S. Reid, The Echo library, 2007. This short book is built on the refutation of four charges made against old age, namely 1) old age withdraws men from active life, 2) it weakens the physical powers, 3) it takes away capacity for enjoyment, and 4) it involves the anticipation of death.

[19] Excerpts taken from Wayne C. Booth, op.cit., p. 31.

[20] Plato, *Republic*, translated by Benjamin Jowett in 1873 reprinted by Agora Publications, Millis, MA, 2001. Book I, p.3-4. Available at http://classics.mit.edu/Plato/republic.html

[21] Richard A. Posner, *Aging and Old Age*, University Press, Chicago, 1995, in particular p. 105-107.

[22] Aristotle, *Nicomachean Ethics*, Translated by W. D. Ross. Excerpts taken from the Internet Classics Archive by Daniel C. Stevenson, http://classics.mit.edu/Aristotle/nicomachaen.mb.txt

[23] Artistotle, Rethoric, Book II, Part 12 on youth, and Part 13 on the elderly.

[24] Ibid. Book II, Part 13.

positively. They are cynical; that is, they tend to put the worse construction on everything...' And so on.

As we will see briefly, Shakespeare's King Lear vibrates between the edges of normalcy, folly, and power. Dickens and Marx describe disfranchised old men as by-products of industrial city suburbs. Oscar Wilde trashes the wounds of age on Dorian Gray's portrait...Losses, fears, and lamentations; cures, consolations, and celebrations. [25] And all at the same time. This is what ageing seems to be about.

From our review, the first impression is that older people do not constitute a group having any common interests, but chronological age. Older persons' life are characterised by heterogeneity of values, education, habits. Good writers avoid giving lessons about what ageing is and about the best way to go about it. Trying to give a sense of getting old, Norberto Bobbio, professor in legal doctrines, was eighty when he published his '*De Senectude.*' [26] Bobbio offers a division between elderly of the 'rhetoric tradition', the satisfied old men and women proposed by the media, and the lonesome, retired and secluded elders, who withdraw from active life. Yet, as Bobbio admits, this is an overly simplified, unrealistic picture. It can't be helped. There are many shades of grey. They both withdraw from the world, says Bobbio, but the *tedium vitae* of the misanthrope is quite another thing from the *contemptus mundi* of the mystic.[27] As *The Economist* quips, 'someone in his 70s may be in frail health and living in an old folks' home; or he may be running for president of the United States, as John McCain did last year.'[28] 'Darker purposes' underpin old age decisions of Kind Lear.[29] There are many shades of grey. Withdrawal from the world may be a deliberate act; or be imposed upon by disease, retirement, widowhood, solitude. There are many shades of grey in acting life too, roles, missions, jobs, tasks, paths different than before.

2. ... AND COMMONALITIES

If one thinks about the many ways to ageing exist one would conclude that it makes little sense to treat elderly people as a homogeneous group sharing common interests. And yet, there are some key commonalities about ageing. As Mordini points out[30], our passage through earthly time and space is pinpointed by a series of age-graded roles. Each role has its own social clock for adjudging the age-appropriateness of various role performances, such as the 'right' time for getting married, starting a family, 'peaking' in one's career, retiring and so on. 'Different societies differ in how they value age and how they categorise age given a certain context.'[31] What Mordni suggests is that ageing in a chronological sense is accompanied by age-dependent roles and positions which are culturally determined. Passing of time and cultural context are strictly linked. As time goes by, soon or later one enters, *volentis or nolentis*, the role of senior in the eyes of his or her family, of his or her friends and of

[25] W.C. Booth, *The art of growing older, op.cit.*
[26] N. Bobbio, *De Senectude,*op.cit., p.26-27.
[27] N. Bobbio, op.cit., p.17-20.
[28] *The Economist*, op.cit., Title of the article 'The silver dollar', 25 June 2009.
[29] W. Shakespeare, *King Lear*, see *infra*.
[30] SENIOR, *Ethics of e-inclusion of elderly people*, Discussion paper for the workshop on ethics and e-inclusion, Bled (Slovenia), 12 May 2008. The background paper was subsequently turned into Mordini E., *et al.*, Senior citizens and the ethics of e-inclusion, *Ethics and Information Technology* (2009) 11: 203-220.
[31] Ibid., p.13.

his or her community or network. The role of being old in society thus obtains on the peculiar 'timing' of ageing, which is fixed - time goes by - but culturally determined. For example, in the lost world described by Peter Laslett, the British historian, seniors would sometimes cheat on their age claiming they are older in order to enhance their social status and authority.[32] Different cultures and societies may 'play' differently with passing of time, yet plain and simple passing of time does matter and ageing is, cool it or heat it, about time passing by. Two thousands years ago in ancient Rome, a man would be in *puerita*, up to age fifteen; in *adulescentia*, from fifteen to thirty; in *iuventus*, from thirty to forty-five; he would be a *senior*, from forty-five to sixty; and then he would enter *senectus*, from sixty until…death.[33] It is telling to recall that the Romans called '*senectus*' also '*extrema aetas*'; where the adjective 'extrema' indicates that '*senectus*' is the last period of life. *Senectus* is also tellingly called '*atra senectus,*' where '*atra*' means dark, constrained between life and death.' Nothing has changed in two thousands years concerning the period of life called *senectus*. At the time of Cicero as well as today older persons have more years of life spent on their back than other fellows, and older persons live the last years of their lives and are biologically closer to death. Longer life span means old age is, depending on the perspective adopted, extended or postponed.

II. PASSING OF TIME AND POWER RELATIONS

1. PASSING OF TIME

The theme of ageing as passing of time is nicely portrayed by a young poet, Dylan Thomas (1914-1953), in the poem 'Youth calls to Age.' Thomas writes:

> '...Youth calls to Age across the tired years:
> 'What have you found,' he cries, 'what have you sought?'
> 'What you have found,' Age answers through his tears,
> 'What you have sought' [...] '[34]

    In these lines, the passage from youth and age hinges around two verbs, 'to find' and 'to seek.' Old age is seen as the time to find what youth has garnered. The poet seems to refer to a reserve of skills, knowledge, and experiences one has been willing and able to collect 'through the years', and from which Age can draw from and make use of. Thus put, perhaps the intention of Thomas was to draw an admonishment for himself and the youth in general: live intensely, take advantage, for there comes a time one stops tilling the soil. Take Cato, the elder. Would he be studying Greek at eighty had he not 'sought' during his life?
    The poem can also be read through elderly eyes. The reading Bobbio gives in his *De Senectude,* mentioned above, is that, say, Cato – but Bobbio is clearly talking about himself - is not studying in the real sense of the word. His reading of Greek

---

[32] P. Laslett, *Il mondo che abbiamo perduto*, Jaca Books, 1979, p. 134-135. (Original title, *The World We Have Lost: English Society before the Coming of Industry* (1965)) See also P.Laslett, John M. Eekelaar, David Pearl (eds), *An aging world: dilemmas and challenges for law and social policy*, Clarendon Press, Oxford, 1989.
[33] M. Harlow, R. Laurence, 'Old Age in Ancient Rome', in *History Today*, April 2003, Vol. 53, Issue 4, p.22-27.
[34] Dylan Thomas, *Collected Poems*, edited by Walford Davies and Ralph Maud, Phoenix, London, 2003.

letters has less to do with appropriation and assimilation than it has to do with past-time, what the Romans called '*otium*.' The same can be said about Cicero. Cicero wrote *De Senectude* when, aged 60, was forced to retire into private life; his short book is a superbly drafted exercise in self-indulgence, or self complacence.

Philosopher Jean Amery contends that there comes a time in life when one does not stop living actively, but stoops to the 'impossibility of going beyond oneself in cultural terms.' Amery calls this moment 'cultural ageing.'[35] This is a deep way of looking at the world, philosophical ideas but also habits and petty practical things which become awfully hard to change. How many masters and ideas can be, not just discovered and stock-piled, but studied and assimilated in a life time?[36] Time is scarce by default, says Amery; when one gets old, he or she naturally shelters behind what he or she learnt holding on his or her 'spirit' of time.

Bobbio, Amery and Thomas' views on ageing echo in the studies of Emily Grundy, a social-scientist, on old age and vulnerability.[37] Grundy, more pragmatically, holds out to describe the 'processes and circumstances that create vulnerability among older people.'[38] Grundy starts from the observation that in old age some resources fade out and are difficult to replenish. Calling them 'reserves', she lists and describes few important ones, namely: income and material resources; family, family links, and wider social networks; social support; living arrangements and living alone; health and autonomy. The social scientist suggests that some of the physical and psychological challenges which people face as they age cannot be modified, but others can.[39] One of the salient points she makes is that the determination of the most important challenges, as well as how they can be effectively replenished, depend in large part on social and cultural constructions of ageing. Societal factors, or 'the ambient', influence the degree of power of the old age citizen thus playing an important role in determining the 'reserves' people need to live as elderly persons at any given time in any given society. As we saw above, with Mordini, different societies differ in the way they value and categorise old age. The determination of the reserves of older people depend on the degree of power that elderly people enjoy, given a certain society and given the role such a society recognises to old age.

We therefore need to ask two questions: first, what is peculiar about getting old and what are the power relations at work? Second question, what is the relation between ageing, power struggles and the fixtures of the society in which we live and age, which, in our study, are constituted by the European Union's information society? Let us turn to the first question.

2. AGEING AND POWER

To understand the relationship between ageing and power we need to dispose of a theory which can explain the nature and the extent to which power relations change when individuals age. As Chapter VIII will make clear at length, power is not an

---

[35] J. Améry, *Über das Altern: Revolte und Resignation*, Klett-Cotta, Stuttgart, 1997. Amery suggests that that time may come at fifty.
[36] N. Bobbio, *De Senectude*, p. 20.
[37] E. Grundy, 'Ageing and vulnerable elderly people: European perspectives', in *Ageing & Society*, Cambridge University Press, vol. 26, 2006, p. 105–134.
[38] Ibid., p. 106-107
[39] Ibid., p.128.

inherent quality of the person (no one is powerful per se), but it is rather a possession, which can be present at different degrees, and can decrease or increase according to several variables, age included. Ageing, for its part, always implies – at least to a certain extent and from certain viewpoints – a form of weakening of the individual.

The notion of *power relation* is used in a descriptive sense to illustrate the balance of power or the power struggles between different parties competing to achieve the same ends, in a particular context. Power relations are always relative to a specific situation. With age, for instance, abilities diminish; one looses physical strength, visual and hearing acuity, memory and learning capacities, dexterity, sexual appeal, reproductive capacity, and so on. In addition, these changes produce different effects in urban or rural environments, in pre-industrial, industrial, and post-industrial societies, in diverse social groups.

Crucially, therefore, social roles and social contexts can either mitigate or emphasise age related impairment, resulting in major or in minor losses of social power. For instance, the increasing dependence from others, which is often a consequence of the ageing processes, has very different outcomes in societies with strong community ties, or in societies, which highly value independent living and the lonely search for the meaning of life. This holds true not only in terms of social interactions, but also in psychological terms, as people used to considering isolation as a sign of liberty and autonomous power, will probably feel age-related dependence as a humiliating and degrading experience.

Starting from these premises, it is possible to develop a theoretical framework which can help disentangling the relationship between ageing and power. This is the task and object of chapter VIII. In this paragraph we endeavour to become more familiar with the above mentioned premises on ageing and power by drawing from another literary source, the play. This genre offers the opportunity to observe ageing and power in flesh and in a concrete context; although a fiction, the play, thanks to its repertoire of metaphors and similes, allows us to learn something about the social and psychological dynamics of ageing and power. The play we have in mind is, of course, Shakespeare's King Lear.[40]

When the play begins we are in the hall of the throne of the king of England. The room is crowded when Lear, old and 'every inch a king', enters. The old king intends to divide its kingdom between his three daughters and announces that with this act he is abandoning public life and retire, in the expectancy of death. Shakespeare famously appraises a ceremony to mark the day the old king hands over royal power. Each daughter will, according to the rite, speak words of thanks and love to the father and king.[41] Hyperbolic and obsequious the two elder daughters viciously praise the father and king for convenience, while the third one, Cordelia, does not. Her 'Nothing, my lord' is a brutal staccato which spoils Lear's rite ('Nothing will come out of nothing!, he swears), and precipitates the tragedy. 'Nothing will come out of nothing', Lear rebukes and angrily disclaims paternity over Cordelia. But he remains firm in his intent: he gives away 'cares and business' and only keeps the name and 'additions' of being king. Without power, and having banned the only ones who loved him truly,

---

[40] W. Shakespeare, *King Lear*, 1605-6, edited by R.A. Foakes, The Arden Shakespeare, Thomson Learning, London, 2005. For commentary see Nicholas Brooke, *Shakespeare. King Lear*, Edward Arnold publisher, London, 1963. See also William R. Elton, King Lear and the gods, Kentucky: University Press, 1988. Victor Kiernan, *Eight tragedies of Shakespeare: a Marxist study*, London: Verso, 1996.

[41] Children and grandchildren may recognise here the need for expressions of love, care, and sense of usefulness of older parents or grand parents.

Cordelia and the earl of Kent, Lear is at the mercy of the greed and power hunger of his entourage.

Representing in theatre these early scenes, some actors have made Lear frail and in dotage. In one representation Lear would even enter leaning on a physician.[42] Most representations have, however, removed signs of senility or folly from the face of the king. It is a vigorous Lear who speaks, gives orders and announces he is departing. Lear is vigorous in authority and power, but he also feels tired or just old. The '*intent*', he says, is '*to shake all cares and business from our age, conferring them on younger strengths, while we unburdened crawl toward death.*'[43] These lines exemplify quite well what social gerontologists design as 'disengagemet theory'.[44] Disengagement theory argues that in order to be well-adjusted in old age, senior citizens must decrease their level of active engagement in society. This process of loss of role and participation is considered natural and positive, being based on the assumption that all senior citizens wish to withdraw from society and instead focus on the self in the anticipation of impending death.[45] Thus spoke Lear. While some commentators have seen in the ceremony a useless comedy and a sign of Lear's impending folly, while others have considered it just a fiction created by Shakespeare, arguably the strange 'rite' *is* Lear and its goal is precisely to mark the passage into Lear's old age role, withdrawal from active life and focus on the self.[46]

We said earlier that roles and social contexts can either mitigate or emphasise age related diminution of physical or cognitive abilities and loss of social power. We suggest that Shakespeare's play shows how the weakening of the body and the loss of social power can be exacerbated and emphasised by psychological and social factors.

The psychological question

In psychological terms, Lear represents the powerful person who is undergoing a process of change. Lear epitomises power (he is a king) and this makes the passage into old age role particularly vivid. The position of Lear, however, can be generalised to embrace everyone's experience. The old person realises that it now takes an effort to get on a tram, to go to the supermarket or to ride a bike, and that sense of insecurity now always lingers, while *before* he or she never had to think about it. In Lear's shoes are those individuals who have considered isolation as a sign of liberty and autonomous power. As Lear, those not used to ask for help or favours, to depend on nobody, who proudly manage to satisfy their own needs. As Lear, those individuals may feel age-related dependence as a humiliating and degrading experience.

Back to the play. Lear relinquishes power, he looses the most loved daughter, he keeps only the title and few horsemen. But he is old and alone. Angry, stubborn and proud Lear resists any compromises that in his new position he should concede. He should accept the help of Kent, for instance. As the story goes, when the king

---

[42] J.S. Bratton (ed.), *King Lear. Plays in Performance*, Bristol Classical Press, Bristol, 1987.

[43] Act I, Scene I., lines 35-40. When quoting, the edition we use is the one commented by Foakes (2005), quoted above.

[44] The term 'social gerontology' was first introduced by Clarke Tibitts in 1954 (Donahue, Wilma (1960). Foreword. Pp. v-vii, in C. Tibbitts, Ed., Handbook of Social Gerontology. Chicago and London: The University of Chicago Press).

[45] By contrast, activity theory argues that a high level of activity for senior citizens reinforce adjustment and that the notion of 'having a role' in society is essential for ensuring optimal ageing. See SENIOR project, *Report on the Socio-anthropological workshop on the social and cultural meanings of ageing and ICT*, prepared by Jesper Thestrup and Trine Sørensen, www.seniorproject.eu, p. 7-8.

[46] Nicholas Brooke, *Shakespeare. King Lear, op.cit.*, p.17.

disclaims paternity over Cordelia, the earl of Kent tries to convince him to 'revert his doom'. Kent acts common sense, he proffers to be Lear's physician, he begs to be the true blank of his eye, he even provokes the king *"When Lear is mad What wouldst thou do, old man?*, he asks).[47] What the king is doing is actually foolish, while Kent is acting rational (*'plainness'*) and as spectators or readers we sympathise with his party, not with the king's. Kent is fair and loyal, yet his offer of support triggers a psychological reaction in Lear which prevents him from accepting it. Rather, the king turns down any help or advice in full disdain. The reason is arguably that, in offering assistance and support, Kent insinuates in Lear, though in good faith, the image of incoming senility, dotage, old-age stubbornness. No surprise therefore that, in response, Lear-every-inch-a-king does not see the profession of loyalty and love but he sees the attack on his prestige and person, on his 'sentence', 'power', 'place' and 'nature'.[48]

The social question

This, as far as the psychological factors are concerned. In social terms, the increasing dependence from other people, which often come as a consequence of the ageing process, may have different outcomes depending also on the values attached to social interactions. In the dynamic of power transition the king does not see the weight of his old age. Or perhaps, he does but, for the reasons discussed above, he does not acknowledge or comes to term with it. That is what the fool keeps telling him. Wisely the fool invites him to secure what in human rights language sound like 'adequate resources', for instance proper housing arrangements. Can you tell why a snail has a house? - the fool hot on Lear's heels. That's obvious, to put its head in *'not to give it away to his daughters and leave his horns without a case.'*[49] 'Beware', the fool seems to warn, 'with ageing your power is declining'. And, with it, declines also the social and economic power necessary to bargain one's survival in a world which is greedy and leaves the old and frail behind. Kent, the fool and we as audience see the nexus between social and economic power and ageing, while the king does not. His daughters have the upper hand, they are now more powerful than him, but rather than exercising their increased power in solidarity they exploit it to achieve purely egoistic ends. In this sense, the fool is right to blame the king for being old before the time. Before getting old, Lear should have been wise enough to realise that *'Fathers that wear rags/ Do make their children blind,/But fathers that bear bags/ Shall see their children kind'*[50]. And now Lear is 'in rags'.

The tragic dilemma that, thanks to the character of the fool, Shakespeare puts on us is who is acting fool and who is acting normal or rational? Who's acting rational, the king's entourage who fall on the vacant power and selfishly pursue their personal interest, or the king, who, despite being king and thus knowing about power relations, relinquishes power without securing enough reserves? Who are the fool? Probably the answer depends on the values attached to social interactions. In the world envisioned by Lear, persons moving into an old-age role continue to be respected, even after they

---

[47] Act I, Scene I, lines 146-152.
[48] Act I, Scene I, lines 168, 173. With these words Lear bans Kent from the kingdom. Lear:'Hear me, recreant, on thine allegiance, hear me:/ That thou hast sought to make us break our vow,/ Which we durst never yet, and with strained pride/ To come betwixt our sentence and our power,/ Which nor our nature nor our place can bear, / Our potency made good, take thy reward.'
[49] Act I, Scene V, lines 27-30.
[50] Act II, Scene II, lines 236-245.

decide to give away their money and their power or, as more often happens today, after they have exhausted, as Grundy would say[51], their reserves. Reality is quite different. Lear learns that when power goes away or money becomes scarcer (division of the kingdom), when there is no support of care or affections are lost, and old age frailty kicks in, older persons are helpless against the ravages of greed and power-hunger.[52]

The analysis of Shakespeare's King Lear indicates that as persons grow older and frailer and in need of assistance they are exposed to psychological and social forms of pressures. Psychological pressure derives from the individual acceptance, or lack thereof, of diminishing physical or cognitive abilities which change the horizon of individual agency and the role enjoyed or played in the previous part of life. Social pressure results from the value attached to inter-human and, more precisely, to the purpose of social interactions. When the latter are foundered is the attainment of personal interest those who, like many older persons, are not 'equally cooperating', are fatally pit in a vulnerable position. The two dimensions are strictly related, social norms influencing the individual self-perception of old age normalcy on the one hand, and the individual contributing to shape social norms through the affirmation of his or her way to live old age, on the other. King Lear invites its public to ask, "when we offer assistance to the old and frail, do we give it out of compassion, solidarity, or on the basis of a common good?" As we will see in chapter eight, the theme of ageing interrogates our understandings of human society and the conceptions of justice that a long tradition has bequeathed on us.

III. AGEING, WISDOM, WEALTH AND DEMOCRATIC SYSTEMS

'The ravages of greed and power-hunger' routs the king once old age has weakened body and power. Natural ageing and increased frailty engender an asymmetry in power relations. But, as Cordelia's and Kent's examples indicate, compensation of fading power relations in the context of ageing is possible. Out of metaphor, the effects of health-related limitations on an older person's quality of life can be mitigated by, e.g., family support and social networks.[53] At any rate, Cordelia and Kent, family support and social networks mitigate limitations that arise after reserve capacities have dropped below the threshold needed, in a given society, to carry on. The 'threshold needed to carry on' is in no way fixed, but the result of complex cultural, economic, social, technological processes, which define the level of normalcy that a given society expects its members to live, and to age, in.[54] We will now turn to the second question raised by the theme of passing of time: the relation between ageing, power struggles and the information society. How does the ambient of the information society affect (the power of) elderly people? We will concentrate on two relevant themes *viz.*, transmission of wisdom and accumulation of wealth.

---

[51] Grundy, op.cit.
[52] Barbara A. Mowat and Paul Werstine, *New Folger Library Shakespeare edition*, Folger Shakespeare Library, 1993 http://www.folger.edu/index.cfm
[53] Grundy, op.cit., p.109.
[54] Powell, J., 'Rethinking Gerontology: Foucault, Surveillance and the Positioning of Old Age', Sincronía Summer 2004, http://sincronia.cucsh.udg.mx/verano04.htm

1. ON WISDOM

We have seen earlier with Amery and Bobbio that assimilation of knowledge takes time. Time is necessary for notions to rest, ferment, be filtered and checked against other ideas, events, readings. Experience teaches that older persons embody such a cultural past and, having lived longer, having searched longer, are held wiser.

One of the salient characteristics of the information society concerns the transmission of data, information, knowledge, through electronic means.[55] Information in the context of the information society, according to Berčič and George[56], can be defined as 'data with meaning obtained from context'; while knowledge corresponds, for the same authors, to 'the collection of information for useful intent.' Electronic data do not automatically lead to the creation of information, nor knowledge. Let alone wisdom. Wisdom, according to the definition of the High Level Expert Group on the information society, is "distilled' knowledge derived from experience of life, as well as from the natural and social sciences, from ethics and philosophy.'[57]

Information and communication technologies offer several ways to collect data, information, and knowledge.[58] The time and space it takes to draw information and knowledge from a book or a newspaper are surpassed by faster, abundant, and digital means. Spatial and temporal changes in the acquisition of information and knowledge are likely to change the idea of wisdom as distilled, slow knowledge, that we recognise embodied in older persons, - or maybe not?

In the preface to the book 'Orientalism', Edward Said lamented how the 'book culture based on archival research [...] almost disappeared.' Said contemptuously observed his students making use of 'the fragmented knowledge available on the Internet and in the mass media instead of reading in the real sense of the word.'[59] According to Said, knowledge and information need time to rest and ferment in order to be assimilated, and younger internet natives seem not to have that time. While Said's remark seems sensible, it is worth noting that, before it became the most widespread means for information and knowledge transmission, the written word too was held in suspicion. [60] Plato, in the Phaedrus, compares oral speech with written speech and argues that oral speech is by far a preferred means to attain wisdom, on

---

[55] The launch of the March 2000 Lisbon summit was accompanied by the eEurope initiative. In it, ICT plays a central role in the transmission of data, information, and knowledge in the future knowledge-based society. See Chapter I.

[56] B. Berčič, C.George, 'Investigating the legal protection of data, information and knowledge under the EU data protection regime', *International Review of Law, Computers & Technology*, 23: 3, 189 – 201. The article considers data, information, and knowledge, but not wisdom, in the context of the data protection legal regime.

[57] The HLEG Report, aka *Building the information Society for Us All Report*, p.17, discussed in Chapter 1.

[58] M. McLuhan, *Understanding Media: The Extensions of Man*, McGraw Hill, New York, 1964); S.Papert, *The connected family: bridging the digital generation gap*, Atlanta, Longstreet Press,1996; On human computer interaction M. Friedewald, 'The continuous construction of the computer user: Visions and user models in the history of human-computer interaction', in Buurman, G.M.: *Total Interaction: Theory and practice of a new paradigm for the design disciplines*. Basel: Birkhäuser, 2005, pp. 27-41. See also SENIOR Project, D.2.3 'Intelligent User Interface', prepared by P. De Hert and E. Mantovani, p. 5-6.

[59] Edward Said, Preface to the 2003 edition of *Orientalism*, Penguin Books, London, p. xix, xx.

[60] P. Hadot, 'La figure du sage dans l'antiquité gréco-latine', in P. Hadot, *Etudes de philosophie ancienne*, Les Belles Lettres, Paris, 1998.

two main grounds.[61] First, written speech does not speak, and, second, written speech is nor 'intelligible nor certain', it must be interpreted and most people could be deceived by it or interpret it wrongly. Our reader will bear with us as we report Plato's dialogues. What the Greek philosopher says maybe useful to understand what is at stake with the wisdom of the elderly in the age of the Internet.

First, written speech does not speak. Plato celebrates the art of dialectic as 'far more excellent' than the written word. The art of dialectic is 'the sort of discourse which goes together with knowledge, and is written in the soul of the learner: that can defend itself, and knows to whom it should speak and to whom it should say nothing.'[62] By contrast, written speech seems 'to talk to you as though they were intelligent, but if you ask them anything about what they say, from a desire to be instructed, they go on telling you just the same thing for ever.'[63] The written speech stays to the living speech as the dead body to the living being. The only function Plato concedes to it is as aid to memory, particularly useful in the time 'when age oblivious comes.'[64] Such a function, however, may be of use only to the speaker and, indirectly, to the audience who is going to listen to the speech; but not to the reader, who can not be instructed by written notes.

But why is the written speech not fit to transmit information or advance knowledge? In order to explain his second argument, the 'propriety and impropriety of writing', Plato makes up a story. It is the story of the encounter between a famous god, Theuth, and one of Egypt's wisest pharaohs, Ammon.

> 'Theuth was the inventor of many arts, such as arithmetic and calculation and geometry and astronomy and draughts and dice. But his great discovery was the use of letters. To Ammon came Theuth and showed his inventions, desiring that the other Egyptians might be allowed to have the benefit of them. He enumerated them, and Ammon enquired about their several uses, and praised some of them and censured others, as he approved or disapproved of them. But when they came to letters, 'This', said Theuth, 'will make the Egyptians wiser and give them better memories; it is a specific both for the memory and for the wit.' Ammon replied: 'O most ingenious Theuth, the parent or inventor of an art is not always the best judge of the utility or inutility of his own inventions to the users of them. And in this instance, you who are the father of letters, from a paternal love of your own children have been led to attribute to them a quality which they cannot have; for this discovery of yours will create forgetfulness in the learners' souls, because they will not use their memories; they will trust to the external written characters and not remember of themselves. The specific which you have discovered is an aid not to memory, but to reminiscence, and you give your disciples not truth, but only the semblance of truth; they will be hearers of many things and will have learned nothing; they will appear to be omniscient and will generally know nothing; they will be tiresome company, having the show of wisdom without the reality.'

---

[61] Plato, *Phaedrus*, translated by R. Hackforth, University Press, Cambridge, 1972. 'Phaedrus' was written between 372 and 368 B.C.

[62] Plato, *Phaedrus*, p. 159.

[63] Ibid., p.156 – 158.

[64] *Ibidem.*

Ammon claims that this 'specific' – letters – will create 'forgetfulness in the learners' souls'; written speech accounts for an 'aid to reminiscence'; not 'truth, but only the semblance of truth'. Ammon is concerned that his people will 'trust the external written characters and not remember of themselves', that 'they will be hearers of many things and will have learned nothing.' They will be 'tiresome company, having the show of wisdom without the reality.' Plato's conclusion is that 'he would be a very simple person, and quite a stranger to the oracles of Ammon, who should leave in writing or receive in writing any art under the idea that the written word would be intelligible or certain.' He adds that 'once written down' speeches cannot defend themselves and are at the total mercy of their users and abusers. [65]

These comments sound quite unsettling. With hindsight, the large *written* legacy – in philosophy, oratory, historiography – of ancient political civilisation, of which Plato is such a great a part, had an enormous impact, say, on the construction of democratic states in the XVIII century French Revolution and after. [66] Admittedly, the written words of Athens or Rome dwellers spoke about actual conflicts and interests of social classes of that time (think about the institute of slavery, incompatible with modern time democracy, but normal in Athens). And yet, through the written word, that civilisation elaborated concepts and models which, centuries later, acquired general meaning beyond the concrete reality in which they were uttered and noted down. The foregoing goes to defend the extraordinary importance of the *written* cultural heritage which proved to deliver not 'the show of wisdom without the reality', as Plato claims, but wisdom beyond fortuitous circumstances.

As wise, Ammon's arguments are humbler and the message arguably simpler: 'more literacy' or 'more books' do not, by itself, immediately or automatically, instruct, create or message knowledge, let alone wisdom. This truism is, in fact, not so evident. Being able to read and having access to a written support, such as a book, often meant learning 'formulas.' It is known, for instance, that the early versions of the printed Bible were read and interpreted literally; that the Puritans who fled to the Americas in the early XVII century would all read the Bible and learn, or be instructed by, what it was literally written in it: for instance, if the book says that one day 'the sun came to a halt', it flows that the sun usually moves around the earth, and so on. Ammon's warning that giving too much 'trust to the external written characters' would endow men with 'the show of wisdom without the reality' seems sound.

Ammon's tale can be used to discuss the abundance of sources of information and knowledge, one the principal characteristics of the modern knowledge based society energised by ICT, and the possibility of being instructed by it. A man living in the XVII century, two centuries after Gutenberg and Luther, could already notice the abundance of printed books in circulation. [67] He or she would have marvelled to know that in XXI century it would take less than a year to have as many books published in

---

[65] Plato, Ibid.: '[…]And when they have been once written down they are tumbled about anywhere among those who may or may not understand them, and know not to whom they should reply, to whom not: and, if they are maltreated or abused, they have no parent to protect them; and they cannot protect or defend themselves.'

[66] L. Canfora, *Democrazia. Storia di una ideologia,* Laterza, Bari, 2004, p. 70. In English, *Democracy in Europe: A History of an Ideology,* Malden, 2006.

[67] Tommaso Campanella pondered how 'this century has seen more books published than in fifty centuries'. Tommaso Campanella, *La citta' del sole,* 1602, p.71. '…che maggior numero di libri furono pubblicati in questo secolo che nei conquanta passati', ('this century had more books published than in the past fifty centuries', our translation).

his century.[68] Since the end of the XX century, to the written word in paper format is juxtaposed the written word in electronic and multi-media format.[69] Cloud computing and handy memory sticks offer 'almost endless' storage capacity[70]; widespread terminals or 'clients' enable online access almost everywhere; 'it is not unreasonable to assume', writes Pierre Lévy, 'that in a few years' time the majority of households could be equipped with cyber-gates.'[71] Ammon's reservations on the possibility to be instructed by the written speech are now addressed to the possibility to be instructed by ICT. As Ammon, we need to stay humble.

Individuals in the information society are confronted with a great volume of noise and stimuli unthinkable in the paper or book era, when a person could be 'hit' by a restricted number of encounters, - books, but also individuals and their opinions. Encounters and opinions, in the information society, seem instead to be continuous (think about youtube). It is a great achievement that many of us can read, listen to or watch information, share opinions, learn from others; conversely, it is more difficult to filter information from noise, notably as pieces of information come neat and hard to verify (for instance, on climate change). The information society invites greater personal and social participation, debate and analysis; yet this creates the odd expectation for everyone to have an opinion on everything (leading to the mushrooming of opinion leaders or bloggers). The abundance of information through ICT seems to present many pros and cons. It takes less time than before to consult a library catalogues or to collect an article or a piece of information.[72] On the other hand, a book, or a newspaper, is something one can 'possess': handle, fold, read, sum-up, gloss, forget and find back; or an oral discussion, which is here and now. And in the process, there is time. Time to let information rest, ferment.

Indeed, the spatial and temporal changes in knowledge acquisition in the information society may procure an odd distinction between those who know and those who know less. When the younger generations get older will useful knowledge be the one that can be collected quickly and without much ado? Ammon's utterance is a useful warning to avert the risk that, in a society of older persons, those who hold useful knowledge are the 'hearers of many things who will have learned nothing, omniscient that will generally know nothing, who will be tiresome company, having the show of wisdom without the reality.'

2. ON WEALTH

Changes in the transmission of knowledge in the information society may affect wealth accumulation and transmission. These changes concern in particular the

---

[68] UNESCO, Institute for Statistics, *Book production: number of titles by UDC classes*. Some figures for the year 1996 in Europe: UK: 107 263, Italy: 35 236, Germany: 71 515, Russian Federation: 36 237. http://hypertextbook.com/facts/2009/JianXunZheng.shtml
[69] It is questionable whether digital word is a kind of written word or something new. We assume digital word is a kind of written word. On the role of written word in world's legal traditions see P.Glenn, *Legal Traditions of the World*, Oxford: University Press, 2004, especially chapters I and II. See also P.Lévy, *Collective Intelligence*, Perseus Books, Cambridge (Mass.), 1999, (trasl.: Robert Bonanno). On the relation between technology design and law see M. Hildebrandt, 'A vision of Ambient law', in R. Brownsword & K. Yeung, *Regulating Technologies*, Oxford, Hart Publishers, 2008, p.176-191.
[70] European Data Protection Supervisor (EDPS), Annual report, 2007, p. 56.
[71] P. Lévy, *Collective Intelligence*, op.cit., p.60.
[72] For instance, data about book production in the world in the year 1996 were easily downloadable connecting to the Internet from our offices.

position of older persons in modern economies, and the structure of the information society economy.

As far as the position of older persons is concerned, it is sensible to recall that in the prevalently rural societies of XIX and XX century Europe individual riches and wealth generally incremented with the passing of time. One of the reasons for this was the fact that riches used to be anchored to tangible assets. Also the knowledge, accumulated in a lifetime of work by the farmer or the artisan was a tangible asset an old man could live on. As an old farmer or artisan he would have the *know-how* and the highly important social role of transmitting useful knowledge down through generations. The division of labour in industrialised society (while contributing to advance other areas, such as education) has to some extent reduced the level of know-how possessed by the individual. Even a supporter of the division of labour such as Adam Smith suspected that '[i]n the progress of the division of labour, the employment of the far greater part of those who live by labour, that is, of the great body of the people, comes to be confined to a very few simple operations: frequently to one or two. But the understandings of the greater part of men are necessarily formed by their ordinary employments. The man whose life is spent on performing a few simple operations…has no occasion to exert his understanding, or to exercise his invention…He naturally looses, therefore, the habit of such exertion, and generally becomes as stupid and ignorant as it possible for a human creature to become.'[73]

In addition, highly technological societies are characterised by the rapid obsolescence of the know-how which requires a continuous effort to acquire or update a greater number of notions. Yet, just as means of production become rapidly obsolete, so do men and women when they age.[74] As a result, being old, it is more difficult to survive on the 'know-how' accumulated in a life-time. Often older persons are in need of financial and social support and must rely on external resources, *viz.* social security schemes, transfers and returns on investments, pension-funds and so on.[75] The latter, at their turn, are at risk of 'shocks' that may occur on account of the economy.

This second point takes us to consider the pattern of wealth accumulation prevalent in information society economies. Unlike economies where assets and wealth are anchored in the ground, in the information economy assets and wealth are volatile, 'virtual'. The virtualisation of economies seems to be in line with an established trend and characteristic of modern economies since the eighties of the last century: the 'financiarization' of capitalist economies, in which ICT plays an important enabling role.[76] The idea behind the 'financiarisation' of capitalist economies rests, in essence, on the production of money by other money, a process

---

[73] A. Smith, (1776), *An Inquiry into the Nature and Causes of the Wealth of Nations*, The Glasgow Edition, Oxford, Clarendon Press, 1976, p. 758-88.

[74] For historian Cipolla 'The old man in the rural-agriculture society is the wise man: in the industrial society is a relict.'C. M. Cipolla, *Storia economica dell'Europa pre-industriale,* Il Mulino, Bologna, 1980, p. 303. (Our translation).

[75] One in six older people lives in poverty, with elderly women particularly exposed to low pensions as a result of incomplete careers, COM(1999) 221 final, p.5. See Chapter 1.

[76] On the role of financial market in capitalistic economies see J. Huffschmid, *Politische Ökonomie der Finanzmärkte*, Vsa Verlag, Hamburg 2002; E. Cohen, *Le Nouvel Âge du Capitalism. Bulles, krachs et rebonds*, Fayard, Paris, 2005; K. Knorr Cetina, A. Preda (eds.), *The sociology of Financial Markets*, Oxford: University Press, 2005. On financial de-regulation in the US see R. Weissman, J. Donahue, 'Wall Street's best investment: ten deregulatory steps to financial meltdown', in *Multinational Monitor*, n.1, January-February 2009. See also R. Abdelal, 'le consensus de Paris: la France et les régles de la finance mondiale', Champ Libre, 2005, on financial deregulation in France and Europe.

that has replaced the secular pattern of production of goods from other goods.[77] This process begins, explains Gallino, during the seventies and the eighties of the last century when companies in industrial societies register a drastic slowdown in profits, demand for goods of mass consumption decline, and the so called 'Fordist compromise between capital and labour lead, in many countries, to reduction of working time, adoption of national social security systems, particularly in the area of health and employment.[78] As a consequence, or reaction to the stalemate, market economies have turned *en masse* to more remunerative financial global markets. The 2007 financial crisis showed the size of the wealth so exchanged. According to Gallino[79], in 2007 financial markets traded products amounted to a figure included between 53 and 63 trillion dollars. In the eighties, they were limited to a few trillions. As Gallino notes, in 2007, the registered GDP of the world amounted to ca. 57 trillion dollars.

There is a relation between financial markets and ICT. The relation between financial markets and ICT rests on the 'spatio-temporal fixes and accumulation' that information and communication technologies make – technically- possible.[80] According to Dan Schiller, information and communication technologies create the conditions to craft, move and transit financial products and capitals across frontiers and across markets, with a mere click.[81] As a result, the Information Society economy speeds up the evolution of monetary economies from a goods-based system to a virtual money based system. ICT makes it easier to separate wealth from the real economy. Electronic money can be invested and re-invested and re-invested again and again through myriads of financial products, etc… a process that gets further and further from both concrete wealth and from individual control. Jean-Claude Trichet, President of the European Central Bank, recognized in March 2009 that '[in] the last ten years, we saw a dramatic shift in influence away from entrepreneurship in the real economy to speculation and gambling in the financial sector. […]The assumption and the hedging of genuine economic risk gradually ceased to be the main concern of international finance. [...]. Over time, the creation and assumption of financial risk became the core activity of the financial industry. […] At some point, the financial

---

[77] L. Gallino, 'La crisi e i suoi colpevoli', in *Micromega*, vol. 5, 2009, p.141-166, p.160. See D.T. Bazelon, *The Paper Economy*, Random House, New York, 1963. In the 'paper economy', explains Bazelon, money is not invested on concrete assets or products, but on…other money. See also G. Rimmel, *Filosofia del denaro*, UTET, Milan, 1984. V. Mathieu, *Filosofia del denaro*, Armando, 1985. Financial markets trade financial products. Such 'products' are, in fact, promises of credit, traded and re-traded as 'future' assets, called titles, derivatives, credit default swaps (Cds), Collaterised debt obligations (Cdos) and so on. See N. Prins, *Other's People Money: The Corporate Mugging of America*, The New Press, New York, 2004. The author was for fifteen years consultant at Chase (then J.P. Morgan), Lehman Brothers, and Bear Stearns.

[78] See Chapter 1. Compare with L. Gallino, *L'impresa irresponsabile*, Einaudi, Torino, 2005.

[79] Gallino, Ibid., p.161.

[80] D. Harvey, *The New Imperialism*, Oxford University Press, 2003. Harvey shows that the most effective vehicles for capital accumulation are financial instruments.

[81] Professor Dan Schiller calculated that since 1980 multinational corporations have invested in ICT infrastructures, including software and services, some 1.750 billion dollars since 1980. Schiller indicates that, before accepting 45 billion dollars in state aid by the US government, the bank Citigroup employed 25.000 software engineers and invested 4.9 billion dollars in ICT – excluded the operational costs. Similarly, before falling apart in September 2008 the bank Leham Brothers used 3000 softwares installed in some 25.000 servers spread over the world. Dan Schiller, 'Internet enfante les géants de l'après-crise', in Le Monde Diplomatique, December 2009, n.669, p.1 and p.18. From the same author How to think about information, University of Illinois press, Chicago, 2006.

system seemed to be no longer there primarily to hedge existing economic risks, but more and more to create and propagate risks on its own.'[82]

Such a systemic way to accumulate wealth may have adverse consequences for all citizens, but may hit older persons harder. The reason why elderly persons are particularly vulnerable to the financiarisation of the economy is at least threefold. First, in modern societies the assets and incomes of older individuals almost invariably diminish as they age.[83] Second, as Grundy observes, older people must rely on third external resources to survive, e.g., social security schemes, transfers and returns on investments, pension-funds and so on.[84] Third, as the incumbent financial crisis has made clear, money-based wealth is vulnerable, not just to financial 'shocks,' isolated cases of mismanagement, or exceptional market swings or frauds[85], but to the characteristic features of 'e-' monetary and financial economies, which is based on risk speculation. Few years ago, for instance, the sale of trust units by respectable banks whisked off the savings of many Argentinean nationals, in particular pension funds of older persons, throwing hundreds of them on the street.[86]

3. NOTES ON THE IDOLATRY OF YOUTH (IN HISTORICAL MEMORY AND DEMOCRATIC SYSTEMS)

There is eventually a third element, or fixture of modern information society that is worth investigating as it affects older persons. It concerns the attitude towards historical memory and the effects that such attitude have on democratic systems. While a deeper study in this direction would eschew the scope of this paper, it makes sense annotating a series of short reflections.

As far as historical memory is concerned[87], historian Tony Judt notices a paradox between the abundance of literature and documentaries and the 'burgeoning ignorance and disinterest about where we come from.'[88] Psychologist Frank Furedi agrees with Judt in noting the triumph of myth-making over understanding in the recurrent publicity that surrounds anniversaries, places or days of memory. In his view, the need to be aware that we are part of an ongoing transformative process, history, [...] is progressively abandoning the cultural milieu of the layman.[89] Furedi seems to suggest that the lack of interest in the past is a consequence of the fact that institutions and policy makers, instead of buttressing the link with the past as they should, try to

---

[82] Jean-Claude Trichet, President of the European Central Bank, Introductory remarks to 'What lessons can be learned from the economic and financial crisis?, '5éme Rencontres de l'Entreprise Européenne', organised by La Tribune, Roland Berger and HEC, Paris, 17 March 2009. http://www.bis.org/review/r090318b.pdf

[83] COM(1999) 221 final, p.5., on poverty in old age.

[84] E. Grundy, op.cit., p.110-112.

[85] *Ibidem.*

[86] U. Mattei & L. Nader, *Plunder. When the rule of law is illegal*, Blackwell, Malden (Mass.), 2008, p. 35-42.

[87] What do we mean by historical memory? At least two things: historical memory as *historia,* the narration of events through time and space. Historical memory is also a series of traces which can be recomposed in the present to explain the present or justify policy decisions.

[88] T. Judt, *Reflections On The Forgotten Twentieth Century*, The Penguin Press, 2008.

[89] F. Furedi, *Therapy Culture*, Routledge, London, 2004. Furedi contends that while 'the glorious past' events populate most public authority narratives (the New Britain, the European tradition, the freedom tradition in the state etc..), they are, in fact, 'maquillage', a form of 'public entertainment'. Likewise WWII commemorations, consumption of nostalgia, stories about the past reveal a superficial interest in the past.

divest themselves from it. This view is vigorously defended by another psychologist, Philip Rieff. Rieff is of the opinion that 'the death of culture begins when its normative institutions fail to communicate ideals in ways that remain inwardly compelling, first of all to the cultural elites themselves.' History and, in general, the past, represent to politics and for politicians a 'moral demand system.' Its rejection in favour of less demanding morals, he surmises, represents a cultural revolution with far-reaching consequences.[90]

Philosopher Alain Badiou has linked the rejection and removal of the past to the structure of democratic systems.[91] Alain Badiou reads in the absence of a 'discipline of time' the main characteristic, the emblem, of the (modern) individual living in democratic states. The absence of a discipline of time rests, according to Badiou, on three elements: 'immediateness', 'trend' or 'fashion' and 'movement in the same place.'[92] 'Immediateness', 'trend' and 'movement in the same place' are characteristic features of a society where everything is commodifiable and substitutable.[93] The substitutability happens not only through space, via the appropriation of goods in free and abundant circulation, but also through time: in fact, this happens through the absence of a discipline of time. Growing up or ageing does not mean a diachronic take up of roles and responsibilities, but the continuous reproduction of a youth free of fetters. Badiou calls this reproduction 'idolatry of youth.' The idolatry of youth and the absence of a discipline of time are characteristic features of democracies, he says. Ageing therefore is compromised with a consumption cycle that continues unaltered from cradle to death-bed.[94] Badiou seems to espouse the idea that democracy levels differences of status. Old age thus looses the status and authority derived from being older than others in 'justice and moral endurance.'[95]

IV. THE EXPECTANCY OF DEATH

In the introductory paragraphs of this chapter, we associated ageing as passage through time with ageing as the last years of a person's life and a prelude to death. Focussing on ageing as passing of time, in the previous section we discussed the power of older persons in the information society's areas of knowledge transmission and accumulation of wealth. Now the focus will shift forward, towards death.

---

[90] P. Rieff. , *The Triumph of the therapeutic: uses of faith after Freud*, ISI Books, Wilmington (Del.), 2007.

[91] A. Badiou, 'L'emblème democratique' in Collectif, *Démocratie, dans quel état?*, La Fabrique, Paris, 2009, p. 15-26. On democracy see L.Canfora, *Demoracy. A history of an ideology*, op.cit.

[92] A. Badiou, Ibid., p.23.

[93] Ibid., p.20.

[94] A. Badiou, Ibid., talks about 'abstraction monétaire comme organisation de la pulsion de mort.'

[95] 'The Spartans, the story goes, were about to vote in favour of [a] motion, there came forward one of the Elders – whom they both respect and fear, and the office, called after their age, they regard as the greatest, and they appoint men to it [the office], from those who have been self-controlled from boyhood to old age: one of them came forward, it is said, and denounced them in term like this, they they would not for a long time inhabit an unravaged Sparta, if they used in their assemblies advisers like that [...] At the same time he [one of the Elders] called forward another of the Spartans, a man not well favoured at speaking, but conspicuous in war and remarkable for justice and moral endurance, and commanded him to express the same sentiments, as best as he could, which the former speaker had expressed [...] The old man of self-controlled life from boyhood gave his advice to his fellow citizens[...]' Aeschines (346/5 BC), *Against Timarchos*, translation with introduction and commentary by N. Fisher, Oxford: Clarendon Ancient History Series, 2001.

In the past, senior citizens, being closer to death, were believed to be less vulnerable to losses. As a person aged, the expectancy of death made him or her somewhat stronger. '*Una salus victis nullam sperare salutem*', sums up Virgil in the Aeneid.[96] Modern societies register a marked change in the attitude in front of death and towards conditions such as decadence, morbidity, slowliness and disease. This social attitude affects older persons, who are biologically closer to demise. In the next, and last, paragraphs of this chapter we endeavour to look at the attitude modern highly technological societies place on death.

1. ON DEATH

In his seminal essays on the history of death in the West, Philippe Ariès[97] demonstrates how the 'way of dying', after remaining substantially the same for centuries, has, since the second half of the XX century, changed. In the past, explains Ariès, the characteristic feature was that the dying person, even when it was a child, chaired its death.[98] They could 'chair' death because men and women were very familiar with it. And they were familiar with it for the simple reason that they had seen, crossed it and lived it many times. They knew they would summon, salute, and bless the circle of the living individually, taking *congedo*.[99] Ariès calls this way of dying 'mort apprivoisée.' Since the second half of the XX century, by contrast, *la mort est interdite*. Death gets out-of-the-stage, ob-scene, removed even from the face of the dead.[100] This removal starts with taking the dying individual to hospitals or houses where professional carers assist the body, but know little or nothing about the person. As a result, instead of chairing the last days or months of its life, the person who is dying is isolated. The removal or falsification of death from social discourses contrast with the images and records history and art consigns to us. Records of moves, acts, words of persons who, in the imminence of death, either share their death, or turn their back, turn face to the wall, some looking east (to Jerusalem), some just remaining silent.[101] 'Non sans emotion,' Ariès observes it also in modern hospitals.[102] Yet, he observes how these signs are not intercepted. In this context, the dying

---

[96] Virgil (70 -19 BCE), The Aeneid, liber 2, 334.

[97] P. Ariès, *Essais sur l'histoire de la mort en Occident du moyen age à nos jours* , Seuil, Paris, 1975.

[98] The person feared death would come abruptly and deprive him or her of the possibility to live the last moments. Recall '*a improvisa et morte libera nos, o domine*.'

[99] 'Le mourant présidait [sa mort]. Il présidait et il ne trébuchait guère, car il savait comment se tenir, tant il avait été de fois témoin de scènes semblables. Il appelait un à un ses parents, ses familiers, ses domestiques 'jusqu'aux plus bas' [...]. Il leur disait adieu, leur demandait pardon, leur donnait sa bénédiction. Investi d'une autorité souveraine, surtout aux XVIII et XIXème siècles, par l'approche de la mort, il donnait des ordres, faisait des recommandations, même quand le moribond était une très jeune [...], Ariès, *Ibid.*, p. 169.

[100] Consider, *e.g.*, pratices such as the embalming or, in the US, funeral parties. 'And it is the first time in history,' says Ariès, 'that a community honours its dead by depriving them of the quality of being dead.' Gorer draws a comparison between death and sex. He remarks that once we told children that babies are born under cauliflowers. Today we tell them grandparents have gone to rest amongst the flowers. G. Gorer, 'The Pornography of Death' (revised), in Gorer, G. *Death, Grief and Mourning in Contemporary Britain*, London, Cresset Press, 1965.

[101] 'Il arrive aussi que des malades se tournent vers le mur et ne bougent plus. On reconnaitra là, non sans émotion, l'un des gestes les plus anciens de l'homme quand il sentait la mort venir. Ansi mouraient les juifs de l'Ancien Testament, et, encore au XVIème siècle, l'Inquisition espagnole reconnaissait à ce signe les marranes mal convertis. Ainsi mourut Tristan [...] Ariès, *op.cit.*, p. 175.

[102] Drawing from O.G.Brim, S. Levine, H.E.Freeman, *The dying patient*, New Brunswick, N.J.: Transaction books, 1982.

person's actions create embarrassment, disorder, put medical teams and relatives in disarray; what the French historian sees as something familiar to human kind becomes 'embarrassing.'[103] Ariès suggests that we are no longer familiar with death and that we fear it much more than in past. Therefore we remove it from society and isolate it. Crucially, isolation and removal do not only concern the death and the moments that anticipate or follow it.[104] Isolation and removal clinch to the sick bed and beyond; signs of decadence, fading beauty or fitness, diminishing cognitive capacities become 'embarrassing' as well. Such a trend affects ageing. As Powell suggests, the removal of death tallies well with the value modern societies attach to *non conformity* to discourses of senescence, lowliness and deterioration, morbidity, or dependency.[105]

2. ON CONTRASTING AGEING

2.1. Narrative

Old age, we said, is inevitably *extrema aetas*, the last years of a person's life and a prelude to death. '*Senectus ipsa est morbus,*', old age is a disease, ponders Terence in the comedy *Phormio*. But unlike diseases, from which is possible to recover, old age is a disease one cannot recover from. In fact, Seneca famously corrects him, '*enim insanabilis morbus est.*'[106]

Since technological developments in the field of biotechnology have worked their way into the nano-scale of the human body, a growing narrative in popular media suggests that old age may be treated as a disease; and that it may be possible to technically contrast the cropping up of age-related conditions, such as frailty. The perspective of postponing, decelerating or arresting senescence is fondly, socially acclaimed. As early as the second century BC, Pausanias signalled the existence of a fountain called *Calatos,* where Juno would bath to look always-young and beautiful to Jupiter. At the beginning of the XVI century two infamous conquistadores, Ponce de Leon and Fernando de Soto, ventured on the search of the fountain of youth in the new continent, America.[107] Dorian Gray trashed the wounds of age on his self-portrait. Drinking from the Holy Grail could give eternal youth to the Nazis and the hero Indiana Jones in a famous movie-play of the 1980s. Science fiction author and futurist Ben Bova recently wrote a book predicting that molecular biology and genetics will reveal the secrets of cellular immortality, freeing people of the

---

[103] O.G.Brim, S. Levine, H.E.Freeman, Ibid., p. 63 talk about 'An embarrassingly graceless way of dying'.

[104] For Ariès the removal of death emerges from the use of phrases and expressions such as 'the departed' or 'passing away'. Funeral corteges have almost disappeared from our cities (unless it is a VIP's, in which case the funeral becomes an 'event'); Periods of mourning too. Periods of mourning, he explains, are social mechanisms through which a community protects the circle of the defunct. They have the social function of supporting, shielding, offering them and the community itself the best way to get past the possibly traumatic event. Today to be in mourning, to go into and to come out of mourning, let alone to wear mourning, are rarer and rarer. A sense of guilt seems to affect those visited by death.

[105] J. Powell, 'Rethinking Gerontology: Foucault, Surveillance and the Positioning of Old Age', *Sincronia*, Summer 2004. http://sincronia.cucsh.udg.mx/powell04.htm. See also B. Ehrenreich, *Smile or Die: How Positive Thinking Fooled America and the World,* Granta books, 2009. Enrenreich illustrates the rise of positive thinking - the assumption that one only has to think a thing or desire it to make it happen.

[106] Quoted from M.Fini, *Ragazzo*, Marsilio ed., Venezia, 2006, p.28.

[107] J-P. Bois, *Les vieux: de Montaigne aux premières retraites*, Fayard, Paris, 1979, Chapter I 'La mode et l'angoisse'.

'threescore years and ten.'[108] Media are populated by cosmetic surgery, sports medicine, tissue engineering, bio-electronics, nano-robotics and software resident intelligences, stem cell research and germ line genome modification and so on... technology and science hold out different possibilities for contrasting senescence.[109] News reports about a 'Viagra for the brain' that promises to reverse the age-related memory loss and memory disorders that may occur as one ages[110]. What's more, the show, in the media, of technological sophistication in the field of ageing seems to speak for itself, somehow guaranteeing its own effectiveness and nourishing the belief that a fix always exists.[111]

In the field of medical research, in the 1970s Nobel price laureate doctor Roger Guillemin and his team pioneered studies about how to prevent pathological conditions leading to states of dementia in later age.[112] More recently, the team of Dr H. Lee Sweeney of the Pennsylvania Muscle Institute developed a synthetic gene that, when injected into the muscles cells of mice, makes muscles grow and prevent them from deteriorating with age.[113] Recent developments in regenerative medicine have spurred intellectual excitement about the possibility of decelerating or arresting senescence. Eric Juengst and others described four possible outcomes of anti-ageing medicine: prolonged senescence, compressed morbidity, decelerated ageing, and arrested ageing.[114] Glannon nicely summed up their main features, as follows:

1) *Prolonged senescence* would merely extend lives without mitigating the degenerative effects of ageing. 2) *Compressed morbidity* would shorten the length of time between the onset of ageing-related diseases and death. It would allow us living relatively long lives free of chronic disease and disability and to die quickly from an acute condition. Compressed morbidity may involve accelerated ageing but only for a brief period before death to preclude or at least minimize any disease, pain, or suffering. 3) *Decelerated ageing* would retard but not significantly alter senescence. It would postpone the onset of degenerative diseases, control their progression and result in a moderate extension of the human life span. 4) *Arrested ageing* would involve complete control over the ageing process and could prevent many of its deleterious effects. It would negate the effects of senescence by continuously repairing damage to tissues and organs that is the by product of cell metabolism. Arrested ageing could result in a substantial extension of the lifespan.[115]

Compressed morbidity and arrested ageing as possible outcomes of anti-ageing medicine is particularly interesting. They echo in one of the most vibrant pages of Aldous Huxley's fiction, Brave New World. Huxley's is noteworthy because it gets

---

[108] B. Bova, *Immortality: How Science Is Extending Your Life Span--and Changing The World*, Avon Books, 1998.
[109] *The Telegraph*, 'Long life super pill to help people live past 100 'in development'', by Kate Devlin, 3 February 2010.
[110] *Forbes,* 'Viagra for the brain', by R. Langreth, 4 February 2002.
[111] *The Economist, op.cit.,* reports about 'technological dependence' in America: 'The trouble with health care in America, says Muriel Gillick, a geriatrics expert at Harvard Medical School, is that people want to believe that 'there is always a fix.'
[112] Nobel prize for medicine in 1977 for his work on neurohormones.
[113] The results of the research bode well for curing the immobility which afflicts many elderly. M. Sandel, *The case against perfection*, Harvard: University Press, 2007, p. 10.
[114] E.T. Juengst *et al., Biogerontology, 'Anti-ageing medicine' and the Challenges of Human Enhancemen*t, Hastings Center Report 33 (July-August): 21-30.
[115] W. Glannon, 'Decelerating and arresting human ageing', in B. Gordijn & R. Chadwick (eds.), *Medical Enhancement and Posthumanity*, Springer, Dordrecht, 2008, p. 175-190.

our bearings on what compressed or arrested ageing may look like in a dystopian ageing society.

> 'Oh!' She gripped his arm. 'Look.'
>
> An almost naked Indian was very slowly climbing down the ladder from the first-floor terrace of a neighboring house – rung after rung, with the tremulous caution of extreme old age. His face was profoundly wrinkled and black, like a mask of obsidian. The toothless mouth had fallen in. At the corners of the lips, and on each side of the chin, a few long bristles gleamed almost white against the dark skin. The long unbraided hair hung down in grey wisps round his face. His body was bent and emaciated to the bone, almost fleshless. Very slowly he came down, pausing at each rung before he ventured another step.
>
> 'What's the matter with him?' whispered Lenina. Her eyes were wide with horror and amazement.
>
> 'He's old, that's all,' Bernard answered as carelessly as he could. He too was startled; but he made an effort to seem unmoved.
>
> 'Old?' she repeated. 'But the Director's old; lots of people are old; they're not like that.'
>
> 'That's because we don't allow them to be like that. We preserve them from diseases. We keep their internal secretions artificially balanced at a youthful equilibrium. We don't permit their magnesium-calcium ratio to fall below what it was at thirty. We give them transfusion of young blood. We keep their metabolism permanently stimulated. So, of course, they don't look like that. Partly,' he added, 'because most of them die long before they reach this old creature's age. Youth almost unimpaired till sixty, and then, crack! the end.'
>
> But Lenina was not listening. She was watching the old man. Slowly, slowly he came down. His feet touched the ground. He turned. In their deep-sunken orbits his eyes were still extraordinarily bright. They looked at her for a long moment expressionlessly, without surprise, as though she had not been there at all. Then slowly, with bent back the old man hobbled past them and was gone.' [116]

2.2. Science

Technological developments hold out the promise to intervene technically to arrest, decelerate, or compress old age diseases. The 'promise' of contrasting ageing is part of our imaginary since very long; the show of technological sophistication in popular media seems to be guaranteeing its own effectiveness or nourishes the belief that a fix exists. Biology and cognitive sciences have indeed been able to 'see deeper' into biological processes and to intervene in the 'limes' of organic life. [117] As a result, the mere possibility of intervening at the nano-scale is there, it has entered our sub-

---

[116] A. Huxley, *Brave New World*, New York: Harper and Row, 1965, chapter 7. Available http://www.huxley.net/bnw/index.html

[117] '...all at once science is now delivering a diverse range of information technology, nanotechnology and biotechnology, with a speed and convergence that we could never have even predicted a decade ago', Baronesss Susan Greenfield, House of Lords, April 2006. In R. Brownsword, *Rights, regulation, and the technological revolution*, Oxford: University Press, 2008. Browsword adds neurotechnology to the list of converging technologies.

conscious, and it nourishes fears and hopes.[118] Having illustrated the narrative on contrasting ageing, it is sensible to pause on what we actually know, in science, about the biological process of ageing, also known as senescence. The discipline of bio-gerontology has advanced knowledge of the biological mechanisms that control human ageing or senescence. According to bio-gerontologists, ageing consist of a (biological) process through which cells stop dividing and all (biological) functions gradually cease.[119] At the state of art of research, we know cells division is controlled by an enzyme called *telomerese*. Located at the ends of chromosomes, telomeres are DNA segments which become shorter as somatic cells divide due to the so called 'the end of replication problem. The 'limes' of cells division, that is, the number of times cells can proliferate, is associated with what is known as the 'Hayflick limit.' Named after biologist Leonard Hayflick, this limit indicates that somatic cells can replicate, in vitro, only a limited number of times.[120] According to Hayflick, after a period of reproductive maturity the level of remaining physiological 'reserve'[121] determines longevity. In particular, 'physiological reserve' does not renew at the same rate that it incurs losses. The reason for this is passing of time: biological molecular disorder increases at a rate greater than the capacity for repair. That's the point with biological ageing: the ageing cell does not divide any longer, but it is still alive, keeping its biological functions, breathing and producing energy, including RADICAL OXIGEN SPECIES (ROS) which can damage the DNA of cells. For Hayflick, 'these are age changes, and they increase vulnerability to predation, accidents, or disease.'[122]

This is how 'deep' as we can see into biological ageing. What we cannot see is how the process of cells replication occurs. According to the theory of *antagonistic pleiotropy*[123] some genes contains multiple 'instructions' which trigger different effects on one or more parts or systems of the body *at different stages in life*. This means that some genes which protect us from diseases in early life may make us more vulnerable to diseases in later life.[124]

---

[118] '[…] les nanotechnologies en tous genres sont tellement plus puissantes et invisibles, imprenables, elles s'insinuent partout. Elles rivalisent dans le microbiologique avec les microbes et les bactéries. Mais notre inconscient y est déjà sensible, il le sait déjà et c'est ce qui fait peur.' Excerpts from J. Derrida & J. Habermas, *Le concept du 11 septembre. Dialogues à New York (octobre-décembre 2001) avec Giovanna Borradori,* Galilée, Paris, 2004.

[119] W. Glannon, Ibid., p.177.

[120] L. Hayflick, P.S. Moorhead, 'The Serial Cultivation of Human Diploid Cell Strains', *Experimental Cell Research*, (Wistar Institute, Philadelphia (USA)), 1961, Dec vol. 25, p. 585-621 describing the degenerative changes occurring as cell strains approach their in vitro lifespan. In their discussion, Hayflick and Moorhead use the term 'senescence' to describe the loss of viability that takes place at the end of a cell strain's in vitro lifespan. See also, L. Hayflick, 'The Limited in vitro life-time of Human Diploid cell strains', *Experimental Cell Research*, 1965, vol. 37, pp. 614-636. By the same author, 'The Cellular basis for biological ageing', in l. Hayflick and C. Finch (eds), *Handbook of the biology of Ageing*, Van Nostrand, New York, 1977, p.159-186; and *How and why we age*, New York: Ballantine Books, 1994.

[121] On the use of term 'reserve' in relation to ageing see E. Grundy, op.cit.

[122] L. Hayflick, 'How and why we age - Origin of the theory', in *Experimental Gerontology*, Elsevier, Volume 33, Number 7, November 1998 , pp. 639-653.

[123] Theory developed by G.C. Williams, 'Pleiotropy, natural selection, and the evolution of senescence', in *Evolution*, 1957, vol. 11, pp.398–411.

[124] For example, high level of testosterone and oestrogen may be favourable for fertility in earlier life, but increase the risk of breast, ovarian, and prostate cancer in later life. W. Glannon, *Decelerating and Arresting Human Ageing*, op.cit., p. 178.

2.3. Crossing Lines

What we have seen are the changes that passing of time spawns below the skin. Above the skin, passing of time spawns changes too. Such age changes result in what gerontologists call 'increased frailty.' Increased frailty can be observed in unintentional weight loss (five kg or more in a year), general feeling of exhaustion, weakness (as measured by grip strength), slow walking speed, and low levels of physical activity.[125] Beyond life sciences, life experience teaches us that, getting old, we are all likely to experience a decline in our ability to see, hear, talk, walk, and in general to interpret signals from the outside world. But age changes have an effect also on the environment we live in as elderly people.[126] Changes in the environment mean that fellow citizens, dependants, spouses, colleagues, relatives, friends, will recognise and adjust to ageing fellows. Passers-by, bus drivers, shop assistants, neighbourhoods, and communities may become aware of one's conditions of frailty. They may talk louder, give priority, offer help, offer a seat, provide specialised training and so on. Therefore if, at the end of the day, it is because cells stop dividing that a person becomes old and frailer, the individual and social experience of frailty depends largely on the way a given society accommodates old age needs. As suggested in Chapter 1 (policy context) and as illustrated in Chapter III (legal framework), the ageing of European societies takes on issues such as effective participation, access to services, and enjoyment of rights which take into account the special needs of elderly people. Biotechnology, information and communication technologies for the elderly are part of such a process, they do not replace it. Technological developments, however, seem to hold the promise of putting relief on the vulnerability of old age and do away with the need for solidarity.

This narrative cannot be accepted. One of the reasons why it cannot comes from evidence about the increase in human beings life-span registered in the last decades. There are important economic, social and cultural factors that have given many of us the opportunity to live longer lives in health and comfort. Techno-scientific developments, such as better understanding and insight into alimentation, hygiene conditions, medical treatment, diagnosis, virus contamination and so on, have been possible thanks to better education, health care organisation, working conditions; in this respect the promotion of liberty rights[127] and social rights[128] has been key. These are factors which are related more to the way a society functions than to medical discoveries in a laboratory. This assertion can be defended looking how, in different parts of the world, erosion of social standards, weakening bonds of solidarity, supply-driven consumption strategies, predatory financial practises, low levels of education, and the rationalisation of public health care systems have had a negative impact on

---

[125] Fried, Linda P., Catherine M. Tangen, Jeremy Walston et al., 'Frailty in Older Adults: Evidence for a Phenotype', *Journal of Gerontology: Medical Sciences*, Vol. 56a, No. 3, March 2001, pp. 146-157. http://biomed.gerontologyjournals.org/content/vol56/issue3/#JOURNAL_OF_GERONTOLOGY__ME DICAL_SCIENCES (last visited December 2009), quoted by E. Mordini *et al,* 'Senior citizens and the ethics of e-inclusion', op.cit., p. 18-19.

[126] As it will take us more time to recall a name, to walk the street or to catch the tram, we will devise means (writing down notes, reminders) or prosthesis (a telephone with big dialling bottoms, a remote control, a walking stick) to navigate our way through the day.

[127] Compare A. Sen, *Equality of what?*, in The Tanner Lectures on Human values, ed. S.M. McMurrin, Salt Lake City: University of Utah, reprinted in A. Sen, *Choice, Welfare, and Measurement*, Oxford: Basil Blackwell, 1982, p.353-369. See also, A. Sen, *Inequality Reexamined*, New York, Russell Sage, 1992.

[128] L. Ferrajoli, 'Diritti Sociali e sfera pubblica mondiale', in G. Bronzini (ed.), *Diritti Sociali e Mercato Globale*, Fondazione Lelio e Lisli Basso, Rubbettino Editore, 2007, p. 181-194.

human beings' life span. For instance, since 1991 structural adjustments programs curtailed health care, job security, and social security protection in several countries of the former communist bloc. A US Census Bureau report indicates that over half the decline in male life expectancy at birth in Russia occurred from 1992 to 1994. In 1993 alone, male life expectancy at birth in Russia declined by 3 years, seven years lower than it was some thirty years ago.'[129] In Latin America, expectancy of life in Cuba is six years higher that the average in the rest of the sub-continent.[130] In the same country child mortality (until 5 years old) is 9%, while in the rest of South America the average is 34 %, according to data provided by the 2004 Human Development Report (p.169-171). And in one of the most industrialised and technologically advanced areas of the world, the United States, 'the steady rise in life expectancy during the past two centuries may soon come to an end […] due to obesity.'[131]

V. ACTIVE AGEING: A BLESSING FOR THE AGED?

In the introduction, we pointed out that technology developments are neither neutral, nor inevitable but they are the product of human project and the result of the work of networks of people, scientists, research leaders, companies, sponsors, politician, investors, experts committees, etc…which take decisions and make choices[132]. Small and major decisions mould ICT products and services, check their value, and lead to their final use and commercialisation. An ethical approach to the inclusion of elderly people is therefore first and foremost about taking decisions. Decisions involve specific situations in which conflicting values are present and different solutions are possible. The e-inclusion of the elderly presents conflicts between different policy perspectives, e.g., between industries interested in big scale production and consumption, and individual needs, demands and solutions, between the need to extend working lives and the aspirations of senior citizens wanting to withdraw from active life into something else; between the employment of immigrants as care takers and the opportunity to open up to migrant labour, etc.[133] Conflicts between values also emerge when the implementation of ICT for the elderly requires taking decisions on the intertwined concepts of normality, disease, disability and defect which diverse narratives put forth.

In the EU, the e-inclusion policy framework for elderly people hinges around the notion of active ageing. Active ageing carries the brunt of economic priorities: staying active longer, we said, and postponing the age of retirement, is becoming an economic and social necessity.[134] Staying independent is also considered productive because it

---

[129] W. Ward Kingkade and John E. Dunlop, 'Demographic Developments in Eastern Europe and the Former Soviet Union, Present and Future', *Eurasia Bulletin*, Autumn 1996, p. 13-17. http://www.census.gov/ipc/www/ebaut96c.html (last visited December 2009.)

[130] M. Vandepitte, *De kloof en de uitweg. Een dwarse kijk op ontwikkelingssamenwerking,* EPO, Antwerp, 2004, p.55.

[131] S.J. Olshansky et al., 'A potential decline in life expectancy in the 21st century', *New England Journal of Medicine*, Special Report, 352: 1138-1145, n. 11, March 2005. The authors warn that 'past gains in life-expectancy have largely been a product of saving the young' and maintains that 'since future gains must result from extending the life among the old, another quantum leap in life expectancy can occur only if the future is different from the past.', p. 1142-1145.

[132] S. Gutwirth, *Privacy and the Information Age*, Lanham: Rowman & Littlefield, 2002, p. 65-68

[133] For example, in Italy, restrictive rules enacted in 2009 for the regularisation of migrants were loosen for the category of migrant domestic workers. *ABS-CBN News,* 'Domestic workers, caregivers still in demand in Italy', by Danny Buenafe, 26 August 2009.

[134] *The Economist,* 'Special report on ageing population', 27 June – 3 July, 2009.

relieves society from providing care and from giving support.[135] Active ageing, however, acknowledges the important need for elderly people to participate in society. Sitting idle, being physically fit but without any useful activity to do is psychologically and sociologically distressing. In this sense, e-inclusion and active ageing afford senior citizens the means to actively engage in social, economic and cultural life. In this sense, active ageing could be a blessing for the aged.

The problem with active ageing and the policy of e-inclusion arises when staying active turns out not to be one of many of life's possibilities but 'the' mainstream model for meaningful ageing to which all ageing individuals are expected to adhere by. This chapter underlined some fixtures of the information society which are, in essence, projected towards contrasting natural ageing: transmission of knowledge and *know-how*, accumulation of wealth, idolatry of youth; removal or falsification of death; devaluation of the norm of deterioration and lowliness… Under such circumstances, non-conformity to the discourse of active ageing may become a source for social exclusion. Under such circumstances, old age may be construed as a risk in itself: just like risk 'theft' or risk 'fire' insurance contacts[136], the risk 'old age' would stem from the very condition of being an inactive and unproductive old person. Just as a car may not function well after an accident, so may happen to men when they age. The prospect that old age becomes a risk is suggested by the possibility, propagated by a mediatised scientific community, to get a fix, to mend or to control the insurgence of the deficiencies that put elderly outside the boundaries of active life.

In a context where old age becomes the "risk of old age", active ageing contains social risks for elderly people who, despite all, continue to live in conditions of increased frailty. To these old persons, active ageing may not be a blessing, but a curse and a source of guilt. For the very old, frail, or poor elderly are not only unproductive; they are also weak consumers. Neither productive nor consumers, they are a cost.[137] *The Economist* calculates that 'the bulk of healthcare expenditures concern the last years of a person's life, when he or she needs total assistance. Periods of morbidity may last some years, months, or hours.'[138] Read in the light of the narrative of compressed morbidity and Huxley's dystopia reported above, these lines sound like striking a sinister deal.

Successful e-inclusion and active ageing policies would, instead, harness the empowering aspects of ICT to the 'increased frailty' and asymmetry in power ageing naturally carries with. With the caveat Lear reminds us. No one is forcing king Lear to shake cares and business and to divest himself from power, but 'nature' *and* 'place', yet he pays dear his decision. One ought to keep in mind the vulnerability of old Lear stems from him being old and retired in a greedy context. There is in fact no link of necessity between old age's "tremulous caution" and "toothless mouth" and social exclusion or exploitation. This depends on how society values or devalues ageing, accommodates or less the norm of old age which, *per se,* involves increased frailty

---

[135] Robert N. Butler, *The Longevity Revolution: The Benefits and Challenges of Living a Long Life*, Public Affairs Press, New York, 2008

[136] J-P. Fitoussi, *Il dibattito proibito. Moneta, Europa, Poverta*', Il Mulino, Bologna, 1997, p.43. Original title: J-P. Fitoussi, *Le Dèbat interdit. Monnaie, Europe, Pauvretè*, Paris, Éd. Arléa, 1995.

[137] As we saw in Chapter 1, spending on health is likely to grow faster as patients get older. In the EU, reports the Economist, 'one estimate puts health-care spending on the elderly at about 30-40% of total health spending.' Analysts from the same paper wonder 'whether better health of an ageing population will impose unaffordable costs on public-health budgets. As a rule of thumb, the bulk of spending on an individual's health care is concentrated in the last year or two of life, and particularly in the final six months.' *The Economist*, 'Special Report', *op.cit.*

[138] *The Economist*, Special Report, *op.cit.*, see article 'A world of Methuselahs'.

and diminished power.[139] On the contrary, if old age frailty stumbles against the social ostracism of discourses of deterioration and senescence, old age is forced to go in disguise. Being old becomes consuming, having sex, and in general behaving *as if* young and renouncing to being old. As the story goes, the countess of Castiglione banished mirrors from her palace so she could not see on her face the signs of ageing. A modern countess would invest on sophisticated mirrors reflecting beauty, strength, agility, memory, youth…. 'Youth almost unimpaired... and then, crack! the end', as in Huxley's dystopia. When old age increased frailty means isolation, then the role of technology is to empower elderly people by helping them stay active. This, however, may come at the cost of a generation of misfit, unhappy senior citizens. Those who, after having tried all means to conceal ageing, and notwithstanding the availability of the technology, become older.[140]

REFERENCES

Abdelal, R., *Le consensus de Paris: la France et les régles de la finance mondiale*, Champ Libre, 2005

ACTIVEAGE, *Overcoming the Barriers and Seizing the Opportunities for Active Ageing Policies in Europe*, 30 December 2005(The ACTIVAGE project was funded by the European Community under the HPSE programme 'Improving the Socio-Economic Knowledge Base' (1998-2002)).

Aeschines, *Against Timarchos*, 346/5 BC, translation with introduction and commentary by N. Fisher, Oxford: Clarendon Ancient History Series, 2001.

Améry, J., *Über das Altern: Revolte und Resignation*, Klett-Cotta, Stuttgart, 1997.

Ariès, P., *Essais sur l'histoire de la mort en Occident du moyen age à nos jours* , Seuil, Paris 1975.

Aristotle, *Nicomachean Ethics*, 350 BC, translated by W. D. Ross, Book 6, para 8. Excerpts taken from the Internet Classics Archive by Daniel C. Stevenson, http://classics.mit.edu/Aristotle/nicomachaen.mb.txt

Artistole, *Rethoric*, 350 BC, Book II, Part 12 on youth, and Part 13 on the elderly. http://classics.mit.edu/Aristotle/rhetoric.mb.txt

Badiou, Alain, 'L'emblème democratique' in Collectif, *Démocratie, dans quel état?*, La Fabrique, Paris, 2009.

Bauman, Z., *Liquid Modernity*, Polity Press, Cambridge 2000

Bazelon, D.T., *The Paper Economy*, Random House, New York, 1963.

Berčič B., C.George, 'Investigating the legal protection of data, information and knowledge under the EU data protection regime', *International Review of Law, Computers & Technology*, 23: 3, 189 – 201.

Bobbio, N., *De Senectude*, Einaudi, Torino, 1996.

Booth, Wayne C., *The art of growing older: writers on living and aging*, Poseidon, New York, 1992.

Bova, B., '*Immortality: How Science Is Extending Your Life Span--and Changing The World*', Avon Books, 1998.

Bratton, J.S. (ed.), *King Lear. Plays in Performance*, Bristol Classical Press, Bristol, 1987.

---

[139] Foucault's seminal intuition that 'society exerts its control over individuals not only through conscience or ideology, but also in and with the body' acquires here great significance. See Introduction. See also Foucault, Michel, The Birth of Social Medicine, in James D. Faubion (ed.), *Essential Works of Michel Foucault 1954-1984*, Penguin, London, 2001, pp. 134-156.

[140] Mordini E, Wright D, de Hert P, Mantovani E, Wadhwa K, Thestrup J, Van Steendam G, Ethics, e-Inclusion and Ageing, *Studies in Ethics, Law and Technologies*, 2009, vol.3, issue 1, Article 5.

Brim, O.G., S. Levine, H.E.Freeman, *The dying patient*, New Brunswick, N.J.: Transaction books, 1982.

Brooke, Nicholas , *Shakespeare. King Lear*, Edward Arnold publisher, London, 1963.

Brownsword, R., *Rights, Regulation, and the Technological Revolution*, Oxford: University Press, 2008.

Butler, Robert N., *The Longevity Revolution: The Benefits and Challenges of Living a Long Life*, Public Affairs Press, New York, 2008.

Campanella, Tommaso , *La citta' del sole*, 1602.

Canfora, L., *Democrazia. Storia di una ideologia*, Laterza, Bari, 2004. In English, *Democracy in Europe: A History of an Ideology*, Malden, 2006.

Cicero, Marcus Tullius, *Cato Major De Senectude*, with introduction and notes by James S. Reid, The Echo library, 2007.

Cicero, Marcus Tullius, *Treatises on Friendship and Old Age*, translated by E. S. Shuckburgh. http://ancienthistory.about.com/library/bl/bl_text_cicero_desenec.htm

Cipolla, C. M., *Storia economica dell'Europa pre-industriale*, Il Mulino, Bologna, 1980.

Cohen, E., *Le Nouvel Âge du Capitalism. Bulles, krachs et rebonds*, Fayard, Paris, 2005.

Derrida, J. & J. Habermas, *Le concept du 11 septembre. Dialogues à New York (octobre-décembre 2001) avec Giovanna Borradori*, Galilée, Paris, 2004.

Ehrenreich, B., *Smile or Die: How Positive Thinking Fooled America and the World*, Granta books, 2009.

Elton, William R., *King Lear and the gods*, Kentucky: University Press, 1988.

Ferrajoli, L., 'Diritti Sociali e sfera pubblica mondiale', in G. Bronzini (ed.), *Diritti Sociali e Mercato Globale*, Fondazione Lelio e Lisli Basso, Rubbettino Editore, 2007, p. 181-194.

Fini, M., *Ragazzo*, Marsilio, Venezia, 2006.

Fitoussi, J-P. *Le Dèbat interdit. Monnaie, Europe, Pauvretè*, Paris, Éd. Arléa, 1995.

Foucault, Michel, *Dits et écrits*, Paris 1994, vol. III.

Foucault, Michel, 'The Birth of Social Medicine', in James D. Faubion (ed.), *Essential Works of Michel Foucault 1954-1984*, Penguin, London, 2001.

Fried, Linda P., Catherine M. Tangen, Jeremy Walston et al., 'Frailty in Older Adults: Evidence for a Phenotype', *Journal of Gerontology: Medical Sciences*, Vol. 56a, No. 3, March 2001, pp. 146-157. http://biomed.gerontologyjournals.org/content/vol56/issue3/ #JOURNAL_OF_GERONTOLOGY__MEDICAL_SCIENCES (last visited December 2009)

Friedewald, M., 'The continuous construction of the computer user: Visions and user models in the history of human-computer interaction', in Buurman, G.M.:, *Total Interaction: Theory and practice of a new paradigm for the design disciplines.*, Basel: Birkhäuser, 2005, pp. 27-41.

Furedi, F. *Therapy Culture: Captivating Vulnerability in an Uncertain Age*, Routledge, New York, 2004.

Gallino, L.,'La crisi e I suoi colpevoli', in *Micromega*, vol. 5, 2009, p.141-166, p.160.

Glannon, W., 'Decelerating and arresting human ageing', in B. Gordijn & R. Chadwick (eds.), *Medical Enhancement and Posthumanity*, Springer, Dordrecht, 2008, p. 175-190.

Glenn, P., *Legal Traditions of the World*, Oxford: University Press, 2004.

Gorer, G., 'The Pornography of Death' (revised), in Gorer, G. *Death, Grief and Mourning in Contemporary Britain*, London, Cresset Press, 1965.

Grundy, E., 'Ageing and vulnerable elderly people: European perspectives', in *Ageing & Society*, Cambridge University Press, vol. 26, 2006, p. 105–134.

Gutwirth, S., *Privacy and the Information Age*, Lanham: Rowman & Littlefield, 2002.

Hadot, P., 'La figure du sage dans l'antiquité gréco-latine', in P. Hadot, *Etudes de philosophie ancienne*, Les Belles Lettres, Paris, 1998. Trad. B. Carnevali, "La figura del saggio nell'antichità greco-latina", in Micromega, 4/2009, p.151-174.

Harlow, M., R. Laurence, 'Old Age in Ancient Rome', in *History Today*, April 2003, Vol. 53, Issue 4, p.22-27.

Harvey, D., *The New Imperialism*, Oxford University Press, 2003.

Hayflick L., and C. Finch (eds), *Handbook of the biology of Ageing*, Van Nostrand, New York, 1977.

Hayflick, L. , P.S. Moorhead, 'The Serial Cultivation of Human Diploid Cell Strains', *Experimental Cell Research*, (Wistar Institute, Philadelphia (USA)), 1961, Dec vol. 25, p. 585-621.

Hayflick, L., 'The Limited in vitro life-time of Human Diploid cell strains', *Experimental Cell Research*, 1965, vol. 37, pp. 614-636.

Hayflick, L., 'How and why we age - Origin of the theory', in *Experimental Gerontology*, Elsevier, Volume 33, Number 7, November 1998 , pp. 639-653.

Hildebrandt, M., 'A vision of Ambient law', in R. Brownsword & K. Yeung, *Regulating Technologies*, Oxford, Hart Publishers, 2008, p.176-191.

Huffschmid, J., *Politische Ökonomie der Finanzmärkte*, Vsa Verlag, Hamburg 2002;

Huxley, A., *Brave New World*, New York: Harper and Row, 1965.

Judt, T., *Reflections On The Forgotten Twentieth Century*, The Penguin Press, London, 2008.

Juengst, E.T., et al., *Biogerontology, "anti-ageing medicine" and the challenges of human enhancement*, Hastings Center Report 33 (July-August): 21-30.

Kiernan, Victor , *Eight tragedies of Shakespeare: a Marxist study*, London: Verso, 1996.

Kingkade, W. and John E. Dunlop, 'Demographic Developments in Eastern Europe and the Former Soviet Union, Present and Future', *Eurasia Bulletin*, Autumn 1996, p. 13-17.

Knorr Cetina, K., A. Preda (eds.), *The sociology of Financial Markets*, Oxford: University Press, 2005.

Laslett, P. , *Il mondo che abbiamo perduto*, Jaca Books, 1979. (Original title, *The World We Have Lost: English Society before the Coming of Industry* (1965))

Laslett, P., John M. Eekelaar, David Pearl (eds), *An aging world: dilemmas and challenges for law and social policy*, Clarednon Press, Oxford, 1989.

Lévy, P., *L'intelligence collective: pour une anthropologie du cyberspace*, Paris : La Découverte, 1994. English version: *Collective intelligence*, Perseus Books, Cambridge (Mass.), 1999, (trasl.: Robert Bonanno).

Mathieu, V., *Filosofia del denaro*, Armando, 1985.

Mattei U., L. Nader, *Plunder. When the rule of law is illegal*, Blackwell, Malden (Mass.), 2008.

McLuhan, M., *Understanding Media: The Extensions of Man*, McGraw Hill, New York, 1964 Papert, S., *The connected family: bridging the digital generation gap*, Atlanta, Longstreet Press,1996.

Mordini E, et al., Ethics, e-Inclusion and Ageing, Studies in *Ethics, Law and Technologies*, 2009, vol.3, issue 1, Article 5)

Mordini E., et al., Senior citizens and the ethics of e-inclusion, Ethics and Information Technology (2009) 11: 203-220.

Mowat, B.A., and Paul Werstine (eds), New Folger Library Shakespeare edition, Folger Shakespeare Library, 1993

Olshansky S.J., et al., 'A potential decline in life expectancy in the 21st century', *New England Journal of Medicine*, Special Report, 352: 1138-1145, n. 11, March 2005.

Plato, *Phaedrus*, translated by R. Hackforth, University Press, Cambridge, 1972. 'Phaedrus' was written between 372 and 368 B.C.

Plato, *Republic*, translated by Benjamin Jowett in 1873 reprinted by Agora Publications, Millis, MA, 2001. Book I, p.3-4. http://classics.mit.edu/Plato/republic.html

Posner, Richard A., *Aging and Old Age*, University Press, Chicago, 1995.

Powell, J., 'Rethinking Gerontology: Foucault, Surveillance and the Positioning of Old Age', *Sincronia*, Summer 2004, http://sincronia.cucsh.udg.mx/verano04.htm

Prins, N., *Other's People Money:The Corporate Mugging of America*, The New Press, New York, 2004.

Rieff., P., *The Triumph of the therapeutic: uses of faith after Freud*, ISI Books, Wilmington (Del.), 2007.

Rimmel, G., *Filosofia del denaro*, UTET, Milan, 1984.

Rooke, C. ,'Oh What a Paradise It Seems: John Cheever's Swan Song', in Anne M. Wyatt-Brown and Janice Rossen (eds), *Aging and Gender*, Studies in Creativity, University Press of Virginia, Charlottesville and London, 1993, pp. 204-225.

Said, Edward, *Orientalism*, Penguin Books, London, 2003.

Sandel, M., *The case against perfection*, Harvard: University Press, 2007.

Schiller, Dan, *How to think about information*, University of Illinois press, Chicago, 2006.

Schrödinger, E., *What is Life? The Physical Aspect of the Living Cell*, Cambridge: University Press, 1944.

Sen, A., *Equality of what?*, in The Tanner Lectures on Human values, ed. S.M. McMurrin, Salt Lake City: University of Utah, reprinted in A. Sen, *Choice, Welfare, and Measurement*, Oxford: Basil Blackwell, 1982.

Sen, A., *Inequality Reexamined*, New York, Russell Sage, 1992.

Shakespeare, King Lear, 1605-6, edited by R.A. Foakes, The Arden Shakespeare, Thomson Learning, London, 2005.

Smith, A., (1776) , *An Inquiry into the Nature and Causes of the Wealth of Nations*, The Glasgow Edition, Oxford, Clarendon Press, 1976.

Thomas, Dylan , *Collected Poems*, edited by Walford Davies and Ralph Maud, Phoenix, London, 2003.

Trichet, J.C. ,President of the European Central Bank, at the '5e Rencontres de l'Entreprise Européenne', organised by La Tribune, Roland Berger and HEC, Paris, 17 March 2009. http://www.bis.org/review/r090318b.pdf

Vandepitte, M., *De kloof en de uitweg. Een dwarse kijk op ontwikkelingssamenswerking*, EPO, Antwerp, 2004, p.55.

Virgil (70 -19 BCE), *The Aeneid*.

Weissman, R., J. Donahue, 'Wall Street's best investment: ten deregulatory steps to financial meltdown', in *Multinational Monitor*, n.1, January-February 2009.

Williams, G.C., 'Pleiotropy, natural selection, and the evolution of senescence', in *Evolution*, 1957, vol. 11, pp.398–411.

SENIOR Project, D.2.3 'Intelligent User Interface', prepared by P. De Hert and E. Mantovani.

SENIOR project, 'The Inclusion of Senior Citizens in the Information Society', Expert meeting on Ubiquitous communication', Presentation by Birgit Jæger, 22 September 2008, Brussels.

SENIOR project, 'The competent Seniors: Aging and use of digital media – conflict or happiness?', 6 June 2008, presentation by Øyvind Nøhr, Lillehammer University College,.

SENIOR project, Work Package 1 final, prepared by D. Wright

SENIOR project, D.2.3, 'Intelligent User Interface', prepared by P. De Hert & E. Mantovani

SENIOR project, Report on the Socio-anthropological workshop on the social and cultural meanings of ageing and ICT, prepared by Jesper Thestrup and Trine Sørensen, www.seniorproject.eu

SENIOR project, Text analysis report, D.1.2, prepared by Guido Van Steendam, 30 September 2008.

SENIOR, Ethics of e-inclusion of elderly people, Discussion paper for the workshop on ethics and e-inclusion, Bled (Slovenia), 12 May 2008.

Forbes, 'Viagra for the brain', by R. Langreth, 4 February 2002.

Le Monde Diplomatique,Schiller, Dan, 'Internet enfante les géants de l'après-crise', in, December 2009, n.669.

L'Echo, 'Colruyt se lance dans le marketing personnalisé', 27 January 2010.

ABS-CBN News, Italy, 'Domestic workers, caregivers still in demand in Italy', by Danny Buenafe, 26 August 2009.

The Economist, 'Special report on ageing population', 27 June – 3 July, 2009.

Science Daily, Obituary Photos Suggest Growing Bias Against Aging Faces, 18 May 2009. http://www.sciencedaily.com/releases/2009/05/090513121059.htm. Check powell

The Telegraph, 'Long life super pill to help people live past 100 'in development'', by Kate Devlin, 3 February 2010.

I-Cat research community http://www.hitech-projects.com/icat/index.php

UNESCO, Institute for Statistics, Book production: number of titles by UDC classes. Some figures for the year 1996 in Europe: UK: 107 263, Italy: 35 236, Germany: 71 515, Russian Federation: 36 237. http://hypertextbook.com/facts/2009/JianXunZheng.shtml

European Commission, *Towards a Europe for all ages - Promoting prosperity and intergenerational security*, Communication from the Commission, Brussels, 21 May 1999, COM (1999) 221 final.

European Data Protection Supervisor (EDPS), *Annual report*, 2007.

CHAPTER THREE. THE EU LEGAL FRAMEWORK FOR THE E-INCLUSION OF OLDER PERSONS

By Paul De Hert and Eugenio Mantovani

INTRODUCTION

Chapter three illustrates the EU legal framework relevant for older persons and e-inclusion. At the level of European Union, the main sources include human rights law, provisions on equality, and on the information society. Human rights law is arguably the most important body of law encompassing a large body of soft law commonly known as 'international framework on ageing' and, in the European context, a set of detailed provisions included in the European Convention of Human Rights (1950), the Revised European Social Charter (1996) and the EU Charter of Fundamental Rights of the European Union(2000). Concerning equality, the Treaty of Lisbon in article 9 recognises as one of the policies and activities of the Union 'adequate social protection, the fight against social exclusion, and a high level of education, training and protection of human health.'[1] In the European Union *acquis*, discrimination on grounds of age is forbidden in the context of employment. Old age discrimination, however, is increasingly treated as a horizontal equality matter. Eventually, a growing body of rules regulates the area of information society. We will follow the SWAMI[2] method to list and illustrate some relevant areas such as interoperability, e-health, consumer protection, product safety which we deem important for ICT and the aged.

I. HUMAN RIGHTS AND THE ELDERLY

Human rights law in the twentieth century has been characterised by a momentum of inflation of rights. More rights, more subjects entitled to have these rights, and more duties imposed upon persons, the state and private actors to respect these rights. Rights became more coloured. Rights of disabled, of children, of soldiers, of internet users, of women and patients have come to replace or supplement the traditional rights of Man. Our century seems to prolong this tendency. The identification of possible new subjects for rights entitlement seems to be fuelled by sensibilities that develop over time. In the essay 'Human Rights and society', Norberto Bobbio describes the proliferation of human rights and the relation with social change.[3] According to the Italian professor, proliferation of human rights during the second half of the XX century occurred a) because of the increase in the number of assets considered worthy of protection; b) because of few typical rights have been extended to entities other than human beings; and c) because human beings themselves are no longer considered a generic entity or abstract man, but are seen in their specific or concrete situation in society.

---

[1] Consolidated versions of the Treaty on European Union and the Treaty on the Functioning of the European Union Official Journal C 115 of 9 May 2008.
[2] D. Wright et al., *Safeguards in a World of Ambient Intelligence,* Springer, 2008.
[3] Norberto Bobbio, *The Age of Rights*, Policy Press, Oxford, 1994, p. 47-61.

The first point refers to the demands addressed to the state not only to refrain from interference (negative rights), but also to intervene (positive rights) to ensure, *e.g.*, a sufficient level of education, or adequate standard of living, minimum health or a basic income.[4] The second point underlines a shift in attention from the person (the Man) to entities other than the person, such as the family, ethnic minorities, linguistic minorities and also the environment, future generations and the whole world.[5] The third point interests us more closely and refers to the *status* of the human being in human rights law. While the subject of human rights has remained for long time an abstract, generic person, in the last decades human rights law has considered mainly the specifics of the person. His or her concrete characteristics, as a child, old person, sick person etc., the statuses he or she embodies on the basis of criteria for differentiation such as sex, age, physical conditions.[6] This 'proliferation through specification' has concerned social rights and it led to the adoption of human rights conventions on the rights of women (1979), children (1989), persons with disabilities (2006). According to Bobbio, the first world assembly on ageing, celebrated in 1982, was prodromic of the unfolding, in the future, of a treaty on the human rights of the older persons.

1. THE INTERNATIONAL FRAMEWORK ON AGEING

At the international level, the theme of ageing is considered in a large body of soft law and in provisions of positive human rights law. As far as soft law is concerned, three main policy documents, mentioned in chapter I, mark the shaping of an 'international framework or guidelines on ageing (or aging).'

The first policy initiative is the 1982 First World Assembly on Ageing, to which Bobbio refers. Celebrated under the aegis and later endorsed by the UN General Assembly[7], the summit adopted a Plan of Action, the *Vienna International Plan of Action on Ageing.*[8] The first international instrument on ageing endorsed by the UN invited states to protect and promote the rights of older persons as part of the International Bill of human rights (the 1948 UDHR, and the 1966 twin Conventions[9]) and comprises sixty-two recommendations designed to guide their application on elderly people. Recommendations include guidelines on health and nutrition (n. 1-17); protection of elderly consumers (18); housing and environment (19-24); on family (25-29); social welfare (30-35); income security and employment (36-43); and on

---

[4] Consider, e.g., article 34.2 of EU Charter (social security) W. Chiaromonte, *La Protezione dei soggetti piu' bisognosi e le indicazioni dell'UE: spunti giurisprudenziali e considerazioni a margine di tribunale di Napoli 22 Aprile 2009*, in www.europeanrights.com

[5] Compare Article 225 of the Constitution of Brasil, Right to an ecologically balanced environment.

[6] The 'constitutionalisation' of the person is its concrete vicissitudes and problems is one of the main results of the 2000 European Union Charter of Fundamental Rights for S.Rodotà , *Social ethical and privacy needs in ICT for older people: a dialogue road map*, Opening lecture to the launching event of SENIOR, 3 March 2008, p.1. www.seniorproject.eu.

[7] U.N. General Assembly, 37th Session (1982). Resolution 37/51. *Question of Aging.* A/RES/37/51. http://www.un.org/documents/ga/res/37/a37r051.htm

[8] U.N. General Assembly, *Report of the World Assembly on Ageing*, Vienna, 26 July to 6 August 1982 (United Nations publication, Sales No. E.82.I.16).

[9] The International Bill of human rights is formed of three core human rights conventions, the 1948 Universal Declaration of Human Rights (UDHR), the 1966 International Covenant on Economic, Social and Cultural Rights (ICESCR), and the 1966 International Covenant on Civil and Political Rights (ICCPR).

education (44-51), on data collection and analysis (n. 52-53), training and education (54-59), and on research (60-62).[10]

Second, in 1991, the UN General Assembly adopted the *United Nations Principles for Older Persons.*[11] Under the formula 'life added to years added to life' the Principles asked governments to incorporate in their national policies eighteen principles relating to independence, participation, care, self-fulfillment, and the dignity of older persons. 'Independence' refers to access to adequate food, water, shelter, clothing and health care, remunerated work and access to education and training. 'Participation' concerns broadly active participation in the formulation and implementation of policies, the opportunity of sharing their knowledge and skills with the younger generations, and to form movements and associations. The section headed 'care' is concerned with the concrete possibility for older persons to benefit from family care, health care and be able to enjoy human rights and fundamental freedoms when residing in a shelter, care or treatment facility. With regards to 'self-fulfillment', the Principles ask governments to create conditions necessary for older persons to pursue their full development and potential through, e.g., access to educational, cultural, spiritual and recreational activities. Last, the section titled 'Dignity' recommends older persons remain free from want, exploitation, physical and mental abuse; that they are treated fairly, no matter their age, gender, racial or ethnic background, disability, financial situation or any other status, and be valued independently from their economic contribution. In the year 1992, the General Assembly annexed to Resolution 47/5 a Proclamation on Aging[12], which set a series of targets and of priority policy areas.[13]

Third, and last, in 2002 the second World Assembly on Aging took place in Madrid. On that occasion, United Nations members approved the *Madrid International Plan of Action on Aging (MIPAA)*[14] with the stated goal of 'ensur[ing] that older persons are 'mainstreamed' into overall policy, not treated as a separate group in need of remedial care.' Designed to facilitate the assessment, planning, and evaluation of national policies affecting older persons,[15] the MIPAA identifies four main social areas: 1) poverty and sustainable livelihoods, family and culture; 2) health and active life, food security and nutrition, housing and physical amenities, conflicts and disaster management; 3) education, communication and training, employment and

---

[10] Adopted by the U.N. General Assembly, A/RES/37/51. Recommendations are available at http://www.un.org/esa/socdev/ageing/vienna_intlplanofaction.html.

[11] U.N. General Assembly, 46th Session (1991). Resolution 46/91, *Implementation of the International Plan of Action on Ageing and related activities.* A/RES/46/91

[12] U.N. General Assembly, 47th Session (1992). Resolution 47/5, *Proclamation on Ageing.* A/RES/47/5.

[13] See the 1992 global targets (A/47/339) endorsed by the General Assembly in its Resolution 47/86. U.N. General Assembly, 89th Plenary Meeting (1992). Resolution 47/86, *Implementation of the International Plan of Action on Ageing: integration of older persons in development.* A/RES/47/86. Women should be given adequate support for their largely unrecognized contributions to society. Older persons in general are encouraged to develop social, cultural and emotional capacities, which they may have been prevented from developing during breadwinning years; families should be supported in providing care and all family members are encouraged to cooperate in caregiving etc.

[14] United Nations, *Report of the Second World Assembly on Ageing Madrid*, 8-12 April 2002. A/CONF.197/9. Available at http://www.un.org/swaa2002/documents.htm. The text of MIPAA is available at http://www.un.org/esa/socdev/ageing/documents/building_natl_capacity/guiding.pdf

[15] *Ibid.*,p.12: '…making older persons' concerns and experiences an integral dimension of the design, implementation, monitoring and evaluation of policies and programmes in all political, economic and societal spheres.'

income security, social security, social welfare; and 4) Institutional framework and implementation of laws targeting older persons, *e.g.*, preparation for retirement).[16]

In pursuance of the MIPAA, a number of regional strategies were adopted; in Europe, the Regional Strategy for the Implementation (RIS) of the Madrid international Plan of Action on Ageing. On 5-8 November 2007, the United Nations Economic Commission for Europe (UNECE) held a ministerial conference on ageing in Leon, Spain.[17]

Among its recommendations, the UNICE suggested setting up a working group within the UN Human Rights Council mandated to draw up 'a Convention on the Rights of Older Persons and mainstream age in the agenda of the Council.' A further step was made more recently by the advisory committee to the Human Rights Council which explicitly called for a treaty on the human rights of the older person.[18]

2. THE RIGHTS OF ELDERLY PEOPLE IN POSITIVE HUMAN RIGHTS LAW IN EUROPE

The sixty-two guidelines which accompany the 1982 Vienna Plan on Ageing, the 1991 UN Principles for Older Persons and the mainstreaming guidelines of the 2002 MIPAA constitute the "International Framework on Ageing." In legal terms, none of these instruments is binding; however, together they offer ample and concrete guidance to traditional international human rights law in relation to the special needs of elderly people. As such, these three international instruments can be practically used by international, regional or national organisms in shaping 'hard' legislation. The most prominent example and reference is the General Comment 6 of the supervisory committee to the UN International Covenant on Economic Social and Cultural Rights (ICESCR). Drafted in 1995, 'General Comment 6 on the economic, social and cultural rights of older persons' provides for a fresh re-reading of the articles of the Covenant - and also of other International Human rights law instruments - in the light of population ageing.[19] In its review of economic, social and cultural human rights, the Committee makes explicit reference to the 1982 recommendations and the 1991 Principles.[20]

While to date there is not any specific human rights treaty on them, positive human rights law encompasses, internationally, a great number of provisions on older persons. Even a cursory review of the status of elderly people in positive human rights

---

[16] A. Sidorenko, & A. Walker, 'The Madrid International Plan of Action on Ageing: From conceptualization to implementation', in *Ageing & Society* 24 (2): (2004) 147-165.

[17] U.N. Economic Commission for Europe, *Main Conclusions and Recommendations of the Research Forum on Ageing*, 5-8. 11.2007, http://www.un.org/esa/socdev/ageing/documents/2007LeonFinal.pdf

[18] Human Rights Council. Advisory Committee, Fourth Session, *Working paper*, A/HRC/AC/4/CRP.1, 25-29 January 2010.

[19] Office of the High Commissioner for Human Rights, *Economic, Social and Cultural Rights of Older Persons: General Comment 6,* U.N. ESCOR, Econ., Soc., & Cultural Rts. Comm., 13th Sess., para. 1, UN   Doc.   E/C.12/1995/16/Rev.1   (1995)   .http://www.unhchr.ch/tbs/doc.nsf/(Symbol)/482a0aced8049067c12563ed005acf9e?Opendocument

[20] See the excellent research paper of D. Rodriguez-Pinzon and C. Marin, 'The International Human Rights status of elderly persons', in *American University Inernational Law Review*, 2003, vol. 18, number 4, p.916-1007. See also P. De Hert, E. Mantovani, *The Rights of the Elderly in the Age of Rights*, (forthcoming).

law would exceed the scope of this chapter.[21] We restrict the focus to the European continent.

In Europe, sources of human rights of older persons are found in the three principal human rights law instruments, namely the 1950 European Charter of Human Rights (ECHR), the 1996 Council of Europe Revised European Social Charter, and the 2000 EU Charter of Fundamental Rights. We are going to review the main features of these three instruments and pause on some relevant provisions.

II. THE EUROPEAN CONVENTION OF HUMAN RIGHTS (ECHR)

The Convention for the Protection of Human Rights and Fundamental Freedoms (ECHR) was adopted under the auspices of the Council of Europe in 1950 to protect human rights and fundamental freedoms in Europe. All EU member states are party to the Convention and new members are expected to ratify the convention. With the entry into force of the Lisbon Treaty, the EU as a whole is expected to accede to the ECHR. The Convention consists of three sections. Rights and freedoms are enshrined in Section I, articles 2 to 18, and have similar structure. The first period sets out a basic right or freedom (such as Article 8(1) - the right to private life and correspondence), while the second (such as Article 8(2)) provides for the possible exceptions or limitations.

1. ARTICLE 3: PROHIBTION OF TORTURE, INHUMAN OR DEGRADING TREATMENT OR PUNISHMENT

Article 3 of the European Convention for the Protection of Human Rights and Fundamental Freedoms states that 'No one shall be subjected to torture or to inhuman

---

[21] There is a large body of human rights law on older persons. Older persons are mentioned in other UN conventions or declarations such as the 1979 Convention on the rights of women (article 10), the 1951 Convention on the status of refugee (article 24), the 1969 Declaration on social progress and development (article 11), the 2007 Declaration on the rights of indigenous people (article 22). Other non UN instruments include ILO conventions and international Humanitarian Law. Extremely variegated is the status of older persons under regional human rights instruments. Different legal traditions differ in the way they categorise age and protect older persons. In the Americas, the American Declaration of Rights and Duties of Man (1948), the American Convention of Human Rights ('Pact of San Jose') (1969), the Additional Protocol to the American Convention on Human Rights in the area of Economic, Social, and Cultural Rights (known as the 'Protocol of San Salvador') (1988, and the Andean Charter for the promotion and protection of human rights (2002) recognize the status of older persons. In Africa, mention of older people's rights is made in the African (Banjul) Charter on human and peoples' rights (1981) and in the Protocol to the African charter on human and peoples' rights on the rights of women on Africa (2000). In Asia, the Declaration of the basic duties of ASEAN peoples and governments (1983) and the Asian Charter of human rights (1997) refer to older persons and their special needs of protection. The Islamic Legal Tradition foresees provisions on the aged in the Universal Islamic Declaration of human rights (1981) and in the Cairo Declaration of Human rights in Islam (1990). Eventually, in Europe, a helicopter view of human rights law relevant for older persons include the Revised European Social Charter (1961 and 1996, when the charter is revised), the European convention on human Rights (1950), and the Charter of Fundamental Rights of the European Union (2000). In addition, the constitutions of some EU member states directly or indirectly refer to the older persons. D. Rodriguez-Pinzon and C. Marin, op.cit., 952-972.

or degrading treatment or punishment'(Prohibition of torture).[22] 'No one' also mean elderly people, in particular those living in institutions or retirement homes. Under article 3, a state owes its citizens not only a negative obligation to refrain from inflicting such treatment but also a positive obligation to protect people from it. In *Mouisel v. France*[23], the Court of Strasbourg found the detention of a person who is ill may raise issues under Article 3 of the Convention […]. In *Papon v. France*[24] the Court observed that the detention of an elderly sick person over a lengthy period could fall within the scope of Article 3. 'Age', held the judges, [together with health, and severe physical disability] 'is now among the factors to be taken into account under Article 3 of the Convention.'[25]

The Committee of Ministers of the Council of Europe drew the attention to the relation between article 3 and senior citizens conditions in 1994 when it reminded member states that, pursuant to article 3, '…elderly people should be able to live in security, wherever they are, free from fear of exploitation or of physical or mental abuse'. Confronted with an increasing number of cases of ill-treatment against older persons, in 2002 the Commissioner for human rights indicated that the protection of article 3 was in fact rarely activated when the victim was an elderly person.[26] One of the reasons for this is that the Convention lacks a legal instrument to obtain report from national authorities, which could help to identify and prevent conditions likely to lead to cases of ill-treatment. We will see below that the European Social Charter disposes of a reporting-supervisory mechanism. There is also very little training for staff in this area and a lack of prevention policies, observes the Commissioner.

2. ARTICLE 5: RIGHT TO LIBERTY AND SECURITY

Article 5 of the European Convention of Human Rights recognises to everyone the right to liberty, but for a restricted number of cases foreseen in law and which must be interpreted narrowly. Under paragraph 1, sub-paragraph (e) ('the lawful detention of persons for the prevention of the spreading of infectious diseases, of persons of unsound mind, alcoholics or drug addicts, or vagrants'), the detention of patients is justified only when the latter represent a danger to themselves or to others. As pointed out in the 2002 report, mentioned above, elderly people may infringe the rights of others, for example carers, family or neighbours; older persons may also become a danger to themselves, as in cases of attempted self-mutilation, or they may become incapable of looking after their basic personal needs.[27]

In determining when a person of unsound mind represents a danger to himself or herself or to others to justify compulsory detention or treatment, cooperation between law and medical science is as key as delicate. In *Winterwerp v. the Netherlands*[28], the

---

[22] See ECtHR, *Merczegfaluy v. Austria* of 24.09.1992, A series No. 244. and *Price v. The United Kingdom,* in Human Rights Case *Digest*, Volume 12, Numbers 7-8, 2001 , pp. 529-532(4) relating to the detention of a paraplegic person

[23] ECtHR, *Mouisel v France* [2004] 38 EHRR 34.

[24] ECtHR, *Papon v. France* (no. 1) (dec.), no. 64666/01, ECHR 2001-VI. The application concerned Mr Papon's continuing detention following his conviction despite his age and state of health. The Court rejected the complaint as being manifestly ill-founded.

[25] ECtHR, *Mouisel v France* [2004] 38 EHRR 34, para. 38.

[26] Commissioner for Human Rights, *Second Annual Report April 2001 to December 2001' to the Committee of Ministers and the Parliamentary Assembly*, Comm. DH (2002)2, p.119-131.

[27] Commissioner for Human Rights, *Second Annual Report,* p. 125.

[28] ECHR, *Winterwerp v. the Netherlands* (1979) 2 EHRR 387.

Court made it clear that article 5 paragraph 1, sub-paragraph (e) 'cannot be taken as permitting the detention of a person simply because his views or behaviour deviate from the norms prevailing in a particular society.'[29] The determination of 'unsound mind' must be established before the competent national authority and involve objective medical expertise. The mental disorder must be of a kind or degree warranting compulsory confinement and continued confinement depends upon the persistence of such a disorder.[30] In *H.L v. UK,* the Court ruled that the absence of procedural rules warranting the regular verification of persistence of the disorder leading to confinement violates article 5.1 of the ECHR. [31] The Court held that states are under the obligation to put in place the procedures and guarantees so the admission and protracted stay of a patient who lack legal capacity can be submitted to scrutiny and review. In the *H.L.* case, which concerned an autistic person admitted to hospital following an outburst of self-inflicted violence, the Court ruled that 'the permanent monitoring of the applicant and the impossibility of leaving the hospital did constitute deprivation of liberty.' While the mental disorder the applicant suffered did justify confinement for the duration of his stay at the hospital, the necessity of absence of arbitrariness to ensure the lawfulness of deprivation of liberty was not met because of the lack of procedural guarantees related to the admission and detention of patients who lack legal capacity (e.g., rules on who can propose admission, list of the causes, reasons, purpose and duration of the admission, clinical evaluation of the relevance of the detention, and who can nominate a representative etc.).[32]

The case *Aerts v. Belgium*[33] clarified that there must be a reasonable relationship between the ground of permitted deprivation of liberty and the place and conditions of detention. Living arrangements must be appropriate to the mental and physical conditions of a person. A mental health patient cannot be lawfully detained, for the purposes of sub-paragraph (e) of paragraph 1, but in places such as a hospital, clinic or other appropriate institution.[34]

Eventually, according to article 5 (elderly) individuals may only be moved to a specialised institution if they give their free consent.[35] When it is not possible to rely on consent, compulsory placement order must always foreseen a right to appeal, regular revisions of the decision, the right to appear before a judge, to take proceedings, to have a prompt ruling, to be informed, and to obtain compensations.[36]

3. ARTICLE 8: RIGHT TO RESPECT FOR PRIVATE AND FAMILY LIFE

The right to private and family life under article 8 of the European Convention of Human Rights (1950) has proved to be one of the most fertile provisions of the Convention.[37] Through the case law of the European Court of Human Rights, article 8

---

[29] ECHR, *Winterwerp v. the Netherlands* (1979) 2 EHRR 387, paragraph 37.
[30] ECHR, *Winterwerp v. the Netherlands* (1979) 2 EHRR 387, paragraph 39.
[31] ECrHR, *H.L. v. United Kingdom* (2004) ECHR 471.
[32] ECrHR, *H.L. v. United Kingdom* (2004) ECHR 471, para. 5.1.
[33] ECrHR, *Aerts v. Belgium*, (1998) ECHR 64.
[34] ECrHR, *Aerts v. Belgium*, (1998) ECHR 64, paragraph 46.
[35] Commissioner for Human Rights, *Second Annual Report,* op.cit., p.125.
[36] See below, chapter 5 on consent.
[37] Article 8 (Right to respect for private and family life):
1 Everyone has the right to respect for his private and family life, his home and his correspondence.

has grown to include the notion of non-interference (the right to be left alone), and also the notion of positive obligation on the state to create or remove the conditions that hinder the fulfilment, or *épanoussiment*, of personal and social development. As we will see below when we deal with 'privacy and data protection', these two functions are tightly interwoven. For the moment, we intend to review the emergence of the shielding and empowering dimensions of article 8 in the case law of the European Court of Human Rights.

The jurisprudence of Strasbourg shows that in the last decades the protection of private life has moved beyond the realm of the household to embrace social life, work-life, leisure and social relations in general. In *Niemietz* and in *Halford*[38] the Court held that there was 'no reason of principle why [...] the notion of 'private life' should be taken to exclude activities of a professional or business nature.'[39] As a result, sending private e-mails from the workplace is a personal matter in Europe, unlike what happens, e.g., in the US. With *Peck* v. *UK*, disclosure of private data retained by a public institution is prohibited when it constitutes a serious interference with the right to respect for the individual's private life.[40] In *Amann* v. *Switzerland,* the Court specified that 'private life' must be interpreted to comprise the right to establish and develop relationships with other human beings.[41]

In *Botta* v. *Italy* the Court clarified that the notion of 'private life' had to be expanded to 'ensure the development, without outside interference, of the personality of each individual.'[42] Accordingly, Article 8 imposes positive obligations on the state to facilitate popel with daisabilities' access to essential economic and social activities. In *Kutzner* v. *Germany*, the Court stated that article 8 creates obligations upon states to provide support to disabled parents in order to maintain their right to a 'family life'.[43] Other positive measures were required by the ECHR to facilitate access to services[44] or of care-takers to social service files.[45] In *X and Y against The Netherlands*[46] the Court made clear that the notion of private life may put states under the obligation to guarantee that effective means necessary to vindicate private life interests are in place. We could go on. The Strasbourg judge has turned to article 8 right to private life to hear individual claims for self determination in cases involving access to personal files (*Gaskin v. the United Kingdom*[47]); it has recognised the right to delete personal data from public files (*Leander v. Sweden*[48], *Segerstedt-Wiberg v.*

---

2 There shall be no interference by a public authority with the exercise of this right except such as is in accordance with the law and is necessary in a democratic society in the interests of national security, public safety or the economic well-being of the country, for the prevention of disorder or crime, for the protection of health or morals, or for the protection of the rights and freedoms of others

[38] ECtHR, *Halford v UK*, (1997) ECHR 32, para. 44; *Niemietz v. Federal Republic of Germany* , 251 Eur. Ct. H.R. (ser. A) (1992), para. 32. I.

[39] ECtHR, *Niemietz* v. *Germany*, para. 29.2.

[40] ECtHR, *Peck v United Kingdom,* (2003) 36 EHRR 41*, para.* 85.

[41] ECtHR, *Amann v. Switzerland, 30 Eur. Hum. Rts. Rep. 843 (2000)*, para. 65-67.

[42] ECtHR, *Botta* v. *Italy* (1998) 26 EHRR 241*,* para. 31.

[43] ECtHR, *Kutzner* v. *Germany* (2002) *E.H.R.R.* 653.

[44] ECtHR, *Gaskin* v. *UK* (1989) 12 EHRR 36.

[45] ECtHR *, R (S)* v. *Plymouth City Council* (2002) 5 CCLR 251.

[46] ECtHR, *X and Y* v. *Netherlands* (1985) 8 EHRR 235.

[47] ECtHR *Gaskin v. the United Kingdom,'*(1989) 12 EHRR 36.

[48] ECtHR, *Leander v. Sweden*, (1987) 9 EHRR 433. In this case there was a breach of article 8.1 because the use of the secret police files, coupled with a refusal to allow L access to this information, amounted to an interference with the applicant's right to private life. However, the breach of Article 8(1) was justified by the legitimate aim under 8(2) of protecting national security. (para. 74)

Sweden[49] and the recent *Marper v. United Kingdom*); it has heard cases regarding the change in 'official sex data' (*Goodwin*); it has recognised the right to access information about the environment in the choice of residence (*Guerra v. Italy*[50]); it has recognised the right to live in a society which put limits on secret surveillance systems (*Klass v. Germany*[51], *Leander v. Sweden*[52] and *Rotaru v. Romania*[53]) etc…

This case law indicates that the protection of private life may, depending on the circumstances of the case, call to the fore other fundamental rights and individual liberties, such as article 14 (non discrimination), article 9 (thought, conscience and religion), article 10 (freedom of expression), article 11 (assembly and association), article 12 (right to found a family). These rights protect interests that affect directly the way individuals develop their life, and must therefore be afforded to all individuals. This conclusion on the right to private life bears important indications for the development and implementation of ICT for older persons, which we are going to discuss in Chapter IV. Before turning to this key aspect of the European legal framework, we need first to complete the review of positive European human rights law on ageing.

III. THE REVISED EUROPEAN SOCIAL CHARTER

The European Social Charter was drawn up under the auspices of the Council of Europe in 1961 and came into force in 1965. In the year 1988, an additional protocol was added and subsequently incorporated into the 'Revised' European Social Charter, signed in 1996. Thus, today we refer to the 1996 (Revised) European Social Charter.[54] The Charter was born to promote common, decent, labour and social standards across Europe in response to concerns for social justice and peace which stemmed from differences in levels of economic development across Council of Europe countries. Some provisions of the European Social Charter served as model and reference to the provisions included in the equality and solidarity titles of the 2000 EU Charter of Fundamental Rights, notably article 25 'The rights of elderly people.'

The aims of the Social Charter are laid down in Part I of the Charter which consists of thirty-one propositions or principles such as: 'All workers and their dependents have the right to social security' (n. 12), 'Everyone has the right to housing' (n. 31), All workers have the right to dignity at work (n.26), 'Every elderly person has the right to social protection' (n. 23). State parties must only 'accept' the principles listed in Part I and 'commit' to realizing them in their planning of social policies, 'by all appropriate means.' Part II's structure is symmetric to Part I. It contains thirty-one rights which correspond to the thirty-one propositions or principles enunciated in Part I, such as: Article 12 (The right to social security), Article 31 (The right to housing), Article 26 (The right to dignity at work), Article 17 (The right of children and young persons to social, legal and economic protection), article 23 (The right of elderly persons to social protection), and so on. Part III ('Undertaking') regulates participation of member states to the Charter through a peculiar mechanism. States accessing the Charter have to choose to be bound by six

---

[49] ECtHR, Segerstedt-Wiberg v. Sweden, application no. 62332/00, judgement of 6 June 2006.
[50] ECtHR, Guerra v. Italy, (1996) 26 EHRR 357.
[51] ECtHR, Klass v. Germany, (1978) 2 EHRR 214.
[52] ECtHR, Leander v. Sweden, (1987) 9 EHRR 433.
[53] ECtHR, Rotaru v. Romania, Application no. 28341/95 judgement of 4 May 2000.
[54] Council of Europe - ETS no. 163 - European Social Charter (revised).

out of nine articles included in Part II.[55] In addition, states have to endorse other articles or numbered paragraphs included in Part II so, in total, each state party is signed up to no less than sixteen articles or no less than sixty-three numbered paragraphs.

The Charter does not foresee a judicial mechanism. The Charter, however, does comprise a supervisory mechanism. The European Committee of Social Rights (ECSR) is responsible for monitoring compliance of states parties to the articles of the Charter, notably to those they have chosen. States are under the obligation to submit annual reports on their implementation and show the progress made towards their realisation. This mechanism allows the ECSR to monitor, scrutinise, and support contracting states as they undertake important reforms in their social security systems.[56] In addition, a 1995 Protocol to the Charter introduced a system of collective complaints for NGOs or interest groups.[57]

In Part I, point 23, state parties agree to pursue by all appropriate means the realization of the right of every elderly to social protection. This principle was added to the Social Charter by the 1998 Additional Protocol, where it was enshrined with the same wording in article 4. Article 23 (in Part II, which corresponds to principle number 23 I of Part I) is not one of the nine articles which contracting parties have to choose. However, article 23 may be chosen in order to attain the minimum number of sixteen rights or sixty-three numbered paragraphs, as requested by Part III. As of April 2009 the EU member states which are also member of the European Social Charter having accepted to be bound by article 23 are Finland, France, Ireland, Italy, Malta, The Netherlands, Norway (EEA member), Portugal, Slovenia, and Sweden.[58]

1. ARTICLE 23: THE RIGHT OF ELDERLY PERSONS TO SOCIAL PROTECTION

According to article 23, states undertake to adopt appropriate measures designed to a) 'enable elderly persons to remain full members of society for as long as possible', b) 'enable elderly persons to choose their life-style freely and to lead independent lives in their familiar surroundings for as long as they wish and are able', and c) 'to guarantee elderly persons living in institutions appropriate support, while respecting their privacy, and participation in decisions concerning living conditions in the institution.'[59]

---

[55] The nine articles are: Articles 1 (right to work), 5, 6 (the right to bargain collectively), 7 (The right of children and young persons to protection), 12 (The right to social security), 13 (The right to social and medical assistance), 16 (The right of the family to social, legal and economic protection), 19 (The right of migrant workers and their families to protection and assistance) and 20 (The right to equal opportunities and equal treatment in matters of employment and occupation without discrimination on the grounds of sex).

[56] Consider, e.g., the comments delivered to Italy regarding article 23 (The right of elderly persons to social protection). 'The Committee also asked Italy to explain how it intended to reconcile the decision to gradually increase the contribution period for qualifying for old-age benefit with its international obligations, in particular Article 4 of the Additional Protocol.' Available at http://www.humanrights.coe.int/cseweb/GB/GB2/Conclusions_XV-2/Italy%20XV-2.doc (last visited 15 October 2009).

[57] Council of Europe, ETS no. 158, Additional Protocol to the European Social Charter Providing for a System of Collective Complaints, Strasbourg, 9 November 1995.

[58] http://www.coe.int/t/dghl/monitoring/socialcharter/Presentation/ProvisionTableRev_en.pdf

[59] Article 23 (The right of elderly persons to social protection):

To attain the first objective of article 23 - enable elderly persons to remain full members of society for as long as possible – state parties undertake to adopt appropriate measures, in particular by providing *a) adequate resources enabling them to lead a decent life and play an active part in public, social and cultural life;*and b) *provision of information about services and facilities available for elderly persons and their opportunities to make use of them.*

The expression 'full members' means that elderly persons must suffer no ostracism on account of their age. The preoccupation of the Charter is to avoid that the right to take part in social life be restricted, not granted or refused, 'depending on whether an elderly person has retired or is still vocationally active, or whether he or she is still of full legal capacity or is subject to some restrictions in this respect.'[60] For this reason, article 23, paragraph 1, point a), puts it on states to afford 'adequate resources enabling them [elderly persons] to lead a decent life and participate actively in public, social and cultural life.' The expression 'adequate resources' must be read in the light of article 12 and article 13.[61]

Article 12 (the right to social security) pursues the attainment of similar levels of social security across the Council of Europe area.[62] It invites states to maintain their social security system at a satisfactory level, in particular by index-linking pension benefits.[63] In order to assess whether elderly person have enough resources, the Committee of Social Rights compares pensions with the average wage levels and the overall cost of living; it also takes into consideration costs of transport, of medical

---

With a view to ensuring the effective exercise of the right of elderly persons to social protection, the Parties undertake to adopt or encourage, either directly or in co-operation with public or private organisations, appropriate measures designed in particular:
– to enable elderly persons to remain full members of society for as long as possible, by means of:
a. adequate resources enabling them to lead a decent life and play an active part in public, social and cultural life;
b. provision of information about services and facilities available for elderly persons and their opportunities to make use of them;
– to enable elderly persons to choose their life-style freely and to lead independent lives in their familiar surroundings for as long as they wish and are able, by means of:
a. provision of housing suited to their needs and their state of health or of adequate support for adapting their housing;
b. the health care and the services necessitated by their state;
– to guarantee elderly persons living in institutions appropriate support, while respecting their privacy, and participation in decisions concerning living conditions in the institution.
[60] Council of Europe, *Digest of Case law of the European Committee of Social Rights*, 1 September 2008, p.147-148, http://www.coe.int/t/dghl/monitoring/socialcharter/Digest/DigestSept2008_en.pdf . Another important source is the explanatory report to the 1988 additional protocol to the European Social Charter. *Explanatory report to the Additional Protocol to the European Social Charter*, E.T.S. no. 128, available at http://conventions.coe.int/Treaty/EN/Reports/HTML/128.htm
[61] 'It is moreover understood that there is no inconsistency between the concept of 'social assistance' used in Article 13 of the Charter and the concept of 'social protection' embodied in Article 4 of the Protocol' [which becomes article 23 of the Revised Social Charter]. *Explanatory report*, op.cit., para 55.
[62] Article 12(4) '…a equal treatment with their own nationals of the nationals of other Parties in respect of social security rights.'
[63] See Conclusions 2003, on France, p. 186, quoted in *Digest*, op.cit., p.149. Where the Committee invites France to give information about whether pension benefits are index linked. And the Conclusion of the Committee two years after where 'the Committee notes that old age pension benefits in France are index linked by taking into account inflation and the purchasing power of the pension benefit.' See also Conclusions 2005, France, p. 248, Ibid.

care and medicine, as well as 'the existence of a carer's allowance for family members looking after an elderly relative.'[64]

Article 13 can be read as *lex specialis* to the norm of protection established in article 12. Article 13 (The right to social and medical assistance) addresses those persons who, although they have a pension, are unable to cover the costs of assistance or care. The attention paid to the least advantaged is particularly clear in paragraph 2, where the Social Charter's preoccupation is that senior citizens who are in need of assistance are not exploited or discriminated - 'diminution' - in the full enjoyment of 'their political and social rights', as compared with others. The foregoing suggests that the Charter, through the architecture of article 23, article 12 and article 13 devotes special attention and protection to those elderly persons who are most needy and vulnerable in society. These persons should always be afforded the resources and services necessary to remain full members of society.

As far as article 23, paragraph 1, point b) is concerned ('b. provision of information about services and facilities available for elderly persons and their opportunities to make use of them'), the observations issued in two national reports clarify that providing 'information about service and facilities' is not enough. What matters, and what the Social Charter supervisory committee wants to know, is the existence of the services and facilities for the aged, from home care to cultural and social participation, how they are organized, their costs and eventual barriers hindering their implementation.[65]

The second objective of article 23 is '*to enable elderly persons to choose their life-style freely and to lead independent lives in their familiar surroundings for as long as they wish and are able.* This objective shall be pursued by means of:

a) provision of housing suited to their needs and their state of health or of adequate support for adapting their housing; and
b) the health care and the services necessitated by their state'

This paragraph encourages states to adopt measures in the field of housing and in the field of health care. Moving out from familiar surroundings should be a measure of last resort, indicates the Committee of Social Affairs[66]; the Committee therefore invites states to take into account the 'special needs of this group' in their national or local housing policies, in particular by giving assistance to the adaptation of homes and by organising services such as food delivery, day-care, and transport.[67]

Regarding paragraph 'b) the health care and the services necessitated by their state', private and/or public health programmes and health services should be integrated. They 'must exist together with' guidelines on health care for elderly persons, in particular mental health programmes and adequate palliative care services.[68]

---

[64] Council of Europe, *Digest*, op.cit., p.148.

[65] *Digest*, op.cit., p.149 referring to Conclusions 2003, France, p. 186. Conclusions 2005, Slovenia, p. 659. In the France report the committee sought to know about: home help services, community based services, cultural leisure and educational facilities for elderly, specialised day care provision for persons with dementia and related illnesses and services such as information, training etc..... The Committee also invites information about respite care or services for families who provide care for highly dependent persons.

[66] *Digest*, op.cit., p.149.

[67] *Digest,* op.cit., p.149 referring to Conclusions 2003, Slovenia, p. 530.

[68] *Digest,* op.cit., p.149 referring to Conclusions 2003, France, p. 189.

Eventually, article 23 calls upon states to *'guarantee elderly persons living in institutions appropriate support, while respecting their privacy, and participation in decisions concerning living conditions in the institution.'*

This paragraph, specifically concerned with elderly persons living in institutions, should be read in conjunction with the other paragraphs of Article 23.[69] The measures advocated in paragraphs 1 (adequate resources and services for full membership and decent life) and 2 (housing facilities and health care necessary to lead an independent life) are valid and apply to persons living in institutions as well, 'in so far as this mode of life living in an institution does not render their implementation impossible or manifestly irrelevant.'[70] The context 'living institutions', however, is different and should be given enhanced attention and protection. The Committee of Social Rights lists a series of rights which ought to be carefully scrutinized, namely the right to appropriate care and adequate services, the right to privacy, the right to personal dignity, the right to participate in decisions concerning the living conditions in the institution, the protection of property, the right to maintain personal contact with persons close to the elderly person and the right to complain about treatment and care received in institutions.[71] A specific indent is dedicated to the respect of privacy (*'while respecting their privacy'*). As the explanatory report clarifies, the reference to privacy refers and should be interpreted according to article 8 (respect for private life) and the case law developed on it, which applies fully also to living institutions.[72] The Committee does not provide insight on the special requirements of the right to private life in these closed settings, but limits itself to indicate that special measures may be necessary to identify the situations that may lead or conceal assaults on personal dignity and privacy, for instance through the creation of independent inspection mechanisms.[73]

IV. THE EU CHARTER OF FUNDAMENTAL RIGHTS

The EU Charter of Fundamental Rights represents the first human rights document of the new millennium and the first fully fledged human rights treaty adopted by the European Union since its foundation in 1957.[74] With the entry into force of the Lisbon Treaty (1 December 2009), the EU Charter became part of the EU *acquis.*[75] Until

---

[69] *Explanatory report*, op.cit., paras 58-59.

[70] Ibid.

[71] The Committee of Social Rights adds that 'There should be a sufficient supply of institutional facilities for elderly persons (public or private), care in such institutions should be affordable and assistance must be available to cover the cost.' And 'all institutions should be licensed, subject to a declaration regime, to inspection or to any other mechanism which ensures, in particular, that the quality of care delivered is adequate.' Respectively, Conclusions 2003, Slovenia, p. 530; Conclusions 2005, Slovenia, p. 659, quoted in *Digest, op.cit.,* p.148-149.

[72] *Explanatory report*, para 59 and Conclusions 2003, France, p. 189. On privacy, see below, chapter IV.

[73] *Explanatory report*, para 59 and Conclusions 2003, France, p. 189

[74] European Parliament, the Council and the Commission, *European Charter of Fundamental Rights*, 2000/C 364/01, December 2000. http://www.europarl.europa.eu/charter/default_en.htm

[75] Article 1(8) of the Lisbon Treaty provides that Article 6(1) of the Treaty on European Union is to be replaced by the following: 'The Union recognises the rights, freedoms and principles set out in the Charter of Fundamental Rights of the European Union of 7 December 2000, as adapted at Strasbourg, on 12 December 2007, which shall have the same legal value as the Treaties.' The provisions of the

now, the Charter, though not yet binding, was referred to in decisions of national courts and of the European Court of Justice.[76] While it is too soon to evaluate the impact of the Charter on the EU's community of rights and on elderly persons, information society and inclusion, it is already possible to ponder on this new human rights treaty in general, and on elderly people in particular.

Gutwirth and De Hert suggest that the EU Charter reflects two types of constitutions, codifying and transformative.[77] Codifying constitutions preserve essential tenets of the constitutional or legal culture in which they are enacted and aim at protecting them against changes in the future, whereas transformative constitutions or transformative amendments to existing constitutions aim at changing essential aspects of the constitutional or legal culture in which they are enacted.[78] These two types of constitutions are at work in the EU Charter. 'There may be no doubt about the codifying character of the EU Charter', contend the authors, 'preserving a European human rights heritage and being the result of a merely 'technical' exercise.' Gutwirth and De Hert, however, defend the less well-known side of the Charter, the transformative side. This side of the Charter is well illustrated by diverse provisions, e.g., the right to data protection (article 8), the right to good administration (article 41), a general prohibition on discrimination on the grounds of gender, race and colour...and also genetic features (article 21); bioethics, individual consent and the right to integrity of the person (article 3); workers' right to information and consultation within the undertaking (article 27) and the right of access to placement services (article 29), family and professional life (article 33), environmental protection (article 37), consumer protection (article 38) and so on. The emblem of the transformative character of the Charter is perhaps the codification of human dignity which is 'taken from the German constitution, as the mother right of the EU Charter, proudly occupying the royal throne of the Charter in its first article, but absent as a concept in almost all Member State constitutions, except for the German one.'[79]

The EU Charter therefore not only incorporates most of previous human rights instrument, notably Council of Europe Conventions such as the ECHR, but purposely proclaims additional rights. It is quite interesting to observe, with Lessig, that of the two constitutional options, the transformative constitution is clearly the most difficult to realise. A codifying regime at least has inertia on its side; a transformative regime must fight. From a legal point of view, suggest Gutwirth and De Hert, this invites

---

Charter, however, shall not extend in any way the competences of the Union as defined in the Treaties. (Article 6.1, paragraph 2, Lisbon Treaty).

[76] The Charter was first mentioned by the Court of Justice in T-54/99, *Max.mobil Telecommunications Service GmbH v. Commission*. See also C-279/99 P, *Z v Parliament* [2001] ECR I-9197 and C-353/99 P, *Council v Hautala et al* [2001] ECR I-9565. The European Court of Human Rights referred to the EU Charter in ECtHR, *Goodwin v United Kingdom*, (2002) 35 EHRR 18, para. 100.

[77] De Hert Paul, Gutwirth Serge, 'Data protection in the case law of Strasbourg and Luxemburg : constitutionalisation in action', in *Reinventing data protection ?*, Springer, 2009, p. 3-45; L. Lessig, *Code and Other Laws of Cyberspace*, New York, Basic Books, 1999, p. 213.

[78] 'For Lessig (L. Lessig, op.cit., p. 214) the US Constitution of 1789 qualifies as a transformative constitution, since it initiated a new form of government and gave birth to a nation, whereas the US Constitution of 1791—the Bill of Rights— qualifies as a codifying constitution, entrenching certain values against future change. The Civil War amendments were transformative, since they aimed to break the American tradition of inequality and replace it with a tradition and practice of equality.', De Hert and Gutwirth, op.cit. p.12.

[79] Gutwrith and De Hert, op.cit., p.13.

prudence when enforcing rights and duties that have not been properly internalised by the legal subjects.'[80]

1. ARTICLE 25: THE RIGHTS OF THE ELDERLY

The codifying – transformative description offers a useful way to read the provision contained in article 25 'The rights of the elderly,' which states:

The Union recognises and respects the rights of the elderly to lead a life of dignity and independence and to participate in social and cultural life.

The explanatory report indicates in article 23 of the 1996 Revised European Social Charter, discussed above, the archetype of article 25.[81] Following Gutwirth and De Hert, the reference to dignity represents one of the innovative, transformative elements introduced by the Charter. It should be read in combination with article 1: 'Human dignity is inviolable. It must be respected and protected' and with the preamble of the Charter, which states: 'The Union places the individual at the hearth of its activities.' The reference to article 1 implies that in order to make dignity effective, a static attitude ('must be respected') is not enough. It also requires a positive obligation to intervene (protected).[82] The protection of dignity, one could retort, is better served by article 23 of the European Social Charter, which is more detailed and impose positive measures: a) adequate resources and services to enable elderly persons to remain full members of society for as long as possible; b) housing and health care lead preferred life-style and to lead independent lives in familiar surroundings; and c) higher protection of elderly persons living in institutions appropriate support.[83] Article 25 of the EU Charter rather parsimoniously rephrase them in 'to lead a life of dignity and independence and to participate in social and cultural life.' On the other hand, as Baer indicates[84], article 25 and its reference to dignity acquires great significance if we bear in mind the threats to human rights posed by modern highly technological societies, a perspective that features prominently in EU Charter[85], while it is totally absent from the European Social Charter.

---

[80] 'The codifying regime has a moment of self-affirmation; the transformative regime is haunted with self-doubt, and vulnerable to undermining by targeted opposition. Constitutional moments die, and when they do, the institutions charged with enforcing their commands, such as courts, face increasing political resistance. Flashes of enlightenment notwithstanding, the people retain or go back to their old ways, and courts find it hard to resist' Gutwirth and De Hert, Ibid., p.13.

[81] But one could look further to other sources of international human rights law, which have devoted increasingly attention to the situation of older persons, in the wake of demographic ageing. See D. Rodriguez-Pinzon and C. Marin, 'The International Human Rights status of elderly persons', op.cit.

[82] S. Rodotà , *Social ethical and privacy needs in ICT for older people: a dialogue road map*, Opening lecture to the launching event of SENIOR, 3 March 2008, p.1. www.seniorproject.eu.

[83] Council of Europe, European Social Charter (Revised), 1996, see above.

[84] S.Baer, 'Il Diritto all'uguaglianza nella Carta dei Diritti Fondamentali dell'Unione Europea', in M.Rossilli (ed.), *I Diritti delle donne nell'Unione Europea: Cittadine, migranti, schiave*, Ediesse, Roma, 2009, p. 47-72.

[85] Amongst the innovations of the Charter is the attention devoted to integrity of the person (article3), the ban on eugenic practices for the selection of persons (article3), the right to non discrimination on ground of genetic features (article 21).

2. ARTICLE 14: THE RIGHT TO EDUCATION

There is, eventually, another consideration to be drawn from the transformative/ codifying character of the EU Charter. In general, the recognition of human rights can have the effect of excluding certain groups; some rights, in particular social rights, can benefit certain groups of persons while others, seen as less concerned, remain excluded from the purview and the force of the law.

The expression "seen as less concerned" indicates that some groups of persons having specific characteristics are recognized entitlements to, e.g., education, health or work, while some groups are excluded. Such recognition can be the result of 1) a deliberate and explicit decision taken when a right is drafted or 2) be the result of norms, attitudes or even stereotypes which influence and orient the implementation of certain rights.

To the first category belongs, e.g., the right to education enshrined in article 14 of the EU Charter, which lends protection in particular to the right and freedom to education of children.[86] Older persons are included as ''Everyone' has the right to education and to have access to vocational and continuing training.' Following De Hert and Gutwirth's analysis of the Charter, mentioned above, one could say that the right to education for older persons has 'to fight' more to be implemented. In this respect, the large consensus on life long learning, described in detail in chapter I, and the recognition of the right to complete a *curriculum studii* in later age may invite the integration of older persons' demands under article 14, for instance through ad hoc educational initiatives or specialised institutes.

On a quite similar string, article 9 of EU Charter states that the right to marry and to found a family shall be guaranteed in accordance with the national laws governing the exercise of these rights. As Baer notes, this provision poses problems to the human right of same-sex couples to marry or found a family, which some Member States, such as Italy, do not recognise.[87] Social norms, in this case, delimit the purview of the right through a statutory reserve directly included in the provision.

In other cases, which pertain to the second category described above, social norms, or market pressure, or widespread prejudices or attitudes can intervene after a right is formally established. For instance, under the imperative of cutting costs and rationalise care in the wake of demographic change, well established universal rights, such as the right to health care, can be restricted by practises which jeopardise the enjoyment of, say, high quality health care by older persons affected by chronic diseases. Similar reasoning can apply to other rights, such as the right to work or to play, whose implementation may exclude groups, such as older people, which are considered as less concerned.

---

[86] Article 14 (Right to education):
1. Everyone has the right to education and to have access to vocational and continuing training.
2. This right includes the possibility to receive free compulsory education.
3. The freedom to found educational establishments with due respect for democratic principles and the right of parents to ensure the education and teaching of their children in conformity with their religious, philosophical and pedagogical convictions shall be respected, in accordance with the national laws governing the exercise of such freedom and right.
[87] Baer, op.cit., p.62.

V. OLD AGE AND DISCRIMINATION

Article 9 of the 2009 Treaty of Lisbon states that '[i]n defining and implementing its policies and activities, the Union shall take into account requirements linked to the promotion of a high level of employment, the guarantee of adequate social protection, the fight against social exclusion, and a high level of education, training and protection of human health.'[88] As pointed out in chapter 1, the EU's e-inclusion policy brings together social and economic objectives. Although social policy objectives can be favored as well as be hindered by certain aspects of economic policy, admittedly EU social policy often merely supplements economic integration.[89] If social Europe plays, as it does, a secondary role in the architecture of the EU integration, this is imputable not only to internal market priority focus, but also to the lack of agreement about *which* entitlements or rights should be part of the European social model, and *how* to implement them. Old age and discrimination offers a fitting example of this two-edged approach. On the one hand, European Union law treats old-age as anti-discrimination issue and internal market requirement (free movement of workers); on the other hand, old age demands are treated as a horizontal human right issue requiring public policy to intervene across social fields of health, education, housing, and services in general, not only in employment and occupation.[90]

1. LEGAL FRAMEWORK

Until the Treaty of Amsterdam (1997-1999) inserted article 13 into the EC Treaty[91], European Union law could stem only two forms of discrimination, *viz.* discrimination on grounds of nationality[92] and sex discrimination in employment.[93] Article 13

---

[88] Article 9 of Treaty on the Functioning of the European Union (TFEU) summarises the existing Article 2 TEU, and Articles 2, 127, 136, 137, 140, 149, 150 and 152 TEC

[89] M. Bell, 'Anti-discrimination law and the European Union', Oxford: University Press, 2004, p.12.

[90] See European Commission, *For a Europe of civic and social rights. Report by the Comitè des Sages*', Luxembourg: Office Official Publication of the European Communities, 1996. B. De Witte, 'Protection of fundamental social rights in the European Union. The choice of the appropriate legal instrument', in L. Betten and D. MacDevitt (eds), *The protection of fundamental social rights in the European Union*, London: Kluwer Law International, 1996. H. Meenan, 'Reflecting on age discrimination in the European Union—the search for clarity and food for thought', *ERA Forum,* (2009) 10: 107–124.

[91] Now Article 19 of the consolidated version of the Treaty on the functioning of the European Union (ex Article 13 TEC):

1. Without prejudice to the other provisions of the Treaties and within the limits of the powers conferred by them upon the Union, the Council, acting unanimously in accordance with a special legislative procedure and after obtaining the consent of the European Parliament, may take appropriate action to combat discrimination based on sex, racial or ethnic origin, religion or belief, disability, age or sexual orientation.

2. By way of derogation from paragraph 1, the European Parliament and the Council, acting in accordance with the ordinary legislative procedure, may adopt the basic principles of Union incentive measures, excluding any harmonisation of the laws and regulations of the Member States, to support action taken by the Member States in order to contribute to the achievement of the objectives referred to in paragraph 1.

[92] Article 12 TEC provides that 'within the scope of this Treaty, [...], any discrimination on grounds of nationality shall be prohibited.' See Case 15/69 *Württenbergische Milchverwertung-Sudmilchv Ugliola* [1969] ECR 363. See also Case C-187/96 *Commission v Greece* [1998] ECR I-1095, Case C-57/96 *H Meints v Minister van landbouw, Natuurbeheer en Visserij* [1997] ECR-I-6689. Recall the opinion of the Advocate General Jacobs in Case C-274-96 *Bickel and Franz* [1998] ECR I-7637, para 24: 'Freedom from discrimination on grounds of nationality is the most fundamental right conferred by the

provided the possibility for the Council to 'take appropriate action to combat discrimination on different grounds.' To date, the EU legislator made use of this Treaty provision three times. Under article 13 of the Treaty, the EU *acquis* acquired:

a) Directive 2000/43 outlawing discrimination on grounds of racial and ethnic origin in employment, occupation and training, goods and services[94];
b) Directive 2000/78 or the 'Employment Framework directive' outlawing discrimination on grounds of religion or belief, disability, age or sexual orientation in employment, training and occupation[95];
c) Directive 2004/113 on equal treatment between men and women in the access to and supply of goods and services.[96]

In July 2008, the European Commission issued a proposal for a new directive based on article 13 TEC (now article 19 Lisbon Treaty) designed to give all citizens basic protection in areas of life others than employment, such as housing, education, and health care. However, the implementation of anti-discrimination on grounds of age in these sectors, say, health are or housing, would put member states under the obligation to allocate substantial financial resources, not an easy policy choice.[97]

2. DISCRIMINATION ON THE GROUND OF (OLD) AGE

The cardinal provision in EU law on discrimination based on grounds of age is Article 6 ('Justification of differences of treatment on grounds of age') of the 2000/78 Employment Equality Directive. Pursuant to article 6 of the 2000 European Employment Directive all member states are required to put in place legal and regulatory measures to 'tackle age and disability discrimination' in the workplace. According to a consolidated jurisprudence, this means that a difference in treatment on the ground of age constitutes discrimination when it lacks 'objective and reasonable' justification, or when there is no reasonable relationship or proportionality between the means employed and the legitimate aim sought to be realised. [98] However, differences of treatment on grounds of age do not constitute

---

Treaty and must be seen as a basic ingredient of Union citizenship.' More recently see C-524/06, *Heinz Huber*, on the protection of personal data and the prohibition of discrimination on the basis of nationality.

[93] Article 119 TEC mandates equal pay for men and women. See Case 80/70 *Defrenne v Belgium State* (I) [1971] ECR 445. The case concerned pay discrimination by the (then) Belgian airline, SABENA, between male and female employees. On that occasion, the Court of Justice indicated that article 199 was capable of being given 'direct effect', the principle developed by the Court in the Case 26/62 *Van Gend en Loos v Nederlandse Administratie der Belastingen* [1963] ECR 1.

[94] Council Directive 2000/43 implementing the principle of equal treatment between persons irrespective of racial or ethnic origin, 19 July 2000 OJ L 180.

[95] Council Directive 2000/78/EC establishing a general framework for equal treatment in employment and occupation, 3 December 2000, O J L 303.

[96] Council Directive 2004/113/EC implementing the principle of equal treatment between men and women in the access to and supply of goods and services, 13 December 2004, O J L 373.

[97] European Commission, Proposal for a Council Directive on implementing the principle of equal treatment between persons irrespective of religion or belief, disability, age or sexual orientation, Brussels, 2 July 2008, COM(2008) 426 final.

[98] ECtHR, *Case relating to certain aspects of the laws on the use of languages in education in Belgium, (Belgian Linguistic Case)*, Judgment of 14 July 1968, 1 EHRR 252, para 10. ECJ, Case C-203/86 *Kingdom of Spain v. Council of the European Communities* [1988] ECR 4563, para 25. ECJ, Case C-279/93 *Finanzamt Koeln-altstadt v. Roland Schumacker* [1995] ECR I-225.

discrimination, if, within the context of national law, they are objectively and reasonably justified by a legitimate aim. Article 6.2 contains a long series of exceptions which make it quite easy for the employer to avoid the prohibition of discrimination on grounds of age, which would initially imply higher costs.[99]

In the case *Mangold v. Germany*[100], the European Court of Justice seemed to have broadened the scope of the prohibition beyond work when it held out that 'the principle of non-discrimination on the grounds of age must be regarded as a general principle of Community law.'[101] The Court, however, also stated that the general principle prohibiting all forms of discrimination, including on ground of age, is not found in Community law properly, but 'in various international instruments and the constitutional traditions common to the member states.'[102] One may observe that such principle emerges from the combined reading of article 25 of the 2000 EU Charter, article 23 of the 1996 Revised European Social Charter, discussed above, and in Protocol Twelve to the European Convention of Human Rights (Rome, 4 November 2000), which includes a free standing right to non discrimination.[103]

3. REASONABLE ACCOMMODATION

The role of antidiscrimination law for older persons should, for some authors[104], be reassessed to meet the challenges posed by demographic ageing and to stem mounting anti-ageing attitudes.[105] From a strictly legal point of view, however, the peculiar relation between Self and Other in the field of age makes it totemic the issue of defining a legally workable notion of old age.[106] Legal practice is not interested in drawing up definitions; more simply, anti discrimination law intervenes when a certain social condition or a state measure puts a prejudice or harms a person's rights. Take religion. From a legal perspective is less interesting defining what religion is; what matters is that when someone is affected in his or her say, right to free speech,

---

[99] Article 6.2, Directive 2000/78/EC states: '[...] Member States may provide that the fixing for occupational social security schemes of ages for admission or entitlement to retirement or invalidity benefits, including the fixing under those schemes of different ages for employees or groups or categories of employees, and the use, in the context of such schemes, of age criteria in actuarial calculations, does not constitute discrimination on the grounds of age, provided this does not result in discrimination on the grounds of sex.'

[100] Case C-144/04 *Werner Mangold v. Rudiger Helm* [2005] ECR I-9981.

[101] Case C-144/04 *Werner Mangold v. Rudiger Helm*, para. 75.

[102] Case C-144/04 *Werner Mangold v. Rudiger Helm,* para 74.

[103] While article 14 of the European Convention of Human Rights proscribes discrimination in the 'enjoyment of the rights and freedoms set forth in this Convention', Article 1 of protocol XII introduces a general prohibition of discrimination.
Article 1 – General prohibition of discrimination of Protocol No. 12 to the Convention for the Protection of Human Rights and Fundamental Freedoms:
1 The enjoyment of any right set forth by law shall be secured without discrimination on any ground such as sex, race, colour, language, religion, political or other opinion, national or social origin, association with a national minority, property, birth or other status.
2 No one shall be discriminated against by any public authority on any ground such as those mentioned in paragraph 1.

[104] H. Meenan, 'Reflecting on age discrimination in the European Union—the search for clarity and food for thought', op.cit.

[105] Compare Human Rights Council. Advisory Committee, Fourth Session, 25-29 January 2010, *Working paper*, A/HRC/AC/4/CRP.1. In Chapter 2 we concluded that modern technological societies woo the idea of contrasting ageing.

[106] S. Fredman, *Disrimination law,* Clarednon Law Series, University Press, Oxfod, 2002, p. 59-65. See also M. Bell, 'Anti-discrimination law and the European Union', Oxford: University Press, 2004.

association, housing or education because of her religion (or belief, creed, confession...) anti discrimination intervenes. Likewise it is less crucial to defend the formal equality of all sexual orientations, than to defend the expression of this or that sexual inclination in, e.g., a public office or in family life. Put under this light, anti discrimination law is chiefly about the way individuals interact. It is a tool which can be used to stem distinctions/actions which affect the legal positions of others negatively.[107] Therefore, it is questionable whether a society needs a formal defence of old age, which would require squaring the circle of old age in legal terms and determine what old age is about, what it protects and against whom.

Non discrimination law also plays a crucial role in imposing the duty to overcome problems, remove obstacles or create enabling conditions that hinder individuals' enjoyment of rights. The key notion in anti discrimination law is that of 'reasonable accommodation' or 'reasonable adjustments'. Enshrined in article 5 of Directive 2000/78, reasonable accommodation proved important for persons with disabilities, in employment context. In accordance with article 5, the employer is under the obligation to provide 'reasonable accommodation' if the limitations suffered by an employee fall within the concept of 'disability'[108]. In the context of employment and occupation disability 'must be understood as referring to a limitation which results in particular from physical, mental or psychological impairments and which hinders the participation of the person concerned in professional life.'[109]

The notion of reasonable accommodation may also be relevant to guide developments, including technology ones, in the area of ageing well at home, at work and on the move. The duty of reasonable accommodation can impose the obligation to adopt technology to enable citizens' participation. However, technological solutions, while meeting the obligation of reasonable accommodation, may also be invasive of individual privacy. The tension between individual privacy and technological accommodation may depend on many factors, including the state of the art of technological developments. If new less privacy invasive means are commercialised, they should be introduced.

The duty of reasonable accommodation, eventually, must be carefully assessed against existing organisational structures which may limit the obligation to provide 'reasonable accommodation.' In the workplace, for instance, reasonable accommodation applies to persons suffering from disabilities while does not apply to cases of 'sickness', even when, as it is often the case, the disability is the result of a protracted state of illness suffered by a person. The difference is in the regime of responsibilities. In the case of an employee affected by a form of disability, the employer must provide reasonable accommodation and is prevented from dismissing him or her by paying financial compensation. On the contrary, a person dismissed

---

[107] According to D. Rodriguez-Pinzon and C. Marin, 'The International Human Rights status of elderly persons', p. 938 'any state measure that establishes a differential treatment of individuals must comply with a basic requirement - the distinction cannot be arbitrary.'

[108] Article 5 (Reasonable accommodation for disabled persons):
In order to guarantee compliance with the principle of equal treatment in relation to persons with disabilities, reasonable accommodation shall be provided. This means that employers shall take appropriate measures, where needed in a particular case, to enable a person with a disability to have access to, participate in, or advance in employment, or to undergo training, unless such measures would impose a disproportionate burden on the employer. This burden shall not be disproportionate when it is sufficiently remedied by measures existing within the framework of the disability policy of the Member State concerned.

[109] ECJ, C-13/05, *Sonia Chacón Navas v. Eurest Colectividades SA,* Grand Chambre, 16 March 2006, para 43.

solely on account of sickness does not fall within the protection of article 5 of Directive 2000/78.'[110] In such a case, a person can be dismissed with no duty of reasonable accommodation, but only by paying compensation in kind.

VI. LEGAL AREAS RELEVANT TO E-INCLUSION

1. E-HEALTH

E-health describes the application of information and communications technologies across the whole range of functions that affect the health sector. E-health tools or solutions include products, systems and services that go beyond simply Internet-based applications. They include tools for health authorities and professionals, as well as personalised health systems for patients and citizens.[111] It has been pointed out how healthcare systems face major challenges due to an ageing population.[112] E-health systems and services are believed to reduce costs and improve productivity in areas such as i) billing and record-keeping, ii) reduction in medical error, iii) alleviation of unnecessary care, and iv) savings achieved by business-to-business e-commerce.[113]

In the EU, high-quality health services is a public policy priority recognised in the Charter of Fundamental Rights of the EU (article 35). As the European Court of Justice held, treaty provisions on free movement also apply to health services.[114] The EU legal framework addresses cross-border care, issues related to the interoperability of eHealth systems, reimbursement, liability and also data protection.[115] In the area of data protection, there are three main references.

First, Article 8 of the ECHR. Article 8.2 indicates that public health allows for a reduction of the protection of private life. On a similar tone, Directive 95/46/EC permits derogation from the principled prohibition of processing of health data in article 8 (The processing of special categories of data[116]) and in the preamble,

---

[110] ECJ, C-13/05, *Sonia Chacón Navas v. Eurest Colectividades SA,* Grand Chambre, 16 March 2006, para 47.

[111] European Commission, e-Health – making healthcare better for European citizens: An action plan for a European e-Health Area, Communication from the Commission to the Council, the European Parliament, the European Economic and Social Committee ad the Committee of the Regions, COM(2004) 356 (final), Brussels, 30 Apr 2004.

[112] Chapter 1, paragraph V.3.

[113] Examples include health information networks, electronic health records, telemedicine services, personal wearable and portable communicable systems, health portals, and many other information and communication technology-based tools assisting prevention, diagnosis, treatment, health monitoring, and lifestyle management. Today, at least four out of five European doctors have an Internet connection, and a quarter of Europeans use the Internet for health information. The health sector employs 9 per cent of Europe's workforce. E-health is today's tool for substantial productivity gains. SENIOR project, D1.1 'Environmental scanning report', prepared by David Wright (Trilateral), 6 July 2008 p. 34-36.

[114] SEC (2007) 0811 final, paragraph 2.3.4.

[115] B. Bennett, 'Health law Kaleidoscope. Health law rights in a global age ', Ashgate Publishing: Aldershot, UK, 2008. On the regulation of personal data in e-health see CNIL, La CNIL et l'e-santé, note de synthèse, Paris 8 March 2001.
http://www.cnil.fr/fileadmin/documents/approfondir/dossier/sante/e_sante.pdf

[116] Article 8 The processing of special categories of data, 95/46/EC.
1. Member States shall prohibit the processing of personal data revealing racial or ethnic origin, political opinions, religious or philosophical beliefs, trade-union membership, and the processing of data concerning health or sex life. (bold face added) […]

considerations number 33[117] and 34.[118] These references indicate that e-health initiatives - implying derogation from the general restriction on the processing of health data - should first of all be assessed against the requirement of 'necessity in democratic societies.' The role of micropolitics decisions, mentioned in chapter 2, is here pivotal to decide, e.g., whether to allocate or not financial resourses in e-health or to other initiatives, such as migrant labour.

Second, the legal framework foresees a general regime of protection for personal health data which must be always upheld. The legal reference is provided by article 6 of Directive 95/46 which includes a list of fair processing principles, such as fair and loyal processing, purpose limitation, proportionality, adequacy, security and limited duration of the processing.

Third, the legal framework for e-health must adhere by a regime of formalities overseen and controlled by an independent authority and in place prior to the start of the processing activity. Article 20.2 of Directive 95/46 states that 'prior checks shall be carried out by the supervisory authority following receipt of a notification from the controller or by the data protection official, who, in cases of doubt, must consult the supervisory authority.'[119] In addition, article 28.2 puts member states under the obligation to create an independent system of consultation charged with monitoring the respect of individuals' rights and freedoms with regard to the processing of personal data.[120] Eventually, Directive 2000/31/EC on electronic commerce applies. The Directive regulates information obligations, unsolicited commercial communication from regulated professions, the conclusion of contracts and the placing of orders.[121] The directives applies also to special kind of e-commerce, called e-pharmacy.

2. E-GOVERNMENT

E-government is defined as 'the use of information and communication technologies in public administrations combined with organisational change and new skills in order to improve public services and democratic processes and strengthen support to public policies.'[122] Concretely, most e-Government portals act as intermediaries between the citizens and the public administration units: the portal transfers the requests of the citizens and deposits the documents of the public administration unit until these are recalled by the citizen.

E-government requires that information is shared across departments and different levels of government (e.g. between the local and national level), thus raising

---

[117] (33) Whereas data [....] the processing of these data is carried out for certain health-related purposes by persons subject to a legal obligation of professional secrecy [...] (bold face added)

[118] (34) Whereas Member States must also be authorized, when justified by grounds of important public interest, to derogate from the prohibition on processing sensitive categories of data where important reasons of public interest so justify in areas such as public health and social protection – [...] (bold face added)

[119] Article 20 (prior checking)

[120] Article 28 (Supervisory authority)
1. Each Member State shall provide that one or more public authorities are responsible for monitoring the application within its territory of the provisions adopted by the Member States pursuant to this Directive.

[121] Directive 2000/31/EC, respectively, articles 5, 6, 7, 8, 10, and 11.

[122] European Commission, Communication on the Role of eGoverment for Europe's Future, COM(2003) 567 final, 26 Sept 2003. http://ec.europa.eu/information_society/eeurope/2005/doc/all_about/egov_communication_en.pdf

important questions about trust and confidence in online interaction, access to online services so that no digital divide is created, interoperability for information exchange across organisational and national borders and so on. With the ageing of the population, furthermore, public administrations are expected to do with fewer employees and fewer working taxpayers as well, while still having to provide largely the same number of services and at better quality.

A delicate implication of access to public documents relates to the right not to be forced into inclusion. It is important that public documents remain available to all, including those who sit in the dark side of the digital divide. In the Moniteur Belge case[123], a non-discrimination complaint was brought against a law which limited the publication in paper format of the Belgium Official Journal (*le Moniteur Belge)*, to three copies, and opened up public consultation via an on-line service and database. The Court recognized the objectives pursued by the law as 'objective and reasonable', say, economic, environmental, and in line with the social evolution towards e-communication. The Court went on to analyse the requirement of proportionality. The judges found that, notwithstanding compensatory measures (the intention of the legislator to equip public libraries with the necessary IT support to access the *Moniteur Belge*, and the possibility to obtain a hard copy upon request within 24 hours), the law violated the general principle of non-discrimination and had to be annulled. The law discriminated against those who did not have access to the Internet or enough skills to consult, without excessive effort, the official gazette online as they used to do on paper.

The relevance of the Moniteur Belge case for e-inclusion is the importance attributed by the Court to the capacities prevalent in a community, notably those of non-mainstream groups. The Court made a strong point for the legal equality of individual capacities and stated that, individual capacities being equal, the right to non-discrimination is to ensure that members of society have equal access to goods or services, such as access to rights and duties setting laws, deemed most important to society. The Moniteur Belge case indicates that access to goods or services deemed crucial in a democratic society should not be hampered; thus, as technology spreads in society it should be designed to accommodate all capacities prevalent in the public to access information or services of public interest.

3. CORPORATE SOCIAL RESPONSIBILITY

Underlining the important contribution of the private sector in achieving active ageing goal, the European Council addressed businesses directly launching 'a special appeal to companies' corporate sense of social responsibility regarding best practices in lifelong learning, work organisation, equal opportunities, social inclusion and sustainable development.'[124] In the 2006 Communication on 'Implementing the partnership for growth and jobs: Making Europe a pole of excellence on corporate social responsibility'[125], the Commission stated that Corporate Social Responsibility (CSR) can contribute to reach a 'more integrated labour markets and higher levels of social inclusion'. With this Communication, the Commission launched the *European Alliance for CSR* – an open partnership to make Europe a Pole of Excellence on CSR

---

[123] La Cour d'arbitrage (Belgian Constitutional Court), Arrêt n° 106/2004 du 16 juin 2004.
[124] Green paper on 'Promoting a European framework for corporate social responsibility' COM(2001) 366 final COM(2002) 347 final 116, and COM(2006) 136 final
[125] COM(2006) 136 final

– whose priorities include 'Better responding to diversity and the challenge of equal opportunities taking into account the demographic changes alongside the rapid aging of the European population.'[126]

4. CONSUMER PROTECTION

One of the commitments included in the 1982 of the Madrid International Plan on Ageing mentioned above was to enhance the social, economic, political and cultural participation of older persons.[127] 'Older persons', it was said, 'should be recognized as a significant consumer group with shared and specific needs, interests, and preferences. Governments, service providers and civil society should take into account the views of older persons on the design of products and delivery of *services*.'

In the EU minimum standards of consumer protection have been harmonised by specific regulations and provisions included in various legal texts dealing with other issues (e.g., data protection). The EU legal framework is built on Council Directive 93/13/EEC of 5 April 1993 on unfair terms in consumer contracts,[128] Directive 97/7/EC of the European Parliament and of the Council of 20 May 1997 on the protection of consumers in respect of distance contracts[129], and the 'new' unfair commercial practices directive containing a general ban on unfair commercial practices relating especially to the provision of information, representation, and commercial communication.[130] Directive 93/13 on unfair terms in consumer contracts covers 'the abuse of power by the seller or supplier, in particular against one-sided standard contracts and the unfair exclusion of essential rights in contract'.

Contracts, advertisements, sales techniques and warranties must not confuse, frighten or mislead and older consumers must be given adequate time to consider and reconsider their contractual undertaking. Consumers who use the Internet to purchase goods, such as medicaments, may become increasingly dependent on these services. This will put suppliers of ICT services in a stronger power position, which may lead to abuse. These suppliers, says Directive 93/13 on unfair terms in consumer contracts, should not be allowed to set out requirements that are manifestly not in compliance with the generally applicable privacy rules, or to include contractual conditions that put the consumer in a disadvantageous position, e.g., by unfairly limiting liability for 'security reasons' when providing a service to a consumer. As we will see when dealing with consent (Chapter V), Directive 97/7 on consumer protection in respect of distance contracts determines which information should be provided to the consumer in contexts of distance contracting. The directive imposes limitations to the use of unsolicited marketing and contains an article stemming 'inertia selling.'[131] The

---

[126] COM(2006) 136 final

[127] U.N. Economic Commission for Europe, Regional Implementation Strategy for the Madrid International Plan of Action on Ageing, October 2009, Commitment 2, paragraph 14.

[128] OJ L 095, 21/04/1993, pp. 29–34.

[129] OJ L 144, 04/06/1997, quoted above in Consent.

[130] Directive of the European Parliament and of the Council of 11 May 2005 concerning unfair business-to-consumer commercial practices in the internal market and amending Council Directive 84/450/EEC, Directives 97/7/EC, 98/27/EC and 2002/65/EC of the European Parliament and of the Council and Regulation (EC) No 2006/2004 of the European Parliament and of the Council ('Unfair Commercial Practices Directive'), OJ L 149, 11.6.2005, pp. 22–39.

[131] Article 9 (Inertia selling):
Member States shall take the measures necessary to:
- prohibit the supply of goods or services to a consumer without their being ordered by the consumer beforehand, where such supply involves a demand for payment,

directive has potential to protect older online consumers, in view of the increasing personalisation and intrusiveness of services and communications in ambient intelligence information society. Conversely, this raises the problem of which necessary information must be provided to the consumer.[132]

5. PRODUCT SAFETY AND LIABILITY FOR DEFECTIVE PRODUCTS

An increasing number of actors will be involved in the creation and provision of products in the information society. Many different producers will provide parts of the final product. When a defective product causes damages, it will be very difficult to determine which producer to hold liable for the damages caused and whether this producer has committed a fault that caused the damage. That is why directive 85/374 on liability for defective products stipulates that producers are jointly and severally liable.[133] It also creates a 'liability without fault' clause (or strict liability) because it is the sole means of adequately solving the problem, peculiar to our age of increasing technicality, of a fair apportionment of the risks inherent in modern technological production. The directive does not apply to services and it is unclear whether it applies to software. In many cases, in an AmI world, the general rules on liability will still apply and problems remain.

The directive does not provide that a product is defective when it insufficiently protects against privacy violations or when it easily allows identity theft. The Directive 2001/95/EC of the European Parliament and the Council of 3 December 2001 on general product safety introduces general requirements for product safety, and obligations on manifacturers and distributors obligations. The Directive also introduced a rapid alert system for products which pose a serious risk (RAPEX), and provisions for products to be withdrawn from the market if they are likely to put the health and safety of consumers at risk.

6. E-COMMERCE

A variety of commerce can be conducted electronically. Modern electronic commerce typically uses the Internet at least at some point in the transaction's lifecycle, although it can encompass a wider range of technologies, from e-mail to RFID. The amount of trade conducted electronically has grown dramatically since the spread of the Internet, but many people are still unsure about its reliability, including older persons.

- exempt the consumer from the provision of any consideration in cases of unsolicited supply, the absence of a response not constituting consent.

[132] The European Parliament called for clarification in the existing rights and obligations of consumers in the digital environment. *E-confidence* should not only deal with consumer protection but also set out a coordinated approach to the issue of the digital environment as a whole, including analyses of non-market factors such as the protection of privacy, access by the general public to information technologies ('e-inclusion'), internet security, and so on. European Parliament, *Non-legislative Resolution on Consumer confidence in the digital environment*, INI/2006/2048, Strasbourg, 21 June 2007. http://www.europarl.europa.eu/oeil/file.jsp?id=5319182 . See also below, Chapter V on consent.

[133] Directive 85/374/EC amended by Directive 1999/34 concerning the liability for defective products where it is stated that product includes electricity; see also Directive 98/37 on the approximation of the laws of the member states relating to machinery.

The e-commerce directive 2000/31[134] stipulates important and substantial information obligations for the services provider. It sets out rules concerning unsolicited commercial communications and concerning the liability of the intermediary services provider in case of mere conduit, caching and hosting. In an Ambient Intelligence world, spam and unsolicited communications will become an even bigger problem than they are today and this directive tries to protect consumers from it. The opt-out registers, however, seem to be insufficient and impractical. It is also regrettable that the directive does not contain rules on the liability of intermediary services providers when they violate privacy rules. The e-commerce directive obliges information service providers to stop the distribution of illegal content on their networks (the so-called 'notice and take-down' procedure) but it is not sure whether this notice-and-take down procedure applies also to illegal content concerning personal data.

7. INTELLECTUAL PROPERTY RIGHTS

Directive 91/250 harmonises the copyright protection of software within the European Union.[135] The legal protection regime for software is important for the implementation of standards and the achievement of interoperability. In the EU Directive 96/9 harmonises the legal protection of databases.[136] This is important in situations, such as health care services, requiring linking and integration of several databases at the same time. The directive foresees a double protection for databases: a copyright protection and a *sui generis* database protection. Copyright Directive 2001/29[137] harmonises copyright protection in the European Union in several important aspects and reassesses the exceptions to the exclusive rights of the right holder in the light of the new electronic environment.

8. STANDARDIZATION OF ICT PRODUCTS AND SERVICES

Standardisation plays a significant role in the economy because it ensures a level playing field between different market players and improves the quality of ICT products and services placed on the market. Standards are also the outcome of micro-politics decisions, conflicting interests and perspectives; they are therefore very important to society in general. Technical standards may act as a tool for structuring economic behaviour. Most importantly, standards can also act as a tool of technical regulation to ensure that legal provisions are respected, e.g., as for privacy enhancing technologies.[138] As technology embodies and reinforces values, evaluation

---

[134] Directive 2000/31/EC of the European Parliament and of the Council of 8 June 2000 on certain legal aspects of information society services, in particular electronic commerce, in the Internal Market ('Directive on electronic commerce'), Official Journal L 178 , 17/07/2000 P. 1-16
[135] Council Directive 91/250/EEC of 14 May 1991 on the legal protection of computer programs Official Journal L 122 , 17/05/1991 P. 0042 - 0046
[136] Directive 96/9/EC of the European Parliament and of the Council of 11 March 1996 on the legal protection of databases, OJ L 77, 27.3.1996, p. 20–28
[137] Directive 2001/29/EC of the European Parliament and of the Council of 22 May 2001 on the harmonisation of certain aspects of copyright and related rights in the information society, OJ L 167, 22.6.2001
[138] See above, Privacy by design, chapter IV.

mechanisms for the realisation of standards in ICT for elderly people require making values (and standards procedures) explicit.[139]

EC directives define the 'essential requirements' that goods must meet when they are placed on the market, e.g., protection of health and safety.[140] The European standards bodies (CEN[141], CENELEC[142] and ETSI[143]) have the task of drawing up the technical specifications which meet the essential requirements of the directives, compliance with which will provide a presumption of conformity. Such specifications are referred to as 'harmonised standards'. In the field of ICT, most of the actions undertaken have been described the communication from the Commission on the role of European standardisation in the framework of European policies and legislation[144]and the Commission's staff working document 'The challenges for European standardisation.'[145]

In the field of ICT for elderly people, important standardisation efforts are being put in support to: projects on residential homes and home services; standards and guidelines addressing EU accessibility requirements for public procurement of products and services in the ICT domain; USEM Project: user Empowerment in Standardization; eHealth, notably the eHealth card containing patient's data in electronic format and eHealth systems interoperability; eventually, standards play an important role in the pursuit of e-accessibility for all.[146]

9. STANDARDS AND INTEROPERABILITY

As pointed out in Commission Staff Working Document supporting the Ageing well in the Information Society initiative[147], sensible technological solutions for end-users often require putting together and interconnecting a variety of equipment, services and providers that final users are not capable to seamlessly assemble (e.g. assistive technologies combined with mainstream technologies). Making such interconnection possible is what interoperability is about. A way to realise compatibility is through common standards.[148] These technical standards could, however, also constitute

---

[139] See SENIOR project, *Background paper to the Ministerial conference on e-inclusion*, Bled (Slovenia), 12 May 2008, p.26: 'As technology embodies and reinforces values, evaluation requires making values explicit.'

[140] The most important directives in this area are Council Resolution of 7 May 1985 on a new approach to technical harmonization and standards, O J C 136; Directive 98/34/EC of the European Parliament and of the Council of 22 June 1998 laying down a procedure for the provision of information in the field of technical standards and regulations O J L 8; Directive 98/48/EC of the European Parliament and of the Council of 20 July 1998 amending Directive 98/34/EC laying down a procedure for the provision of information in the field of technical standards and regulations O J L 217 ,; and the consolidated version Council Directive 2006/96/EC of 20 November 2006 adapting certain Directives in the field of free movement of goods, by reason of the accession of Bulgaria and Romania O J L 236.

[141] European Committee for Standardization, www.cen.eu/cenorm/homepage.htm

[142] European Committee for Electrotechnical Standardization. www.cenelec.eu/Cenelec/Homepage.htm

[143] European Telecommunications Standards Institute. www.etsi.org

[144] COM (2004) 674.

[145] SEC (2004) 1251.

[146] A.Gulacsi, *A short inside into Eurpean Standardization: what is CEN?*, SENIOR experts meeting on ubiquitous computing, 22 September 2009. Text available at http://seniorproject.eu/resources/1ExpertMeeting/Gulacsi.pdf

[147] Commission Staff Working Document 'Ageing well in the Information Society', SEC/2007/0811 final, paragraph 3.2.6.

[148] Interoperability manifests itself at three levels: technical, organisational, and semantic. IDABC European Interoperability Framework http://ec.europa.eu/idabc/en/document/3473/5585

barriers to trade within the internal market. That is why Directive 98/34/EC on technical standards and technical regulations in Information Society Services foresees a detailed information procedure.[149]

Standards are also relevant for the respect of privacy and data protection. Working Party 29 Opinion 1/98[150] describes Platform for Privacy Preferences (P3P) and Open Profiling Standard (OPS). The single vocabulary created by P3P might be important: in order to ensure the respect for privacy and data protection, all participants in the information society, suppliers and users, including older users, should have a common understanding of the content of privacy and data protection. The point made by the working party opinion is reaffirmed in the Future of privacy report, discussed below.[151]

Interoperability in the area of e-health commands seamless integration of heterogeneous systems. This will allow secure and fast access to comparable public health data and to patient information located in different places over a wide variety of wired and wireless devices. However, this may depend on the standardisation of system components and services such as health information systems, health messages, electronic health record architecture, and patient identifying services. Work has been launched within European standards organisations to answer this issue partly, but the take-up of e-Health interoperability standards has been slow.[152]

10. E-ACCESSIBILITY

eAccessibility is an importnat element to make plans of an Information Society for all reality, including for people who find it more difficult to use new technologies, such as people affected by a disability.[153] To date, the EU lacks a specific piece of legislation on e-accessibility. The existing legal framework is provided by the EU Directives on Electronic Communications Regulatory Framework[154], which apply to fixed telephony services. The 'framework Directive' asks national authorities to promote accessibility in terms of choice, quality, price and access to universal service for all, including disabled users. However, member states are free to determine the minimum level of access taking in consideration the access circumstances in the territory of the state.

---

[149] This allows the European Commission, the Member States and the economical operators to be aware of technical standards and regulations which the Member States want to install. The information and co-operation procedure foreseen in this directive can help the Commission in harmonising the standards and can even form the basis for the creation of European standards.

[150] Article 29 data protection Working Party, *Platform for Privacy Preferences (P3P) and the Open Profiling Standard (OPS)*, Opinion 1/98, 16 June 1998. http://epic.org/privacy/internet/ec-p3p.html

[151] Chapter IV on privacy and data protection.

[152] See European Commission, *e-Health – making healthcare better for European citizens: An action plan for a European e-Health Area*, Communication from the Commission to the Council, the European Parliament, the European Economic and Social Committee ad the Committee of the Regions, COM(2004) 356 (final), Brussels, 30 Apr 2004.

[153] K. Cullen, L. Kubitschker, and input from P Blanck, W. N Myhill, G. Quinn, P.O Donoghue, and R. Halverson, *Accessibility to ICT Products and services by Disabled and Elderly People. Towards a framework for further development of EU legislation or other co-ordination measures on eAccessibility*, Bonn, November 2008.

[154] Directive 2002/22/EC on universal service and users' rights relating to electronic communications networks and services. ('Universal Service Directive'); Directive 2002/21/EC on a common regulatory framework for electronic communications networks and services. ('Framework Directive')

The Radio and Telecommunications Terminal Equipment (R&TTE) Directive[155] refers to accessibility as a special requirement for people with disabilities.[156] Paragraph 19 adds that 'Whereas it should therefore be possible to identify and add specific essential requirements on user privacy, features for users with a disability, features for emergency services and/or features for avoidance of fraud'. According to article 3.3 the Commission 'may decide that apparatus within certain equipment classes or apparatus of certain types shall be so constructed that....(f) it supports certain features in order to facilitate its use by users with a disability'.

In 2005, a communication[157] from the Commission purported to strengthen industry self-regulation and to encourage co-ordination among the Member States. It also called on stakeholders to co-operate in order to enhance the accessibility of ICT. At the level of research and development, a Web Accessibility Initiative (WAI) develops strategies, guidelines, and resources to help make the Web accessible to people with disabilities in cooperation with the World Wide Web Consortium (W3C)[158].

11. UNIVERSAL SERVICE AND USERS' RIGHTS

Universal service is an economic, legal and business term used mostly in industries, referring to the practice of providing a baseline level of services to every resident of a country. Goals of universal service are, e.g., to promote the availability of quality services at just, reasonable, and affordable rates; to increase access to advanced telecommunications services; and to advance the availability of such services to all consumers, including those in low income, rural, insular, and high cost areas at rates that are reasonably comparable to those charged in urban areas.

Within the EU, Directive 2002/22/EC of the European Parliament and of the Council of 7 March 2002 concerns the provision of electronic communications networks and services to end-users.[159] The Directive's aim is to ensure the availability throughout the Community of good quality publicly available services while

---

[155] Directive 1999/5/EC of the European Parliament and of the Council of 9 March 1999 on radio equipment and telecommunications terminal equipment and the mutual recognition of their conformity OJ L 91.

[156] In the Preamble, it states (paragraph 15): 'Whereas telecommunications are important to the well-being and employment of people with disabilities who represent a substantial and growing proportion of the population of Europe; whereas radio equipment and telecommunications terminal equipment should therefore in appropriate cases be designed in such a way that disabled people may use it without or with only minimal adaptation.'

[157] European Commission, eAccessibility, Communication from the Commission to the Council, the European Parliament and the European Economic and Social Committee and the Committee of the Regions, COM(2005) 425/final, 13 Sept 2005.

[158] Website: http://www.w3.org/WAI/. Rudi Vansnick (Internet Society Belgium, President) 'ICT for an ageing society', presentation delivered at SENIOR final conference, 27 Novembre 2009. 'We are convinced that the entire community can benefit from an 'accessible ICT world,' as people can be permanently or temporarily disabled due to personal, environmental (e.g., a phone call in a noisy environment) or cultural (e.g., spoken language diversity) conditions. Moreover, we will all grow old and lose abilities that we take for granted now, thus enlarging the part of the population that would benefit from accessible communication. We cannot allow isolation of a part of the population due to lack of appropriate functionality that prevents the use of ICT resources by everybody to the fullest possible degree.'

[159] European Parliament and Council, Directive 2002/22/EC of the European Parliament and of the Council of 7 March 2002 on universal service and users' rights relating to electronic communications networks and services (Universal Service Directive), Brussels, 7 March 2002.

respecting effective competition, choice, and the circumstances in which the needs of end-users are not satisfactorily met by the market. The directive defines the minimum set of services of specified quality to which all end-users have access, at an affordable price in the light of specific national conditions and without distorting competition.[160] The snag is whether this regulation can balance contradictory elements of ICT market for elderly persons. In this direction goes the recognition of rights of end-users and of obligations on undertakings to provide publicly available electronic communications networks and services.

11.1. BROADBAND ACCESS

A fundamental requirement of universal service is to provide users on request with a connection to the public communications network at a fixed location and at an affordable price. Most ICT applications for older persons rely on secure and adequate broadband network, mostly wifi. Older persons will have an interest both in having broadband access and that Internet connection is not arbitrarily cut off.

In the year 2009, Finland became the first country in the world to make broadband internet access a legal right. By July 2010, telecommunications companies will be obliged to provide all Finnish residents with broadband lines that can run at speeds of at least 1 megabit per second.[161] Measures taken by Member States regarding end-users' access to, or use of, services and applications through electronic communications networks shall respect the fundamental rights and freedoms of natural persons. The 2009 EU telecoms package and in particular amendment 138 was at the center of vehement debate between the Parliament and the Council. Amendment 138 stressed the need for 'prior ruling by the judicial authorities' for those suspected of illegal downloading. However, any measures regarding end-users' access to, or use of, services and applications through electronic communications networks liable to restrict freedom of access may only be imposed if they are appropriate, proportionate and necessary within a democratic society. For member states to impose a requirement to cut off end-users without a prior hearing would clearly not be permissible.[162] On this point the European Commission's note is quite clear: ''Three-strikes-laws', which could cut off Internet access without a prior fair and impartial procedure or without effective and timely judicial review, will certainly not become part of European law.'[163]

12. ICT IMPLANTS

At the time of writing, the use of ICT implants is limited to active medical devices. In the future information society, however, ICT implants could be used much more frequently, such as for identification and location purposes. With the ageing of the population, a significant number of persons, in particular those reaching very old

---

[160] See Preamble, paragraph 4 and article 2.1 of the Directive.
[161] *The Guardian,* 'Finland makes broadband access a legal right', by Bobbie Johnson, 14 October 2009. See also chapter 1.
[162] This view is defended by P. Brisby, Managing Partner, Towerhouse Consulting LLP, 'The Internet as a Human Right', presentation delivered to the SENIOR final conference, Brussels, 27 November 2009.
[163] Leigh Phillips, 'Reding warns Spain against internet cut-off', EU Observer, 24 November 2009.

ages, may go through long periods of impairing neuropsychiatric conditions.[164] The use of implants which supplemeting enhancinmg immlants may be run together with anti ageing and become more frequent. The opinion of the European Group on Ethics in Science and New Technologies (EGE)[165] sets out some general principles, which shouydl inspire standard meausres and regulation of ICT implants. The governing principle should be the precautionary one: ICT implants should always be avoided when alternative means are available. According to the EGE, there are serious risks for security, privacy and data protection Some of them may be unknown. Thus 'specific research', indicates the group, 'will have to contemplate how ICT implanst affects personal identity, autonomy, and control; how they alter self-perception and how they impact on social interactions.'[166] At the level of European Union, regulation is limited to Directive 90/385 on active implantable medical devices.[167] The directive sets out strict essential safety requirements. The directive, however, does not take into consideration these devices' interplay with questions of privacy and identity. If the use of non-medical implants become frequent this might require even stricter rules, since safety risks are not counterbalanced by effects on health.

13. CLINICAL TRIALS

The development of ICT for people with special needs entails carrying out trials, which are necessary to evaluate whether the technology meets the users needs and concerns. Directive 2001/20 on clinical trials sets out strict conditions to ascertain that a person has given his or her informed consent to the trial.[168] The Directive also specifies which information requirements need to be satisfied. The capable adult must be given the opportunity to understand the objectives, risks and inconveniences of the trial (research activity) and the conditions under which it is to be conducted. The subject must have the opportunity to withdraw from the trial at any time and have a contact point where he or she may obtain information about the trial.

VII. ETHICAL GUIDELINES

One of the characteristic features of the Sixth and, in particular, the Seventh Framework Programmes, research and development policy within the European Research Area[169], is increased attention paid to ethical issues[170]. FP7 places particular

---

[164] See chapter 2. See also P. Bartlett, O. Lewis & O. Thorold, *Mental disabilities and the European Convention on Human Rights,* Martinus Nijhoff Publishers, Leiden/Boston, 2007

[165] Opinion of the European Group on Ethics in Science and New Technologies (EGE) on the ethical aspect of ICT implants in the human body Opinion nr 20on the Ethical Aspects of ICT Implants in the Human Body of 16 March 2005 http://ec.europa.eu/european_group_ethics/docs/avis20_en.pdf

[166] *Ibid.*

[167] Council Directive 90/385/EEC of 20 June 1990 on the approximation of the laws of the Member States relating to active implantable medical devices, Official Journal L 189 , 20/07/1990 P. 0017 – 0036.

[168] Directive 2001/20/EC of the European Parliament and of the Council of 4 April 2001 on the approximation of the laws, regulations and administrative provisions of the Member States relating to the implementation of good clinical practice in the conduct of clinical trials on medicinal products for human use.

[169] See Chapter 6.

[170] This paragraph draws from SENIOR project, Background paper to the Ministerial conference on e-inclusion, Bled (Slovenia), 12 May 2008, p.7-8.

attention to the ethical aspects of e-inclusion, including the inclusion of elderly people[171]. In parallel with FP7, various EC communications (e.g., on RFID, e-Inclusion, privacy-enhancing technologies, i-2010) have advocated the need to promote ICT oriented to social goods and consistent with EU fundamental values.

Recent political decisions have reinforced this need. The 2009 Lisbon Treaty indicates a set of European values, such as human dignity, freedom, democracy, human right protection, pluralism, non-discrimination, tolerance, justice, solidarity and gender equality.[172] These values are stated in the Charter of Fundamental Rights of the European Union[173], which is expected to be a key frame for EU policies, from research to security, from immigration to energy and climate change. The presupposition that EU policies have to be consistent with the fundamental rights as stated in the European Charter implies that ICT research activities and policies also need to address these new dimensions. This means that European policies – beyond their obvious and explicit targets – have the general goal to promote and pursue European ethical principles worldwide, as clearly stated in the Commission's Green Paper on the European Research Area.[174]

Actions 30 and 31 of the Science and Society Action Plan[175] specifically address the need to study the ethical implications of new technologies.[176] The Riga Declaration on e-inclusion, discussed in Chapter 1, explicitly calls for increasing ethical awareness of ICT use.[177]

The inclusion of the elderly in the information society should increase quality of life, autonomy and safety, while also respecting privacy, and dignity. The 'Ageing well in the Information Society' communication pointed out how 'solutions can only bring benefits if users have access to basic ICT facilities, have the appropriate education and motivation, and ethical and psychological issues are properly addressed.' It warns

---

[171] ftp://ftp.cordis.europa.eu/pub/fp7/docs/guidelines-annex5ict.pdf

[172] Treaty of Lisbon amending the Treaty on European Union and the Treaty establishing the European Community, signed at Lisbon, 13 December 2007 http://eurlex.europa.eu/JOHtml.do?uri=OJ:C:2007:306:SOM:EN:HTML

[173] See Chapter 3. http://www.europarl.europa.eu/charter/pdf/text_en.pdf .

[174] European Commission, The European Research Area: New Perspectives, Green Paper, COM(2007) 161 final, Brussels, 4 April 2007, 'European research policy[...]should experiment with new ways of involving society at large in the definition, implementation and evaluation of research agendas and of promoting responsible scientific and technological progress, within a framework of common basic ethical principles and on the basis of agreed practices that can inspire the rest of the world.

[175] European Commission, *Science and Society. Action Plan,* http://ec.europa.eu/research/science-society/pdf/ss_ap_en.pdf

[176] Action 30: An open dialogue will be established between NGOs, industry, the scientific community, religions, cultural groups, philosophical schools and interested groups, stimulating an exchange of views and ideas on a range of critical issues, such as the ethical impact of new technologies on future generations, human dignity and integrity, 'info ethics' and sustainability. A variety of mechanisms will be used (focus groups, polling exercise, e-debates, workshops or institutional forums, etc).
Action 31: The level of awareness among researchers of the ethical dimension of their activities is rather uneven in Europe. Actions to raise awareness of good scientific practices, including the ethical dimension, research integrity and the key elements of European legislation, conventions and codes of conduct should be encouraged.

[177] EU Ministerial declaration, 'Riga declaration', 11 June 2006, Riga, p.2. See also European Commission, 'Ethics and e-Inclusion: best practices in Europe - expert meeting', 16 March 2009, Brussels.

that the task may be totemic: 'there is no specific reference point for ethics in ICT for ageing, for example, in safeguarding human dignity and autonomy where solutions require a degree of monitoring and intervention.'[178]

An approach to ethics and ageing in the information society is proposed by the Commission Staff Working Paper 'Ageing well in the information society.'[179] The paper argues that ICT and ageing raise ethical questions which seem to be influenced by diverse elements and narratives. In the opinion of the commission, 'these questions find their origin in the vulnerability of the user, the changing characteristics of the user population (e.g. more people surviving at high age but also the trend towards more educated and empowered users), economic constraints such as public budgets that are at tension with serving all fully in health and social care and the constant renewal of science and technology.'[180] The 'European i2010 initiative on e-Inclusion - To be part of the information society'[181] discussed in Chapter 1 recalls that 'it is also important to raise awareness of the risks involved in processing personal data through ICT networks and educate users in this field, e.g. risks of identity theft, discriminatory profiling or continuous surveillance.' The importance for an ethics of e-inclusion echoes in the opinions of the European Group on Ethics in Science and New Technologies.[182] The EGE calls for embedding ethics and societal considerations in ICT policy on design and implementation as well as for opening debates on the societal implications. Similar messages have been stated in the eContentplus 2008 Work Programme[183] and the Communication on Radio-frequency identification (RFID) in Europe: steps towards a policy framework.[184]

REFERENCES

Baer, S., 'Il Diritto all'uguaglianza nella Carta dei Diritti Fondamentali dell'Unione Europea', in M.Rossilli (ed.), *I Diritti delle donne nell'Unione Europea: Cittadine, migranti, schiave*, Ediesse, Roma, 2009, p. 47-72.

Bartlett, O. Lewis & O. Thorold, *Mental disabilities and the European Convention on Human Rights*, Martinus Nijhoff Publishers, Leiden/Boston, 2007.

Bell, M., *Anti-discrimination law and the European Union*, Oxford: University Press, 2004, p.12.

Bennett, B., *Health law Kaleidoscope. Health law rights in a global age*, Ashgate Publishing: Aldershot, UK, 2008.

Bobbio, Norberto, *The Age of Rights*, Policy Press, Oxford, 1994.

---

[178] European Commission, Ageing well in the Information Society, Action Plan on Information and Communication Technologies and Ageing, An i2010 Initiative, Communication from the Commission to the European Parliament, the Council, the European Economic and Social Committee and the Committee of the Regions, COM(2007) 332 final, Brussels, 14 June 2007, quoted above.

[179] Commission Staff Working Document, Accompanying document to the Communication from the Commission to the European Parliament, the Council, the European Economic and Social Committee and the Committee of the Regions, Ageing well in the Information Society, SEC(2007) 811, Brussels, 14 June 2007.

[180] SEC(2007) 811, Brussels, 14 June 2007.

[181] COM(2007) 694 final.

[182] Ethical issues of healthcare in the information society, Opinion No. 13, 30 July 1999; Ethical aspects of ICT Implants in the Human Body, Opinion No. 20, 16 March 2005. http://ec.europa.eu/european_group_ethics/avis/index_en.htm

[183]http://ec.europa.eu/information_society/activities/econtentplus/programme/workprogramme/index_en.htm

[184] COM (2007) 96 final.

Chiaromonte, W., La Protezione dei soggetti piu' bisognosi e le indicazioni dell'UE: spunti giurisprudenziali e considerazioni a margine di tribunale di Napoli 22 Aprile 2009, in *www.europeanrights.com*

CNIL, *La CNIL et l'e-santé*, Note de synthèse, Paris 8 March 2001.

Cullen, K.,L. Kubitschker, and input from P Blanck, W. N Myhill, G. Quinn, P.O Donoghue, and R. Halverson, *Accessibility to ICT Products and services by Disabled and Elderly People. Towards a framework for further development of EU legislation or other co-ordination measures on eAccessibility*, Bonn, November 2008.

De Hert Paul, Gutwirth Serge, 'Data protection in the case law of Strasbourg and Luxemburg : constitutionalisation in action', in *Reinventing data protection ?*, Springer, 2009.

De Witte, B., "Protection of fundamental social rights in the European Union. The choice of the appropriate legal instrument", in L. Betten and D. MacDevitt (eds), *The protection of fundamental social rights in the European Union*, London: Kluwer Law International, 1996.

Meenan, H., "Reflecting on age discrimination in the European Union—the search for clarity and food for thought", *ERA Forum* (2009) 10: 107–124.

Fredman, S., *Discrimination law*, Clarednon Law Series, University Press, Oxfod, 2002.

French, Ph., 'What is Disability?', in French (ed), *On Equal Terms - Working with Disabled People*, (Oxford: Butterworth-Heinemann, 1994).

Kayess, Rosemary, and Phillip French, "Out of Darkness into Light? Introducing the Convention on the Rights of Persons with Disabilities", *Human Rights Law Review,* 8:1, Oxford University Press, 2008.

Lessig, L., *Code and Other Laws of Cyberspace*, New York, Basic Books, 1999.

Rodotà, S., Social ethical and privacy needs in ICT for older people: a dialogue road map, *Opening lecture to the launching event of SENIOR*, 3 March 2008, www.seniorproject.eu.

Rodriguez-Pinzon, D., and C. Marin, 'The International Human Rights status of elderly persons', in *American University International Law Review*, 2003, vol. 18, number 4, p.916-1007.

Sidorenko, A. and A. Walker, 'The Madrid International Plan of Action on Ageing: From conceptualization to implementation', in *Ageing & Society* 24 (2): (2004) 147-165.

Wright D., et al., *Safeguards in a World of Ambient Intelligence*, Springer, 2008.

European Union

Charter of Fundamental Rights of the European Union, European Parliament, the Council and the Commission, European Charter of Fundamental Rights, 2000/C 364/01, OJ C 303.

Consolidated versions of the Treaty on European Union and the Treaty on the Functioning of the European Union, Official Journal C 115 of 9 May 2008.

Council Directive 2000/43 implementing the principle of equal treatment between persons irrespective of racial or ethnic origin, Official Journal L 180, 19 July 2000, p. 22–26.

Council Directive 2000/78/EC establishing a general framework for equal treatment in employment and occupation, Official Journal L 303 , 02/12/2000 P. 0016 - 0022.

Council Directive 2004/113/EC implementing the principle of equal treatment between men and women in the access to and supply of goods and services, OJ L 373, 21.12.2004, p. 37–43.

Council Directive 2006/96/EC of 20 November 2006 adapting certain Directives in the field of free movement of goods, by reason of the accession of Bulgaria and Romania, OJ L 363, 20.12.2006, p. 81–106.

Council Directive 90/385/EEC of 20 June 1990 on the approximation of the laws of the Member States relating to active implantable medical devices, Official Journal L 189 , 20/07/1990 P. 0017 – 0036.

Council Directive 91/250/EEC of 14 May 1991 on the legal protection of computer programs

Council of Europe, Official Journal L 122 , 17/05/1991 P. 0042 – 0046.

Council Resolution of 7 May 1985 on a new approach to technical harmonization and standards, Official Journal C 136 , 04/06/1985 P. 0001 – 0009.

EU Ministerial declaration, "Riga declaration", 11 June 2006. http://europa.eu/rapid/pressReleasesAction.do?reference=IP/06/769&format=HTML&aged=1 &language=FR&guiLanguage=fr

Directive 1999/5/EC of the European Parliament and of the Council of 9 March 1999 on radio equipment and telecommunications terminal equipment and the mutual recognition of their conformity, OJ L 91, 7.4.1999, p. 10–28.

Directive 2001/20/EC of the European Parliament and of the Council of 4 April 2001 on the approximation of the laws, regulations and administrative provisions of the Member States relating to the implementation of good clinical practice in the conduct of clinical trials on medicinal products for human use, Official Journal L 121 , 01/05/2001 P. 0034 – 0044.

Directive 2001/29/EC of the European Parliament and of the Council of 22 May 2001 on the harmonisation of certain aspects of copyright and related rights in the information society, Official Journal L 167 , 22/06/2001 P. 0010 – 0019.

Directive 2002/21/EC on a common regulatory framework for electronic communications networks and services (Framework Directive), Official Journal L 108 , 24/04/2002 P. 0033 – 0050.

Directive 2000/31/EC of the European Parliament and of the Council of 8 June 2000 on certain legal aspects of information society services, in particular electronic commerce, in the Internal Market ('Directive on electronic commerce'), Official Journal L 178 , 17/07/2000 P. 1-16.

Directive 96/9/EC of the European Parliament and of the Council of 11 March 1996 on the legal protection of databases, OJ L 77, 27.3.1996, p. 20–28

Directive 98/34/EC of the European Parliament and of the Council of 22 June 1998 laying down a procedure for the provision of information in the field of technical standards and regulations, OJ L 204, 21.7.1998, p. 37–48.

Directive 98/48/EC of the European Parliament and of the Council of 20 July 1998 amending Directive 98/34/EC laying down a procedure for the provision of information in the field of technical standards and regulations, OJ L 217, 5.8.1998, p. 18–26.

European Commission, "For a Europe of civic and social rights. Report by the Comitè des Sages", Luxembourg: Office Official Publication of the European Communities, 1996.

European Commission, Ageing well in the Information Society, Action Plan on Information and Communication Technologies and Ageing, An i2010 Initiative, Communication from the Commission to the European Parliament, the Council, the European Economic and Social Committee and the Committee of the Regions, COM(2007) 332 final, Brussels, 14 June 2007.

European Commission, Communication on the Role of eGoverment for Europe's Future, COM(2003) 567 final, 26 Sept 2003.

European Commission, *eAccessibility*, Communication from the Commission to the Council, the European Parliament and the European Economic and Social Committee and the Committee of the Regions, COM(2005) 425/final, 13 Sept 2005.

European Commission, e-Health – making healthcare better for European citizens: An action plan for a European e-Health Area, Communication from the Commission to the Council, the European Parliament, the European Economic and Social Committee ad the Committee of the Regions, COM(2004) 356 (final), Brussels, 30 Apr 2004.

European Commission, Proposal for a Council Directive on implementing the principle of equal treatment between persons irrespective of religion or belief, disability, age or sexual orientation, Brussels, COM(2008) 426 final, Brussels, 2 July 2008.

Europcan Commission, Scicncc and Socicty. Action Plan, 2002. http://cc.curopa.cu/ research/science-society/pdf/ss_ap_en.pdf

European Commission, Staff Working Document, Accompanying document to the Communication from the Commission to the European Parliament, the Council, the European Economic and Social Committee and the Committee of the Regions, Ageing well in the Information Society, SEC(2007) 811, Brussels, 14 June 2007.

European Commission, The European Research Area: New Perspectives, Green Paper, COM(2007) 161 final, Brussels, 4 April 2007

European Commission, Green paper on "Promoting a European framework for corporate social responsibility" COM(2001) 366 final COM(2002) 347 final 116, and COM(2006) 136 final

European Parliament and Council, Directive 2002/22/EC of the European Parliament and of the Council of 7 March 2002 on universal service and users' rights relating to electronic communications networks and services (Universal Service Directive), Brussels, 7 March 2002.

European Parliament, Non-legislative Resolution on Consumer confidence in the digital environment, INI/2006/2048, Strasbourg, 21 June 2007.

http://www.europarl.europa.eu/oeil/file.jsp?id=5319182

European Group on Ethics in Science and New Technologies (EGE), Ethical issues of healthcare in the information society, Opinion No. 13, 30 July 1999.

European Group on Ethics in Science and New Technologies (EGE), Opinion on the ethical aspect of ICT implants in the human body Opinion nr 20on the Ethical Aspects of ICT Implants in the Human Body of 16 March 2005 http://ec.europa.eu/european_group_ethics/docs/avis20_en.pdf

Article 29 data protection Working Party, Platform for Privacy Preferences (P3P) and the Open Profiling Standard (OPS), Opinion 1/98, 16 June 1998.

European Court of Justice

ECJ, Case 144/04 Werner Mangold v. Rudiger Helm.

ECJ, Case 15/69 Württenbergische Milchverwertung-Sudmilchv Ugliola [1969] ECR 363.

ECJ, Case C-187/96 Commission v Greece [1998] ECR I-1095.

ECJ, Case 26/62 Van Gend en Loos v Nederlandse Administratie der Belastingen [1963] ECR 1.

ECJ, Case 80/70 Defrenne v Belgium State (I) [1971] ECR 445.

ECJ, Case C-144/04 Werner Mangold v. Rudiger Helm [2005] ECR I-9981.

ECJ, Case C-203/86 Kingdom of Spain v. Council of the European Communities [1988] ECR 4563.

ECJ, Case C-279/93 Finanzamt Koeln-altstadt v. Roland Schumacker [1995] ECR I-225.

ECJ, Case C-57/96 H Meints v Minister van landbouw, Natuurbeheer en Visserij [1997] ECR-I-6689.

ECJ, Opinion of the Advocate General Jacobs in Case C-274-96 Bickel and Franz [1998] ECR I-7637

ECJ, C-13/05, Sonia Chacón Navas v. Eurest Colectividades SA, Grand Chambre, 16 March 2006.

Council of Europe

Council of Europe - ETS no.005 – European Convention of Human Rights, 1950

Council of Europe - ETS no. 163 - European Social Charter (revised), 1996.

Council of Europe - ETS no. 158, Additional Protocol to the European Social Charter

Explanatory report to the Additional Protocol to the European Social Charter, E.T.S. no. 128, providing for a System of Collective Complaints, Strasbourg, 9 November 1995.

Commissioner for Human Rights, Second Annual Report April 2001 to December 2001' to the Committee of Ministers and the Parliamentary Assembly, Comm. DH (2002)2, p.119-131.

Digest of Case law of the European Committee of Social Rights, 1 September 2008, p.147-148, http://www.coe.int/t/dghl/monitoring/socialcharter/Digest/DigestSept2008_en.pdf.

ECtHR , R (S) v. Plymouth City Council (2002) 5 CCLR 251.

ECtHR, Aerts v. Belgium, (1998) ECHR 64.

ECtHR, Amann v. Switzerland, 30 Eur. Hum. Rts. Rep. 843 (2000)

ECtHR, Botta v. Italy (1998) 26 EHRR 241.

ECtHR, Case relating to certain aspects of the laws on the use of languages in education in Belgium, (Belgian Linguistic Case), Judgment of 14 July 1968, 1 EHRR 252, para 10.

ECtHR, Gaskin v. the United Kingdom,(1989) 12 EHRR 36.

ECtHR, Gaskin v. UK (1989) 12 EHRR 36.

ECtHR, Guerra v. Italy, (1996) 26 EHRR 357.

ECtHR, H.L. v. United Kingdom (2004) ECHR 471.

ECtHR, Halford v UK, (1997) ECHR 32

ECtHR, Klass v. Germany, (1978) 2 EHRR 214.

ECtHR, Kutzner v. Germany (2002) E.H.R.R. 653.

ECtHR, Leander v. Sweden, (1987) 9 EHRR 433

ECtHR, Leander v. Sweden, (1987) 9 EHRR 433.

ECtHR, *Merczegfaluy v. Austria* of 24.09.1992, A series No. 244. and *Price v. The United Kingdom*, in Human Rights Case Digest, Volume 12, Numbers 7-8, 2001 , pp. 529-532(4) relating to the detention of a paraplegic person

ECtHR, *Mouisel v France* [2004] 38 EHRR 34.

ECtHR, Niemietz v. Federal Republic of Germany , 251 Eur. Ct. H.R. (ser. A) (1992)

ECtHR, *Papon v. France* (no. 1) (dec.), no. 64666/01, ECHR 2001-VI.

ECtHR, Peck v United Kingdom, (2003) 36 EHRR 41.

ECtHR, Rotaru v. Romania, Application no. 28341/95 judgement of 4 May 2000.

ECtHR, Segerstedt-Wiberg v. Sweden, application no. 62332/00, judgement of 6 June 2006.

ECtHR, Winterwerp v. the Netherlands (1979) 2 EHRR 387.

ECtHR, X and Y v. Netherlands (1985) 8 EHRR 235.

La Cour d'arbitrage (Belgian Constitutional Court), Arrêt n° 106/2004 du 16 juin 2004. (The *Moniteur Belge* case)

United Nations

Human Rights Council. Advisory Committee, Fourth Session, 25-29 January 2010, *Working paper*, A/HRC/AC/4/CRP.1.

U.N. Economic Commission for Europe, *Main Conclusions and Recommendations of the Research Forum on Ageing*, 5-8 November 2007.

U.N. Economic Commission for Europe, *Regional Implementation Strategy for the Madrid International Plan of Action on Ageing*, October 2009

U.N. General Assembly, 37th Session (1982), Resolution 37/51. *Question of Aging.* A/RES/37/51. U.N. General Assembly, 46th Session (1991), Resolution 46/91, *Implementation of the International Plan of Action on Ageing and related activities*, A/RES/46/91

U.N. General Assembly, 47th Session (1992), Resolution 47/5, *Proclamation on Ageing*, A/RES/47/5.

U.N. General Assembly, 89th Plenary Meeting (1992), Resolution 47/86, *Implementation of the International Plan of Action on Ageing: integration of older persons in development*, United Nations, Report of the Second World Assembly on Ageing Madrid, 8-12 April 2002. A/CONF.197/9. Available at http://www.un.org/swaa2002/documents.htm.

U.N. General Assembly, *Vienna International Plan of Action on Ageing,* A/RES/37/51. Available at http://www.un.org/esa/socdev/ageing/vienna_intlplanofaction.html.

U.N. General Assembly, *Report of the World Assembly on Ageing*, Vienna, 26 July to 6 August 1982 (United Nations publication, Sales No. E.82.I.16).

Office of the High Commissioner for Human Rights, *Economic, Social and Cultural Rights of Older Persons: General Comment 6*, U.N. ESCOR, Econ., Soc., & Cultural Rts. Comm., 13th Sess., para. 1, UN Doc. E/C.12/1995/16/Rev.1 (1995)

International Human rights law on elderly people

Universal Declaration of Human Rights (UDHR), 1948.
International Covenant on Civil and Political Rights (ICCPR), 1966.
International Covenant on Economic, Social and Cultural Rights (ICESCR), 1966.
Universal Islamic Declaration of human rights, 1981.
Cairo Declaration of Human rights in Islam, 1990.
African (Banjul) Charter on human and peoples' rights, 1981.
Protocol to the African charter on human and peoples' rights on the rights of women on Africa, 2000.
American Declaration of Rights and Duties of Man, 1948.
American Convention of Human Rights ('Pact of San Jose'), 1969.
Additional Protocol to the American Convention on Human Rights in the area of Economic, Social, and Cultural Rights (known as the 'Protocol of San Salvador'), 1988
Andean Charter for the promotion and protection of human rights,2002.
Asian Charter of human rights, 1997.
Declaration of the basic duties of ASEAN peoples and governments, 1983.

Other sources

SENIOR project, Background paper to the Ministerial conference on e-inclusion, Bled (Slovenia), 12 May 2008.
SENIOR project, D1.1 "Environmental scanning report", prepared by David Wright (Trilateral), 6 July 2008 p. 34-36.
SENIOR project, 'The Internet as a Human Right', by P. Brisby, Managing Partner, Towerhouse Consulting LLP, presentation delivered to the SENIOR final conference, Brussels, 27 November 2009.

EU Observer, 'Reding warns Spain against internet cut-off', by Leigh Phillips, 24 November 2009.
ABS-CBN News, 'Domestic workers, caregivers still in demand in Italy', by Danny Buenafe, 26 August 2009
The Guardian, 'Finland makes broadband access a legal right', by Bobbie Johnson, 14 October 2009.

CHAPTER FOUR. ON PRIVATE LIFE AND DATA PROTECTION

By Paul De Hert and Eugenio Mantovani

INTRODUCTION

Privacy needs in e-inclusion of elderly people, we suggest, include both a function of shielding the individual from external pressures and an emancipatory one related to one's need and interest in sharing life experiences with others. Often, in concrete situations, older persons will have both interests and needs at the same time. In the information society, the protective function of privacy boils down to shielding older citizens from unnecessary or excessive categorisation. This may include legislative discriminatory measures and also techniques such as spam, targeted advertisements, commercial profiling, inertia selling, in general all occasions when it is not clear why and for which purpose one person's preferences, tastes etc... need to be opened up and used. The right to private life also recognises the right of individuals to establish relations with others. In order to exercise such a right it is necessary that human networks exist in which the act of sharing personal experiences or information can take place without the individual having to care, or to stay alert, or be anxious about the fact that there is a (data) arms race going on behind his or her back. In this sense, the crucial function of privacy is to protect networks, such as private situations of co-dependency, so sharing can remain a trusted inter – personal exercise.

In the area of data protection, the realisation of ubiquitous environments, in particular in the field of health care and medical surveillance, emphasise the tension between data protection and the requirements of ICT environments, which need extensive data collection and profiling in order to make the user's environment act intelligently. Out of the overall solid data protection regime, we esteem three relevant areas ought to be given consideration from an elderly perspective. They concern the definition and implementation of privacy by design settings and regulations; rules on the transparency and accountability of processors and controllers; and consent requirements.

I. PRIVACY

The case law of the European Court of Human Rights on Article 8 of the ECHR offers good guidance in understanding the relevance of the right to privacy in the e-inclusion of seniors.[1] The active Strasbourg judge has in effect produced a rich repertoire of decisions, illustrated above in Chapter III. Starting from this case law, a prolific fabric of micropolitical operators, jurists, sociologists, decision makers, have perched on the meaning of privacy studying what it protects and promotes in modern highly

---

[1] In accordance with Article 52(3) of the EU Charter, the meaning and scope of this right are the same as those in the corresponding article of the ECHR. Consequently, the meaning is the same and the limitations which may legitimately be imposed on this right are the same as those allowed by Article 8 of the ECHR

technological societies.[2] Article 8 of the European Convention of Human Rights, seen above, entails recognition of the right to be left alone[3] and of 'the claim of individuals to determine for themselves when, how, and to what extent information about them is communicated to others[4], on the one hand;' article 8 also relates to the exercise of personal liberties. Other human rights intervene - article 14 (the right to non discrimination), article 9 (thought, conscience and religion), article 10 (freedom of expression), article 11 (assembly and association), article 12 (right to found a family) – which enable or empower a person to set his or her project of life, without excessive outside interference.'[5]

The 'circular' practice that emerges from the case law, according to which private life relates to personal liberties which are necessary to realise one's private life, lends to contemplation. It indicates that the right to private life acquires concrete significance in relation to the social fabric where an individual can exercise their liberty, rather than in the seclusion of his or her private room. These 'social fabrics' are the networks in which a person normally ages, family, living institutions, workplace, public transport, hospitals, neighbourhoods etc. In fact, article 23 of the 1996 European Social Charter (The right of elderly persons to social protection) discussed above, refers to 'full membership', 'independent life in familiar surroundings, 'community.' Likewise, article 25 of the EU Charter (The rights of elderly people), seen above in Chapter III, protects and promotes 'participation in social and cultural life'. Social and cultural life, living institutions, communities, workplace, public transport, hospitals, neighbourhoods…senior persons exercise within societal networks their right to private life.[6]

1. PRIVACY, NETWORKS AND ACTIVE AGEING

How are the networks in which older persons age constituted? In chapter two, we contended that societal arrangements are characterised by a norm of being old or ageing which determine a series of age-graded roles, such as the 'right' time for getting married, starting a family, 'peaking' in one's career, retiring and so on.[7] We warned, however, that in modern societies the norm of ageing can be 'sheer balance and comparison, without any reference as such to the individual.'[8] Active ageing polices, for instance, while benevolently seeking to empower the individual, may have

---

[2] P. De Hert, and S. Gutwirth, "Privacy, data protection and law enforcement: Opacity of the individual and transparency of power", in E. Claes, A. Duff and S.Gutwirth (eds.), *Privacy and the criminal law*, Intersentia, Antwerp/Oxford, 2006, pp. 61–104.

[3] S. Warren and L. Brandeis, 'The right to privacy', *Harvard Law Review*, Vol. IV, No. 5, 15 Dec 1890.

[4] Alan F. Westin, *Privacy and Freedom*, Atheneum, New York, NY, 1967.

[5] ECtHR, *Botta v. Italy*, seen above.

[6] F. Rigaux, *La protection de la vie privée et des autres biens de la personnalité,* Bruylant, Bruxelles-Paris, 1990, p. 167 ; S. Rodotà, *Tecnologie e diritti,* Il Mulino, Bologna, 1995, p. 122, According to Rodotà privacy protects the right to keep control over one's own information and the right to determine and give shape to one's projects. See also S. Gutwirth, *Privacy and the information age,* Rowman & Littlefield Publishers, Lanham, 2002.

[7] SENIOR project, *Ethics of e-inclusion of elderly people, Discussion paper for the workshop on ethics and e-inclusion*, Bled (Slovenia), 12 May 2008, p.13. SENIOR refers to Lois W. Banner, 'Coming of Age: A Cultural Studies Approach to Aging', *Journal of Women's History*, Vol. 12, No. 4, Winter 2001, pp. 212-214. http://muse.jhu.edu/login?uri=/journals/journal_of_womens_history/v012/12.4banner.html

[8] S. Gutwirth, *Privacy and the information age*, p. 68. See also chapter II, conclusions.

counteracting effects which restrict the liberty to determine one's ageing projects. What to do or how to live the last years of one's life is a matter of social places, activities and inter personal relations. The identification and the protection of the networks where people age, for instance the workplace, or health care, depends on decisions taken by 'micropolitics' operators which allocate budgets, make projects, create new technologies. Who decides what is positive and what is negative for older persons from a public policy perspective? The diversity of older individuals presents specific problems and ambiguities which make it difficult to conceive of the elderly as a group, for instance vis-à-vis state's institutions. A recent report by the advisory committee to the UN Human Rights Council on the human rights treaty for the older person, for instance, enlists as 'good practice' those of 'several EU countries which have raised the age for retirement to encourage older persons to remain in the labour force for longer periods of time.'[9] Raising retirement-age and 'remain[ing] in the labour force longer', however, do not automatically promote and respect the rights of older persons. Although being able to work longer, if one so wishes, is important to pursue one's plans also in later age, it is part of a dominant narrative on ageing, active ageing, which eschews rest, deterioration, *otium,* dependency, withdrawal, and expectation of death as natural outcomes of the coming of age.[10] We tend to forget, legal scholar Martha Nussbaum maintains, that human life cycle brings with it periods of dependency in which our functioning is very similar to people with mental or physical disabilities. In fact, we live long periods of our life time in situations of dependency, e.g., as children, as sick, or as frail elderly persons.[11] These lights invite to avoid thinking about one model of ageing which commends individual independence and productivity only and, instead, lend recognition also to other ways to ageing which genuinely necessitate, in order to flourish, assistance, support, sharing life, in particular amongst the least advantaged.

The right to privacy acquires here great significance, shielding the individual from one model of ageing and giving protection to plural ways of ageing. If the meaning of private life rests also on a genuine need to share, then privacy for older persons cannot be reduced to a commodity which those living in situation of need may have to trade off with something else, such as assistance. The trade off argument reduces the need for assistance and the need for privacy to incommensurability, like 'one cannot have

---

[9] Advisory committee to the Human Rights Council, *op.cit.,* p. 11. The report is drafted with the contribution of Helpage International.

[10] We called this trend 'non conformity to the norm of ageing', that is, removal of the conditions that naturally accompany the biological and biographical process of ageing. Compare Ohio State University (2009, May 18). Obituary Photos Suggest Growing Bias Against Aging Faces. ScienceDaily. Retrieved March 4, 2010, http://www.sciencedaily.com/releases/2009/05/090513121059.htm. The study found that the number of obituary photographs showing the deceased at a much younger age than when he or she died more than doubled between 1967 and 1997. See also B. Ehrenreich, Smile or Die: How Positive Thinking Fooled America and the World, Granta books, 2009

[11] Martha C. Nussbaum, *Frontiers of Justice. Disability, Nationality, Species membership*, The Belknap Press of Harvard University Press, Cambridge (Mass), 2007. Nussbaum studies the concept of dependency/independency from a moral philosophical point of view. At p.131-133 Nussbaum concludes that 'We greatly distort the nature of our own morality and rationality, which are themselves thoroughly material and animal; we learn to ignore the fact that disease, old age, and accident can impede the moral and rational functions, just as much as the other animal functions.' As a consequence, 'we tend to forget that usual human life cycle brings with it periods of extreme dependency, in which our functioning is very similar to that experiences by people with mental or physical disabilities throughout their lives.'

the cake and eat it.'[12] Such a rationale, though a logic one, is untenable in concrete life. Particularly in old age, one is likely to be affected by various forms of mental or physical disorders. There is a positive duty to intervene, accommodate and, e.g., provide care, medical assistance, or develop and implement technology tools which can help older persons 'flourish' and develop their personality. These positive measures, however, may be invasive of privacy. The negative function of the right to privacy intervenes to shield the individual against excessive or disproportionate intrusion, (un)reasonable accommodation or measures, including technological ones, which, for instance, invade aspects of life which he or she retains the capability to manage autonomously, or which could be attained using other less invasive means.

In conclusion, privacy needs for older persons in the information society will be sometimes shielding and sometimes sharing. Often they will be both. The right to privacy lends recognition and protection to both. The protective function shields older citizens from unnecessary or excessive categorisation (including techniques such as spam, targeted advertisements, commercial profiling) when it is not clear why and for which purpose one person's preferences, tastes etc. need to be opened up.[13] The emancipatory function recognises the right to establish relations with others. Here the task of privacy protection for older persons in the information society, in particular for those living in situations of dependency, is to ensure that sharing personal experiences or information takes place without the individual having to care, or to stay alert, or anxious about the fact that there is a 'data arms race' going on behind his or her back. Just as we are not either totally dependent or independent, but both, similarly the protection of privacy contains both a protective and an emancipatory dimension so sharing remains a trusted inter – personal exercise between 'wonderfully independent older human beings.' In this sense, one can conclude that the basic *raison d'être* of privacy in ICT for the elderly is to protect networks, such as private situations of co-dependency.

II. DATA PROTECTION

In the information society, the recognition of a fundamental right to the protection of personal data (article 8 of the EU Charter[14], and article 16 of the Lisbon Treaty) responds to new demands for protection of the private life in the context of the information society. As we saw in chapter 1, the information society is characterised by the presence of new elements, 'data', which are collected, processed and transmitted freely (principle of the free flow of data).[15] While the individual cannot

---

[12] Or maybe it is the opposite: the trade off argument puts them on the same scale- like one for the other, while actually they are incommensurable; such being the case it is not an exchange; they are different-not interchangeable, but both are needed.

[13] P. De Hert, 'The perspective of lawmakers', Presentation delivered to SENIOR final conference, 27 November 2009: 'Privacy law 'protects and promotes' different ways to ageing, not a model of ageing: it is both protection and emancipation or sometimes protection (assistive) and sometimes emancipation (enabling).'

[14] We have already seen that Article 8 on the right to protection of personal data is to be exercised under the conditions laid down in Directive 95/46/EC, and may be limited under the conditions set out by Article 52 of the Charter (Scope of guaranteed rights).

[15] The rapid use of computerised means for identification and profiling is at the root of the demand for protection against automatic data processing. As Gutwirth explains: 'The European Union Directive 95/46/EC of the European Parliament and of the Council of 24 October 1995 on the protection of individual with regard to the processing of personal data and on the free movement of such data aims to harmonise the national legislative systems in an attempt to secure the free flow of personal data, *which*

oppose the circulation of data, which is free by default, he or she, through the right to data protection, can rely on a series of procedures designed to hold accountable government and private record-holders when data about him or her are processed. Data protection's claim is, therefore, for the transparency of data processing.[16]The European legal framework for data protection is first provided by the 1981 Council of Europe Convention for the protection of individuals with regard to automatic processing of personal data (Convention 108).[17] The principles of the Convention are refined in Directive 95/46/EC,[18] which forms the building block of the data protection regime within the EU. The legal framework is complemented by Regulation (EC) No 45/2001 on the processing of personal data by the Community institutions and bodies[19]; Directive 2002/58/EC on privacy and electronic communications[20] and Directive 2006/24/EC on the retention of data[21]; in the area of police and judicial cooperation in criminal matters data protection is provided by the Framework Decision Framework 2008/977/JHA on data protection.[22]

In the last years, the data protection framework has been continuously challenged by the fast pace of technological developments. The realisation of ambient intelligence (AmI) is likely to further emphasise the tension between existing regulation on privacy and data protection and the requirements of the new environment.[23] Ubiquitous computing needs extensive data collection and profiling in order to make the user's environment act intelligently. Regulation that simply prohibits such extensive data collection and profiling practices is likely to interfere with the user-friendliness of an AmI world. The emergence of a market for assisting

---

is an internal market requirement. The Directive develops as the extension of a legislative movement that since the 1970s has sought to deal with the increasing processing of personal data and on the impact that 'telematics' would have on individual liberties.' S. Gutwirth, *Privacy in the Information Age*, p.20

[16] A new subject, the data subject, is the holder of the right to data protection, such as, access, control, modification, security of data, accuracy. Fair information processing principles are the fairness obtaining and processing principle, which includes consent; purpose specification; non-disclosure of personal information unless compatible with fair processing; data must be safe and secure, accurate and up to date; the processing must be proportional, not excessive; the detention period must not exceed the period of time necessary for the processing; an independent supervisory authority is established in each Member State and can hear complaints about compliance with data protection directives

[17] ETS No. 108, 28.01.1981.

[18] Directive 95/46/EC of the European Parliament and of the Council of 24 October 1995 on the protection of individuals with regard to the processing of personal data and on the free movement of such data, OJ 1995, L 281, p. 31.

[19] Regulation (EC) No 45/2001 of the European Parliament and of the Council of 18 December 2000 on the protection of individuals with regard to the processing of personal data by the Community institutions and bodies and on the free movement of such data, OJ 2001, L 8, p. 1.

[20] Directive 2002/58/EC of the European Parliament and of the Council of 12 July 2002 concerning the processing of personal data and the protection of privacy in the electronic communications sector (Directive on privacy and electronic communications), OJ 2002 L 201, p. 37; as revised by Directive 2009/136/EC of the European Parliament and of the Council of 25 November 2009.

[21] Directive 2006/24/EC of the European Parliament and of the Council of 15 March 2006 on the retention of data generated or processed in connection with the provision of publicly available electronic communications services or of public communications networks and amending Directive 2002/58/EC, OJ 2006 L 105.

[22] Council Framework Decision 2008/977/JHA of 27 November 2008 on the protection of personal data processed in the framework of police and judicial cooperation in criminal matters OJ 2008 L 350, p. 60, to be implemented in national law before 27 November 2010.

[23] David Wright, Serge Gutwirth, Michael Friedewald, Paul De Hert, Marc Langheinrich, Anna Moscibroda, 'Privacy, trust and policy-making: Challenges and responses,', in *Computer law & security review* 25(2009)69–83, p. 77.

technologies, including health monitoring technologies or internet based service such as e-pharmacies is relevant for the ageing. However, they also raise difficult issues concerning confidentiality and the protection of personal data. Similar problems are raised in e-government or e-commerce.

In December 2009, the article 29 Working Party or Group[24] issued a consultation document discussing whether 'the current legal framework of data protection meets the challenge [of the Information Society]' and 'the action which is needed to address the identified challenges.'[25] The richly elaborated 'Future of Privacy' report raises, amongst other, three points which are relevant to e-inclusion, namely: a) privacy by design; b) transparency and accountability; c) consent requirement. The first two points are illustrated below. The third one is dealt with in the next chapter.

1. PRIVACY BY DESIGN

As the article 29 Working Party indicates, the concept of privacy by design is not completely new to European data protection regulation. The data protection directive recognises the principle of confidentiality and puts data controllers under the obligation to implement the appropriate technical and organizational measures.[26] The Directive also contains provisions on data processing principles such as lawfulness and fairness, purpose limitation, relevance, accuracy, time limit on storage, and responsibility.[27] Recital 46 of the Directive calls for the implementation of 'appropriate technical and organizational measures', both at the stage of the design of the processing system and at the time of the processing itself.

The problem, contends the Working party, is that the Directive only promotes the concept of privacy by design. Promotion, it says, has proved insufficient to embedding privacy in ICT. The non-implementation of privacy settings in the design and management of technology is problematic because 'users of ICT services – business, public sector and certainly individuals – are not in a position to take relevant security measures by themselves in order to protect their own or other persons' personal data.'[28] The challenge, according to the Working Party, is thus to convert 'the currently punctual requirements into a broader and consistent principle of privacy by design.'[29] Privacy by design principle should be binding both for technology designers and producers as well as for data controllers who have to decide on the acquisition and use of ICT.[30] This recommendation seems useful to create a trusty environment for applications, such as e-health, e-pharmacy or e-government, which largely target seniors.

Also the adoption of privacy enhancing technologies (PETs) should be a default setting of ICT products and services sanctioned by the law (see below accountability

---

[24] The Working Party was set up under Article 29 of Directive 95/46/EC. It is an independent European advisory body on data protection and privacy. Its tasks are described in Article 30 of Directive 95/46/EC and Article 15 of Directive 2002/58/EC.

[25] Article 29 Data Protection Working Party, *The Future of Privacy. Joint contribution to the Consultation of the European Commission on the legal framework for the fundamental right to protection of personal data*, Adopted on 01 December 2009, 02356/09/EN, WP 168. Hereinafter 'Future of Privacy'

[26] Article 16 and article 17, Directive 95/46/EC.

[27] Article 6 Directive 95/46/EC.

[28] Future of Privacy, para. 45.

[29] Future of Privacy, para. 46. See also next paragraph on transparency and accountability.

[30] *Ibid.*

and transparency). This would imply that user interfaces be designed in such a way as to facilitate the use of privacy related functions, in particular by less experienced or occasional users. In general, the processing of personal data should, by design, be engineered according to [31]:

- Data Minimization; the processing of personal data should, by design, be engineered towards the minimization of the amount of data which need to be processed;
- Controllability: an IT system should provide the data subjects with effective means of control concerning their personal data. The possibilities regarding consent and objection could be supported by technological settings;
- Transparency: both developers and operators of IT systems have to ensure that the data subjects are sufficiently informed about the means of operation of the systems.
- User Friendly Systems; User interfaces can play a valuable role in assisting occasional users or non expert users, such as many senior citizens, navigating the risks posed by aggressive spam, malware, phishing, requests for personal data against free services etc....
- Data Confidentiality: by design only authorised entities have access to personal data in IT systems;
- Data Quality: data controllers should support data quality by technical means;
- Use Limitation; data run through connected systems, such as data warehouses, cloud computing, digital identifiers. IT systems should guarantee that data and processes serving different tasks or purposes can be segregated from each other in a secure way.

2. TRANSPARENCY AND ACCOUNTABILITY PRINCIPLE

In order to be implemented, privacy by design (PbD) and privacy enhancing technologies (PETs) require that the legal framework impose a level of transparency and accountability. Transparency ideally gives the data subject the opportunity to understand the consequences of the processing of personal data before the processing begins. However, extensive data collection make it difficult for the user to be informed and aware 'by whom, on what grounds, from where, for what purposes and with what technical means data are being processed.'[32] In order to be effective, transparency needs accountability of technology designers, producers, and data controllers who decide on the acquisition and use of ICT. The latter should be 'obliged to take technological data protection into account already at the planning stage of information-technological procedures and systems.'[33] They should demonstrate that 'they have taken all measures required to comply with these requirements.'[34] Privacy by default settings should become routine in products and services provided to third parties and individual customers, including social networks and search engines. Eventually, data controllers would remain accountable and responsible even in the case the data have been transferred to other controllers outside the EU.[35]

---

[31] *Ibid.*, para para 53.
[32] Future of privacy, para. 63.
[33] *Ibid.*, para 46.
[34] Ibid.
[35] Pursuant to the new provision on accountability 'data controllers would remain accountable and responsible for the protection of personal data for which they are controllers, even in the case the data have been transferred to other controllers outside the EU'. Future of privacy, para 19.

The introduction in the data protection framework of solid transparency and accountability rules invites, according to the Future of Privacy report, a series of regulatory measures, such as[36]:

- Strengthening rules on privacy by setting and PETs: protective defaults and use of standards-compliant privacy enhancing technologies or PETS shoudl be binding on technology designers & engineers, hardware manufacturers and developers as well as data controllers;
- Strengthening rules on data controllers' responsibilities: controllers would be required to carry out the necessary measures to ensure that substantive principles and obligations of the current. Certification of compliance should be signed by top level company executives confirming that they have implemented appropriate safeguards to protect personal data and notified with national data protection authorities (DPAs).
- Strengthening and clarifying data protection authorities' roles and cooperation;
- Drawing up of binding corporate rules (BCRs).

Eventually, in order to allocate responsibility, the distinction between 'controller' and 'processor' should be clarified.[37] The distinction serves to identify the responsibilities of those who are more closely involved in the processing of personal data and to determine who shall be responsible for compliance with data protection rules, and how data subjects can exercise their rights in practice. The article 29 Working explains that it is important to be aware of relevant differences and to clarify responsibilities where required.[38] Due to different reasons, *viz.* i) decentralisation of policy departments and executive agencies; ii) an increasing delivery chains or service delivery across organisations; iii) the use of subcontracting or outsourcing of services; iv) the choices of companies to locate databases in one or more countries, within or outside the European Union, Information society services providers do not always consider themselves responsible or accountable. The introduction of micro-technology – such as RFID chips in consumer products – create similar situations in which the responsibilities on the head of the user do not always clearly interact with clear responsibilities in the client organisation.[39]

---

[36] Future of privacy, paras. 79-80.

[37] Article 2 (d) and (e) of Directive 95/46/EC reads as follows:'
'Controller' shall mean the natural or legal person, public authority, agency or any other body which alone or jointly with others determines the purposes and means of the processing of personal data; where the purposes and means of processing are determined by national or Community laws or regulations the controller or the specific criteria for his nomination may be designated by national or Community law;
'Processor' shall mean a natural or legal person, public authority, agency or any other body which processes personal data on behalf of the controller.'

[38] Article 29 Working Party, *Opinion 1/2010 on the concepts of 'controller' and 'processor'*, 16 February 2010, WP 169, http://ec.europa.eu/justice_home/fsj/privacy/workinggroup/wpdocs/2010_en.htm

[39] The WP 169 document contains a wealth of case studies. We report here one concerning platforms for managing health data. 'For instance, In a Member State, a public authority establishes a national switch point regulating the exchange of patient data between healthcare providers. The plurality of controllers - tens of thousands - results in such an unclear situation for the data subjects (patients) that the protection of their rights would be in danger. Indeed, for data subjects it would be unclear whom they could address in case of complaints, questions and requests for information, corrections or access to personal data. Furthermore, the public authority is responsible for the actual design of the processing and the way it is used. These elements lead to the conclusion that the public authority establishing the switch point shall be considered as a joint controller, as well as a point of contact for data subjects' requests.' *Ibid.*, p.24.

REFERENCES

Banner, Lois W., "Coming of Age: A Cultural Studies Approach to Aging", *Journal of Women's History*, Vol. 12, No. 4, Winter 2001, pp. 212-214. http://muse.jhu.edu/login?uri=/journals/journal_of_womens_history/v012/12.4banner.html

De Hert, P. and S. Gutwirth, ''Privacy, data protection and law enforcement: Opacity of the individual and transparency of power'', in E. Claes, A. Duff and S.Gutwirth (eds.), *Privacy and the criminal law*, Intersentia, Antwerp/Oxford, 2006, pp. 61–104.

Gutwirth, S., *Privacy and the information age*, Rowman & Littlefield Publishers, Lanham, 2002.

Nussbaum, Martha C., *Frontiers of Justice. Disability, Nationality, Species membership*, The Belknap Press of Harvard University Press, Cambridge (Mass), 2007.

Rigaux, F., *La protection de la vie privée et des autres biens de la personnalité*, Bruylant, Bruxelles-Paris, 1990.

Rodotà, S., *Tecnologie e diritti*, Il Mulino, Bologna, 1995

Warren S.,and L. Brandeis, "The right to privacy", *Harvard Law Review*, Vol. IV, No. 5, 15 Dec 1890.

Westin, Alan F., *Privacy and Freedom*, Atheneum, New York, NY, 1967.

Wright, D. Serge Gutwirth, Michael Friedewald, Paul De Hert, Marc Langheinrich, Anna Moscibroda, "Privacy, trust and policy-making: Challenges and responses,", in *Computer Law and Security Review* 25 (2009) 69-83.

Convention for the protection of individuals with regard to automatic processing of personal data (ETS No. 108, 28.01.1981)

Directive 95/46/EC of the European Parliament and of the Council of 24 October 1995 on the protection of individuals with regard to the processing of personal data and on the free movement of such data, OJ 1995, L 281, p. 31.

Regulation (EC) No 45/2001 of the European Parliament and of the Council of 18 December 2000 on the protection of individuals with regard to the processing of personal data by the Community institutions and bodies and on the free movement of such data, OJ 2001, L 8.

Directive 2002/58/EC of the European Parliament and of the Council of 12 July 2002 concerning the processing of personal data and the protection of privacy in the electronic communications sector (Directive on privacy and electronic communications), OJ 2002 L 201, p. 37; as revised by Directive 2009/136/EC of the European Parliament and of the Council of 25 November 2009.

Directive 2006/24/EC of the European Parliament and of the Council of 15 March 2006 on the retention of data generated or processed in connection with the provision of publicly available electronic communications services or of public communications networks and amending Directive 2002/58/EC, OJ 2006 L 105.

Council Framework Decision 2008/977/JHA of 27 November 2008 on the protection of personal data processed in the framework of police and judicial cooperation in criminal matters OJ 2008 L 350.

Article 29 Data Protection Working Party, *The Future of Privacy*. Joint contribution to the Consultation of the European Commission on the legal framework for the fundamental right to protection of personal data, Adopted on 01 December 2009, 02356/09/EN, WP 168.

Article 29 Working Party, Opinion 1/2010 on the concepts of "controller" and "processor", 16 February 2010, WP 169. http://ec.europa.eu/justice_home/fsj/privacy/workinggroup/wpdocs/2010_en.htm

SENIOR project, "The perspective of lawmakers", by P. De Hert, presentation delivered to SENIOR final conference, 27 November 2009

SENIOR project, *Ethics of e-inclusion of elderly people*, Discussion paper for the workshop on ethics and e-inclusion, Bled (Slovenia), 12 May 2008.

CHAPTER FIVE. ON CONSENT

By Paul De Hert and Eugenio Mantovani

INTRODUCTION

Starting from an analysis of consent in human right law we pause on the data processing context, where consent is increasingly a formalised a notion. We surmise that sociological changes in the IT societies, unbalanced relations between user and client organizations, complexity of data processing, and increasing situations of incapacity affecting large sectors of the ageing population, pose challenges to the notion of consent. The snag, from an elderly perspective, is to find solutions that, while not frustrating individual self-determination and liberty, assist, where appropriate, the individual declaration of consent and avoid putting on him or her excessive responsibility.

I. LEGAL FRAMEWORK

The domain field in which the legal notion of consent originates is the bio-medical domain. At supranational level, the guiding provisions on consent in the biomedical area are provided by the 1997 Council of Europe Convention on Biomedicine and Human Rights[1] and Recommendation 99 (4) of the Council of Europe[2]. The 1997 Oviedo Convention recognises and regulates the right of the patient to give his free and informed consent before any medical examination or medical treatment[3], while recommendation 99 (4) of the Council of Europe contains in principles 22 to 28 rules on the consent of incapable adults.

Outside the biomedical domain, positive human rights law codifies consent only in few cases. Indeed, one of the innovations of the 2000 EU Charter of Fundamental Rights is that it mentions informed consent as part of article 3 (right to integrity of the person).[4] In the data protection legal framework, the 'mother' Convention on data

---

[1] Convention for the protection of Human Rights and dignity of the human being with regard to the application of biology and medicine: Convention on Human Rights and Biomedicine CETS No.: 164, Oviedo, 4.4.1997.

[2] Council of Europe, *Recommendation No. R (99) of the Committee of Ministers to Member States on principles concerning the legal protection of incapable adults*, adopted by the Committee of Ministers on 23 February 1999, at the 660th meeting of the Ministers' Deputies.

[3] Article 5 states that health care may usually only be provided if the person concerned gives his or her consent. Article 7 states that, when the patient is suffering from a mental disorder, healthcare personnel are authorised to impose a treatment, but only in such cases where failure to act may pose a serious threat to the person concerned health status, and subject to conditions prescribed by law, including supervisory, control and appeal procedures. Article 8 and article 9 provides exception to the asking consent in case, respectively, of emergency, and where the patient is not in a state to express his or her wishes

[4] Article 3 (Right to the integrity of the person):
1. Everyone has the right to respect for his or her physical and mental integrity.
2. In the fields of medicine and biology, the following must be respected in particular:
- the free and informed consent of the person concerned, according to the procedures laid down by law,
- the prohibition of eugenic practices, in particular those aiming at the selection of persons,

protection, the 1981 Convention ETS No 108 of the Council of Europe, did not contain a provision on consent. Consent was introduced with Directive 95/46/EC as a legitimate, as with the law, source or ground for data processing.[5] To be valid, says the Directive, consent needs to be freely given, it must be informed, specific, and unambiguous.[6] The consent by a user or subscriber in Directive 2002/58/EC, dealing with privacy and electronic communications, corresponds to the data subject's consent in Directive 95/46/EC.[7] Rules on consent are also contained in the numerous EU directives dealing with distance contract[8], electronic commerce[9], and distant financial services.[10] However, the reference provision remains article 7 and 8 of the data protection directive.

The case law of the European Court of Human Rights shows the delicate legal and ethical implications of consent in the biomedical domain. In *Evans v. UK*[11], the Court accepted that a legislature was entitled to adopt a system of regulation which drew a 'bright line' on who is entitled to give consent.[12] The majority of the Court concurred that allowing Evans to override the male donor's consent would have produced 'new and even more intractable difficulties of arbitrariness and inconsistency.'[13] In a joint dissenting opinion, however, judges Traja and Mijović disapproved of what they referred to as a 'contractual' approach taken by the Court. It was necessary, in their opinion, to take 'into account the specific rights in the specific situation balancing the burden and conditions imposed on each party.[14]

- the prohibition on making the human body and its parts as such a source of financial gain,
- the prohibition of the reproductive cloning of human beings.
[5] Article 7 and 8 of Directive 95/46/EC.
[6] Article 2 (h) of Directive 95/46/EC., which states that 'Any freely given specific and informed indication of his wishes by which the data subject signifies his agreement to personal data relating to him being processed.'
[7] Article 2(f) of Directive 2002/58/EC. ('-'consent' by a user or subscriber corresponds to the data subject's consent in Directive 95/46/EC;')
[8] Directive 97/7/EC of the European Parliament and of the Council of 20 May 1997 on the Protection of Consumers in respect of Distance Contracts (also known as Directive 97/7 on distance contract), articles 4 (position of those unable to give consent), 9 (inertia selling), 10 (means of communications).
[9] Directive 2000/31/EC of the European Parliament and of the Council of 8 June 2000 on certain legal aspects of information society services, in particular electronic commerce, in the Internal Market ('Directive on electronic commerce'), OJ L 178, 17.7.2000, p. 1–16. Relevant for provisions on unsolicited commercial communications.
[10] Directive 2002/65/EC of the European Parliament and of the Council of 23 September 2002 concerning the distance marketing of consumer financial services and amending Council Directive 90/619/EEC and Directives 97/7/EC and 98/27/EC (Directive on distant financial services), OJ L 271, 9.10.2002.
[11] ECtHR, *Evans v United Kingdom* (2006) 43 EHRR 21.
[12] In *Evans v. UK* the Court considered whether the British legislation on of in vitro fertilization (IVF), the Human Fertilisation and Embryology Act 1990 ('the 1990 Act'), was compatible with the Convention. The applicant had had her ovaries removed for medical reasons, but she and her partner had frozen six embryos, with the intention of later implanting the embryos in her uterus. However, the relationship broke up, and the applicant's former partner withdrew his consent to the treatment. Under the 1990 Act, the consent of both parties is an essential condition of the treatment, and this consent could be withdrawn at any time. The applicant brought court proceedings to compel the giving of consent, but these were unsuccessful.
[13] *Ibid.*, para. 65.
[14] ECtHR, Evans v. UK, *Joint Dissenting Opinion of Judges Traja and Mijović*, 'Here the differences between, as well as the burden imposed on, each party seem to us of the utmost importance. ... While the applicant has no other way of having a genetic child, her partner, J, may have children with another woman and so satisfy his need for parenthood. exercise might lead to a different conclusion if the applicant had another child or the possibility of having a child without using J's genetic material.' They also argued that 'bright-line' legislation is exceptional in the European context and should therefore, be

In *Pretty v. UK*[15], the Court held that, notwithstanding the consent of the Pretty, husband and wife, the national criminal law legislation prevailed over their decision to terminate one of the partners' lives. The Court ruled that neither article 2 (right to life) nor article 8 (right to private life) of the Convention could be interpreted as to include a right for a person to be assisted in committing suicide.

In *Glass v. UK*[16], the Court re-affirmed that individual consent must be taken seriously by medical experts, also when it is taken on behalf of an incapacitated person. The Court held that the decision of the authorities to override the mother's objections to the proposed treatment on her son, in the absence of an authorisation by a court, violated hers and her son's right to a private life.

The foregoing shows how consent pierces into the *sancta sanctorum* of liberty, *viz.* the nature and the extent of control over our own bodies in times of bio-technological revolution. The foregoing also indicates, however, that consent in not an option when other core rights are involved. Not only criminal law provisions (as in Pretty) can not be consented off, but also other fundamental rights. This includes the right to body integrity, biological life and also daily life situations, such as monitoring of employees at the workplace. In both cases, a fundamental human right, the right to privacy, puts a red light which individual consent cannot circumvent. In many cases, however, when the core human right (e.g., to private life) is protected, consent is admitted, provided that other guarantees are in place. Provided that the core human right to privacy is protected, consent can be also formalized as a general waiver. For instance, privacy policy in standardized machine-readable format can be read automatically by a web browser, which automatically gives consent to, e.g., cookies or access or storage to the user terminal equipment.[17]

The notion of consent thus applies on the whole series of activities and transactions performed via electronic means. In the off line world, consent constitutes the legal form through which expressions of will and obligations are validly exchanged. Specific questions arise when consent is exchanged electronically[18]. Dematerialisation of the exchange, physical distance between the parties, and related risks of counterfeited goods, frauds, liability issues requires a system of protection based on the idea that the user/consumer is in a weaker position than the seller of goods or supplier of services as far as his bargaining power and his level of knowledge are concerned. For the European Court of Justice, this situation may lead

---

strictly scrutinized by the Court.' http://portal.unesco.org/shs/en/files/9513/11453766971Evans_UK.pdf/Evans_UK.pdf
See also M. Ford, 'Evans v United Kingdom: What Implications for the Jurisprudence of Pregnancy?', in *Human Rights Law Review* (2008) 8(1): 171-184. K. Wright, 'Competing Interests in Reproduction: The Case of Natallie Evans', in *King's Law Journal*, Vol. 19, No. 1, 2008. For a broader legal perspective see B. Bennett, *Health Law Kaleidoscope*, Ashgate, London, 2008, especially pages 105-110.
[15] ECtHR, *Pretty v. The United Kingdom*, judgement of 29 April 2002. Diane Pretty asked recognition of the right to die with the assistance of her husband (assisted suicide) on the basis of article 2 and 8 ECHR
[16] ECtHR, *Glass v UK* (2004) 1 FLR 1019.
[17] Compare Article 29 Working Party, *Opinion 1/2009 on the proposals amending Directive 2002/58/EC on privacy and electronic communications (e-Privacy Directive)*, 10 February 2009, WP 159, para. 7.
[18] On electronic consent see H. Jacquemin (CRID- FUNDP), 'Le consentement électronique en droit européen', in *Journal du droit européen*, 2009.

to 'the consumer agreeing to terms drawn up in advance by the seller or supplier without being able to influence the content of those terms.'[19]

Under EU legislation, the right to give or refuse consent is reinforced by a set of procedural guarantees ascribable to the right of the user/consumer to withdraw his or her consent, to the obligation to inform, and to the multiplication of formal requirements.

According to the distance contact Directive 97/07, the right to withdraw or retract[20] gives the buyer the faculty to withdraw from the contract without having to pay any penalty and without having to provide any motive within a period of notice. Such being the case, the provider must reimburse the consumer as soon as possible and no later than 30 days.[21]

As far as the obligation to inform is concerned, as a general rule, a person who concludes an online contract should be able to obtain all relevant information necessary to make a decision.[22] The consumer, in practice, should be able, when he or she wishes so, to contact the retailer to ask questions about the product. The difference between e-contact and human to human contact is here particularly evident, as Article 5.1 of 2000/31/EC states.[23] The Court of Justice, in interpreting article 5.1 [24], reckons that there may be different means, other than electronic ones, to fulfill the obligations of article 5.1.[25] Reasonable accommodation, discussed above, may therefore be required to appraise alternative ways to ask or obtain consent.

Eventually, formal requirements are intended to certify that a person genuinely gave his or her informed consent. Directive 2002/65/EC establishes in article 5 (Communication of the contractual terms and conditions and of the prior information) that 'the supplier shall communicate to the consumer all the contractual terms and conditions and the information [...] on paper or on another durable medium available and accessible to the consumer [...]'. Article 11.1 (Sanctions) obliges member states to set an 'effective, proportional and dissuasive sanction [...] in the event of the

---

[19] European Court of Justice, C-168/05 of 26 October 2006, *Mostaza Claro*, paragraph 25. See also ECJ, Joined cases C-240/98 to C-244/98 of 27 June 2000, *Oceano Grupo*, paragraph 25.

[20] Article 6 of Directive 97/07/EC and article 6 of Directive 2002/65/EC

[21] Article 6(1) and (2) of Directive 97/07/EC provides:
'Right of withdrawal
1. For any distance contract the consumer shall have a period of at least seven working days in which to withdraw from the contract without penalty and without giving any reason. The only charge that may be made to the consumer because of the exercise of his right of withdrawal is the direct cost of returning the goods.
2. Where the right of withdrawal has been exercised by the consumer pursuant to this Article, the supplier shall be obliged to reimburse the sums paid by the consumer free of charge. The only charge that may be made to the consumer because of the exercise of his right of withdrawal is the direct cost of returning the goods. Such reimbursement must be carried out as soon as possible and in any case within 30 days.'

[22] Article 4 and 5 of Directive 97/07/EC; article ' and 4 of Directive 2002/65; article 5, 10, 11 of ecommerce directive 2000/31/EC.

[23] Article 5 (General information to be provided) Directive 2000/31/EC. 'Member States shall ensure that the service provider shall render easily, directly and permanently accessible to the recipients of the service [and competent authorities]' at least information about the name of the provider, address, including email address which 'allow him to be contacted rapidly and communicated with in a direct and effective manner.'

[24] ECJ, C-298/07 of 16 October 2008, *Bundesverband der Verbraucherzentralen und Verbraucherverbände –Verbraucherzentrale Bundesverband eV v. deutsche internet versicherung AG.*

[25] *Ibid.*, para 31. 'There are forms of communication other than by telephone able to satisfy the criteria of direct and effective communication [...], that is, communication without an intermediary which would be sufficiently fluid, such as those established by personal contact at the premises of the service provider with a person in charge or by fax.'

supplier's failure to comply [...] with national provisions adopted pursuant to this Directive', including article 5. Such being the case, however, national measures setting procedural requirements will have to be justified and proportional, least they may be construed as obstacles to free movement and turned down by courts.[26]

II. PROBLEMS

As the above mentioned Article 29 Working Party 'Future of Privacy' report contends, consent requirements should be specified to meet the challenges of the expanding information society. These challenges are illustrated by sociological changes in the attitude towards privacy, informational asymmetry and unbalanced power relations, complexity of data processing systems, and the capacity of persons affected by mental disabilities to give consent.

1. SOCIOLOGICAL CHANGES IN THE INFORMATION SOCIETY

The Future of Privacy report questions the level of empowerment that the EU data protection legal regime grants to the individual. The Group notices a marked change in the behaviour of citizens/data subjects with respect to data protection. As a consequence of sociological changes and new ways of data collection, such as profiling, data subjects 'can be careless with their own privacy' and they are 'sometimes willing to trade privacy for perceived benefits.'[27] On the other hand, individuals still place great expectations on those with whom they do business as more and more users, especially Internet users, are themselves processors of personal data. The Working group is of the view that the data subject should be given a stronger position in the data protection framework so he or she is enabled to play a more active role.[28] One may ask whether consent is sufficient to attain a stronger position or if other measures are necessary.

2. UNBALANCED RELATIONS

There are many cases in which consent can not be given freely, especially when there is a clear unbalance between the data subject and the data controller (for example in the employment context, relations of care, of dependency, or when personal data must be provided to public authorities).[29] While consent is an expression of individual liberty, it is usually entangled in a web of power relations or background conditions, which in fact affect or direct the liberty to give or refuse consent. As article 23

---

[26] ECJ, C-205/07 of 16 December 2008, *Lodewijk Gysbrechts.* The ruling concerned a provision of a Belgian law of 1991 on commerce and consumer protection. Indeed, while member states are free to adopt stringent measures to protect the consent of the weak party in online transactions, such measures must be in line with EU principle of free movements of goods and services. In a recent preliminary ruling, the question was whether the obligation that the law put on suppliers of distance sale to have à la carte means of payment other that the credit card, violated article 23 of the EC treaty on free movement of goods. The Court held that the obligation on suppliers to offer consumers means of payment other than credit card constituted a measure having equivalent effect to a quantitative restriction on exports.

[27] Future of privacy, *op.cit.*, para. 59.

[28] Future of privacy, *op.cit.*, para. 60.

[29] Future of privacy, *op.cit.*, para. 66.

paragraph 3 of the European Social Charter mentioned in chapter III recognises[30], older persons in living institutions or living in conditions of dependence (for instance nursing homes, or poor elderly relying on welfare benefits, persons who live alone, persons affected by chronic diseases…) may find themselves in such a situation where it is assumed that giving consent will be rewarded, while refusal might provoke some retaliation, e.g., reduced benefit or changed living arrangements. It does not matter whether the 'assumption' is verifiable or not. What matters is being in a position susceptible to manipulation or exploitation.

3. COMPLEXITY, INFORMATION ASYMMETRY AND REQUIREMENTS

One of the requirements of consent is that the data subject is in the conditions to make an informed decision about what will happen if he or she decides to consent to the processing of his or her data. However, the abundance and complexities of data collection practices, business models, vendor relationships and technological applications 'in many cases outstrip the individual's ability or willingness to make decisions to control the use and sharing of information through active choice.'[31] In fact, the report warns that 'article 7 of Directive 95/46/EC is not always properly applied, particularly in the context of the internet, where implicit consent does not always lead to unambiguous and explicit consent prior to the processing of personal data.'

4. CAPACITY TO CONSENT

As a general rule, only persons who are legally capable can give consent. For the legally incapacitated, consent can be construed according to procedures established by law.[32] According to the Court of Strasbourg case law, the effects of restrictions to the legal capacity should be limited to the purpose of the measure.[33] The problem with limitations arises when the capacity to consent fluctuates through periods of time or situations. In such a case, it is difficult to ground the conditions for valid consent. Importantly, statistics indicate that, in the wake of demographic changes, there will be a larger number of cases where the capacity to consent is, not absent, but impaired.[34]

---

[30] Article 23 paragraph c) calls upon states to 'guarantee elderly persons living in institutions appropriate support, while respecting their privacy, and participation in decisions concerning living conditions in the institution.'

[31] Future of privacy, para. 67.

[32] In particular 1997 Council of Europe Convention on Biomedicine and Human Rights, articles 5 to 9 and Recommendation 99 (4) of the Council of Europe on the legal protection of incapable adults, principles 22 to 28.

[33] ECHR, *Winterwerp v. The Netherlands*, (A/33): (1979) 2 EHRR 387, discussed above concerning the definition of unsound mind ex. Article 5.1. ECHR..

[34] 'Statistics suggest that one in four of the population will experience mental disorders at some time in their life. For the majority of those people, the disorder will be relatively minor. Nonetheless, one tenth of the population will be subject to a serious neuropsychiatric condition, such as schizophrenia, depression, addictive disorder, and dementia at some time in their life. These figures are relatively constant internationally, and do not appear to vary markedly based on wealth or distinctions between urban and rural environments.' P. Bartlett, O. Lewis & O. Thorold, *Mental disabilities and the European Convention on Human Rights,* Martinus Nijhoff Publishers, Leiden/Boston, 2007, p. 2. See also Chapter I, VI.3; and SENIOR Project, D2.3 'Intelligent User Interface', Report, p. 11, ft. 44.

This may require, as the European Social Charter supervisory Committee holds, the organization of a procedure for 'assisted decision making.'[35]

III. PROPOSAL

1. SETTING THE STAGE

Consent remains an important ground for processing but in an increasing number of cases in which there is a clear unbalance or asymmetry in decision-making power and information, 'consent is an inappropriate ground for processing but nevertheless often falsely claimed to be the applicable ground.'[36] The conclusion of the article 29 Working Group is that 'the new legal framework should specify the requirement of consent.'[37] In the following lines, we take stock of these criticisms and put forth a proposal.

In chapter II we pointed out how many elderly people may live in situations of vulnerability stemming from the combined effect of biological frailty and social attitudes towards the value-power of old age. We surmised, drawing from the example of King Lear, that frail, older persons lacking own means are dependent on the social arrangements they live in. In the context of highly technological societies where active aging prevails as the paradigm of old-age normalcy, ICT for elderly people is accepted and introduced, not only as means to stay independent, but also as a complement, or replacement, to human based health care, lack of trained personnel, lack of financial resources, attitudes towards migrant work, new family structures and so on. These and other factors also play a role in determining the level of privacy that an individual is expected to willingly consent away.

The other element which needs to be taken into consideration is the complexity of ICT systems. Such a complexity makes it tricky for users to control his or her 'electronic body' or personal information. It is evident that modern ICT processing activities are and remain opaque to most users. Even when consent is given, the user might not be able to use his or her data protection rights. It is not only a matter of complexity of operating systems; it is also a question of quantity. In the future, users are likely to receive reiterated requests to use their stored data for new purposes.[38] Even the data controller might genuinely ignore what use of, e.g., health data, future research will require. It is unrealistic to think that the user is equipped, or willing, to understand what the new processing activity is about, whether he or she should trust it or not. The most practical solution is then to sign a waiver. But this solution is dangerous as it might engender a practice of forgoing the right to have a say about future uses of one's data. This unsatisfactory situation is particularly worrisome for individuals in conditions of vulnerability, who may give away personal information for convenience or need.

---

[35] Council of Europe, European Committee of Social Rights, Conclusions 2003, France, p. 186: ' The Committee notes that 'elderly persons at times may have reduced decision making powers or no such powers or capacity at all. Therefore there should exist a procedure for 'assisted decision making'' See also: Council of Europe, *Digest* of Case law of the European Committee of Social Rights, 1 September 2008, p.329).

[36] Future of privacy, para. 68.

[37] Ibid., para 69.

[38] For instance, personal data such as health data or genetic data can be processed for different research purposes.

2. THE SNAG WITH CAPACITY

Concerning the capacity to give consent, questions emerge when the individual who gives consent is cognitively disabled. The challenge lies in the fact that often the capacity to consent is specific to a particular decision, not for all decisions; it can also fluctuate throughout short periods of times. This poses two problems. The first concerns the declaration of legal incapacitation and the second the kind of technological solution that can be applied.[39]

As a premise, it is important to clarify that to give or refuse consent a person must be considered 'capable' by the law.[40] The concept of capacity is, just like the concept of normalcy analyzed in chapter II, difficult to fix. Old age frailty is the result of concurring physical, environmental and social conditions. Even conditions such as dementia, bi-polar disorder, schizophrenia, Alzheimer must be considered not only medically, but also against concurring physical, environmental and social conditions.[41] Social norms and attitudes towards ageing, discussed in chapter II, can exercise great clout. Indeed, given an accepted normalcy-level, society may benevolently want to afford the –increasing number of – people living in various, fluctuating, and changing conditions of dementia, a practical, straight solution. As we have pointed out above, we should also remind ourselves that ICT for elderly people is often accepted and introduced not to empower individuals to stay independent, but to complement, or replace, human based health care, lack of trained personnel, strained financial resources, migrant work, family structures and so on.

In most countries the declaration of incapacitation as based on a medical model of capacity has heavy consequences. For the law of many European countries a legally incapacitated person is almost a non-person: he or she is deprived of the ability to decide upon many aspects of his or her life.[42] This happens regardless of the fact that people suffering from mental disorders may be able to take some decisions and not others. And regardless of the fact that the law requires that interventions be the least restrictive to individual freedom.[43] Similarly, ICT solutions adopted pursuant to a medical-legal model of capacity often offer a one way option. Electronic devices, such as bracelets, which control and monitor individual behaviour may end up trumping functions that the individual retains the capacity to perform, and violate the principle of least liberty restrictive interventions.[44] Legal concerns are complicated by sociological changes and disequilibriums of power, discussed above.

---

[39] Monitoring technological developments offer the possibility, for instance through electronic bracelets, to position, control, support people affected by forms of mild dementia or Alzheimer disease. The decision to wear a bracelet depends on the consent of the person concerned.

[40] In the cases of legally incapacitated the provision of the Council of Europe Convention on Biomedicine must be respected, see *above*.

[41] People affected by these diseases might from time to time get 'high' and develop manic behaviour such as going out and spending all money (bi-polar disorder); start forgetting things and have difficulties to do things like cooking (Alzheimer); develop mild learning difficulties, have hard time doing simple arithmetical operations and so on. See SENIOR project, WP2 report, p. 25.

[42] P. Bartlett, O. Lewis & O. Thorold, *Mental disabilities and the European Convention on Human Rights.*, p.14 ss.

[43] ECHR, *Winterwerp v. The Netherlands*, at paragraph 39: '...In the Court's opinion, except in emergency cases, the individual concerned should not be deprived of his liberty unless he has been reliably shown to be of 'unsound mind'. The very nature of what has to be established before the competent national authority - that is, a true mental disorder - calls for objective medical expertise. Further, the mental disorder must be of a kind or degree warranting compulsory confinement. What is more, the validity of continued confinement depends upon the persistence of such a disorder (.)'

[44] See Chapter 7, 'Ethical guidance on use of wandering technologies in Scotland'.

Having said that, one must still recognise there is a genuine matter of justice which imposes helping frail older adults and to accommodate, as appropriate, the impairments that hinder their personal and social development. Accommodation or help may very well include technological solutions that, while helping the individual, significantly alter his or her informational privacy or threaten his or her dignity. Given the high number of persons who are likely to live well beyond the age of 80, periods of physical and cognitive dependence may become more common. An elderly normal person may be disabled for several years, thirty or even forty years, perhaps longer than the total life span of some people with a lifelong disability. As more people live longer into old age, one can expect that also the distinction between normalcy and non-normalcy, capacity and incapacitation, become problematic.[45]

3. CONCIERGE

Different factors play a role in determining the level of capacity that an individual retains and needs to participate in social life. From the users' perspective, the snag is to find solutions that do not frustrate individual self-determination and assist, where appropriate, the individual declaration of consent without reducing it to a mere form, open to exploitation. In pursuance of principle 22 of the Council of Europe Recommendation No. R (99) 4, consideration should be given to the designation of persons or bodies for the purpose of authorising interventions of different types in contexts such as family, living institutions, workplace or health care.[46] As the Glass case mentioned above suggests, choices on best health treatments gain greater legitimacy when the views of family or networks of people have been taken into account.[47] In the context where there is an evident unbalance in power relations, such as in the workplace, collective agreements are better suited to empower the worker than reliance on the individual and his consent.[48] In the e-health care context, ICT services for seniors involve many actors, nurses, suppliers, providers, industry, technicians. Public policy has to take this complexity into account.[49] New technologies often affect not only the individual user but also caregivers and/or family members.[50] Where care impacts carers and families, they too have rights to dignity

---

[45] Francis Fukuyama suggests that living longer life may alter our conception of human nature. F. Fukuyama, 'Our post-human future: Consequences of the Biotechnological Revolution', Farrar, Straus & Giroux, New York, 2002, chapter 6 and 8.

[46] Recommendation 99 (4) of the Council of Europe on the legal protection of incapable adults, seen above.

[47] ECtHR, *Glass v UK* (2004) 1 FLR 1019.

[48] P. De Hert, 'Reply: The Use of Labour Law to Regulate Employer Profiling: Making Data Protection Relevant Again', in M. Hildebrandt & S. Gutwirth (eds), *Profiling the European Citizen,* Springer, 2008, p. 226-237. According to De Hert 'As a set of rules and guarantees focusing on the individual person, [data protection legal framework] does not fit well in an area of society where power differences between the parties concerned are considerable. The only vocabulary that is accepted and recognised is the one used in collective labour law, where union and employee-representatives discuss most issues, including the ones that concern individual rights'. And concludes saying that '[t]he success of data protection will depend on its ability to find its way into this collectivised vocabulary.'

[49] SEC (2007) 0811 final, paragraph 3.2.1.

[50] Recall the opinion of the European Social Charter's Committee of Social Rights. In order to assess whether elderly person have enough resources to lead a decent life, the Committee takes into account the average wage levels and the overall cost of living, costs of transport, of medical care and medicine, as well as 'the existence of a carer's allowance for family members looking after an elderly relative.' Committee of Social Rights, *Digest*,p.149.

and respect and should therefore be involved.[51] Complex modern ICT processing activities are and remain opaque to most users, including perfectly capable, ICT skilled (older) citizens. The consequences of their wrongful processing, particularly in the field of e-health, may be very relevant for personal dignity. Focussing in the specific area of genetics, Irma van der Ploeg[52] suggests that third natural persons or legal persons, such as charitable trusts, monitor the respect of fair processing principles, and assist, upon authorisation, the data subject or give consent on her or his behalf.

On a similar line, our proposal: a 'concierge' of responsible persons could help older individuals go through the hurdles and obscurities of health, work, or social services (ICT) systems and, where possible, support individual decisions. Just like in a real-life 'concierge', where some responsibilities and decisions which still concern the inhabitants of the building are not taken directly by them, e.g., watching the main door and letting people in, but fall on the concierge. Similarly, older people may find in a concierge help to carry out some tasks or functions, both in the off-line and on-line world.

REFERENCES

Bartlett, P. O. Lewis & O. Thorold, *Mental disabilities and the European Convention on Human Rights*, Martinus Nijhoff Publishers, Leiden/Boston, 2007.

Bennett, B., *Health law Kaleidoscope. Health law rights in a global age*, Ashgate Publishing: Aldershot, UK, 2008.

De Hert, P., "Reply: The Use of Labour Law to Regulate Employer Profiling: Making Data Protection Relevant Again", in M. Hildebrandt & S. Gutwirth (eds), *Profiling the European Citizen*, Springer, 2008, p. 226-237.

Fukuyama, F., *Our post-human future: Consequences of the Biotechnological Revolution*, Farrar, Straus & Giroux, New York, 2002.

Ford, M., "Evans v United Kingdom: What Implications for the Jurisprudence of Pregnancy?", *in Human Rights Law Review* (2008) 8(1): 171-184.

http://www.enisa.europa.eu/act/rm/files/deliverables/being-diabetic-2011

Jacquemin, H., (CRID- FUNDP), "Le consentement électronique en droit européen' , in *Journal du droit européen*, 2009.

Nussbaum, Martha C., *Frontiers of Justice. Disability, Nationality, Species membership*, The Belknap Press of Harvard University Press, Cambridge (Mass), 2007.

Van der Ploeg, I., Genetics, biometrics and the informatization of the body, *Ann. Istituto Superiore della Sanità*, 2007, vol. 43, No. 1: 44-50.

Wright, K., "Competing Interests in Reproduction: The Case of Natallie Evans", in *King's Law Journal*, Vol. 19, No. 1, 2008.

---

[51] According to Madeleine Starr of Carers UK, those providing heavy end care are 'twice as likely than the general population to be in poor health themselves, as a result of caring...[they also experience] significant financial disadvantages; very frequently people have to give up work and therefore give up their income...this affects not only their working lives but it also affects their ability to put into the pension system...[thereby] creating a situation where carers themselves might go into poverty in their own retirement.' SENIOR, D.1.5 WP 1 Report Final, p. 97.

[52] Irma van der Ploeg, *Genetics, biometrics and the informatization of the body,* Ann. Istituto Superiore della Sanità, 2007, vol. 43, No. 1: 44-50.

Directive 95/46/EC of the European Parliament and of the Council of 24 October 1995 on the protection of individuals with regard to the processing of personal data and on the free movement of such data, OJ 1995, L 281, p. 31.

Directive 2002/58/EC of the European Parliament and of the Council of 12 July 2002 concerning the processing of personal data and the protection of privacy in the electronic communications sector (Directive on privacy and electronic communications), OJ 2002 L 201, p. 37; as revised by Directive 2009/136/EC of the European Parliament and of the Council of 25 November 2009.

Directive 97/7/EC of the European Parliament and of the Council of 20 May 1997 on the protection of consumers in respect of distance contracts - Statement by the Council and the Parliament re Article 6 (1) - Statement by the Commission re Article 3 (1), first indent OJ L 144, 4.6.1997, p. 19–27.

Directive 2000/31/EC of the European Parliament and of the Council of 8 June 2000 on certain legal aspects of information society services, in particular electronic commerce, in the Internal Market ('Directive on electronic commerce'), OJ L 178, 17.7.2000, p. 1–16.

Directive 2002/65/EC of the European Parliament and of the Council of 23 September 2002 concerning the distance marketing of consumer financial services and amending Council Directive 90/619/EEC and Directives 97/7/EC and 98/27/EC (Directive on distant financial services), OJ L 271, 9.10.2002.

European Commission, Staff Working Document on Ageing well, SEC (2007) 0811 final

Article 29 Data Protection Working Party, *The Future of Privacy*. Joint contribution to the Consultation of the European Commission on the legal framework for the fundamental right to protection of personal data, Adopted on 01 December 2009, 02356/09/EN, WP 168.

Article 29 Data Protection Working Party, Opinion 1/2009 on the proposals amending Directive 2002/58/EC on privacy and electronic communications (e-Privacy Directive), 10 February 2009, WP 159.

ENISA, *Being diabetic in 2011. Identifying emerging and future risks in remote health monitoring and treatment*, 1 March 2009.

ECJ, C-168/05 of 26 October 2006, *Mostaza Claro*.

ECJ, Joined cases C-240/98 to C-244/98 of 27 June 2000, *Oceano Grupo*

ECJ, C-298/07 of 16 October 2008, *Bundesverband der Verbraucherzentralen und Verbraucherverbände –Verbraucherzentrale Bundesverband eV v. deutsche internet versicherung AG*.

ECJ, C-205/07 of 16 December 2008, *Lodewijk Gysbrechts*.

SENIOR project, D.1.5, WP 1 Report Final, 2008.

SENIOR Project, D2.3 "Intelligent User Interface", by P. De Hert and E. Mantovani, 2008.

SENIOR project, WP 2 Report Final, 2009.

Council of Europe, Convention for the protection of Human Rights and dignity of the human being with regard to the application of biology and medicine: Convention on Human Rights and Biomedicine CETS No.: 164, Oviedo, 4.4.1997.

Council of Europe, Recommendation No. R (99) of the Committee of Ministers to Member States on principles concerning the legal protection of incapable adults, adopted by the Committee of Ministers on 23 February 1999, at the 660th meeting of the Ministers' Deputies.

Digest of Case law of the European Committee of Social Rights, 1 September 2008, p.147-148, http://www.coe.int/t/dghl/monitoring/socialcharter/Digest/DigestSept2008_en.pdf.

Council of Europe, European Committee of Social Rights, Conclusions on France, 2003.

ECtHR, *Pretty v. United Kingdom*, (1997) 24 EHRR 423.

ECtHR, *Glass v United Kingdom*, (2004) 1 FLR 1019.

ECtHR, *Evans v United Kingdom*, (2006) 43 EHRR 21.

ECtHR, *Evans v. United Kingdom*, Joint Dissenting Opinion of Judges Traja and Mijović
http://portal.unesco.org/shs/en/files/9513/11453766971Evans_UK.pdf/Evans_UK.pdf

ECtHR, *Winterwerp v. The Netherlands*, (1979) 2 EHRR 387.

CHAPTER SIX. A SURVEY OF TECHNOLOGY FOR THE ELDERLY

By Kush Wadhwa and David Wright

INTRODUCTION

Information highway. Internet revolution. Digital age. Information society. These familiar phrases are all used to describe the surging leaps in technology experienced over the past two decades. The late 20th and early 21st centuries have seen a driving force of technological change that continues to advance solutions for challenges facing society, as well as open up the collective imagination of what is possible. According to Raymond Kurzweil's Law of Accelerating Returns, the overall rate of technical progress is currently doubling approximately every decade. As a result, the 21st century will see almost a thousand times greater technological change than the 20th century. At a point Kurzweil refers to as 'The Singularity,' technological change will be so rapid and profound, it will represent a rupture in the fabric of human history.[1] He and other futurists predict that the exponential improvement in technological advances will eventually lead to a point at which progress in technology occurs almost instantly.

This acceleration in technological advancement provides extraordinary benefits to society, accompanied by extraordinary challenges. The pace of technological change has sometimes been at odds with the available supportive infrastructure, or the ability of the legal system to provide effective regulation and protection. Beyond this, technological change can highlight differences between the haves and have-nots in society, as financial, cultural, social, gender, disability or age-based issues may act as a determinant in access or adoption of new technologies. In many cases, such as technologies geared towards entertainment applications, these lower adoption rates may not be highly consequential, but as governments and civil society organisations rely upon advances in technology to provide key services to citizens, ensuring access to such technologies is critical to provide for an inclusive society.

This chapter examines technology as it impacts the elderly, though many of technologies mentioned herein also have an impact on other marginalised populations who confront similar challenges (e.g., financial, physical impairments, etc.), and discusses technologies in terms of the impact it has upon several key aspects of the individual within society:

- **In the home.** Emerging technologies are extending the ability of elders to live independently for longer periods of time, reducing the need to live in assisted living facilities or care homes, and reducing reliance upon family or paid caregivers to provide support. Technologies for the home range from those that aid in activities of daily living, that monitor and generate alerts based upon usual (and unusual) behavioural patterns, that improve physical safety, to those that bring essential health care services directly into the home. In

---

[1] Kurzweil, Raymond. 'The Law of Accelerating Returns', KurzweilAI.net, 7 Mar 2001. http://www.kurzweilai.net/articles/art0134.html

addition to efforts by industrial actors under private R&D schemes, governments are investing heavily in programmes to encourage technological breakthroughs to enhance independent living.   One of the primary embodiments of policy in this area can be observed in the level of financial investment that is being made in development projects by governments.   The European Commission continues to encourage development through Framework Programme funding, along with significant private and national level investments through the AAL Joint Programme, which has a six-year planned budget of €700 million through the year 2013.[2] Through NIH (National Institute of Health) grants, the US government funds development in the area of assistive technologies totalling over $ 900 million since 2005.[3]

- **At work.** Workers may decide to stay in the work force for personal satisfaction or for financial reasons, but either way, technology may provide support to these goals.   As use of technology has become a critical requirement in many workplace settings, new technologies and adaptations are being developed to ensure that technologies are accessible for older workers, both in terms of addressing physical impairments commonly associated with ageing (such as hearing or vision losses, impairment of dexterity) and in terms of providing access to training on emerging technologies.   Remote connections to workplace systems from home, enabled by broadband access, provide alternatives to overcoming mobility barriers.

- **In the community.** As technology has changed, so has the notion of community. That is not to say that the physical aspects of community in a city, town, neighbourhood, etc. are threatened, rather, the notion of community is augmented by the virtual, global community that has become available through the reach of the Internet. Social connections with family and friends who live at a distance, with strangers who have similar interests and hobbies, with learning communities, are all enhanced through technologies. Access to these communities as well as to the services available to citizens from public authorities relies heavily upon ensuring access to the Internet for all citizens. In an address to the Internet Governance Forum (November 2009), Viviane Reding, former European Commissioner for Information Society and Media, stated the need to provide an inclusive Internet:

> *An open Internet is also an inclusive Internet. There are billions of people still without internet access. They must not be forgotten, nor must we make decisions now that they will regret in the years to come. We must act now to make sure that the global community can participate fully and equally in the important processes that underlie the development and future of the internet.*[4]

Each technological advance in these areas presents a challenge to ensure that all segments of society are included in the revolution and that these technologies support

---

[2] http://www.aal-europe.eu/
[3] Estimates of Funding for Various Research, Condition, and Disease Categories (RCDC), http://report.nih.gov/rcdc/categories
[4] Reding, Viviane, 'Why the Internet must be open, global and multilingual', Opening speech at the Internet Governance Forum Sharm El Sheikh, 15 November 2009.

the goals of independence and inclusion. This Chapter[5] surveys technologies that provide solutions supporting this independence and e-inclusion, and offers a glimpse into the future needs of society at large. This survey shows what is possible today and in the near future, and in doing so, gives examples of recent research and development projects as well as products available on the open market.

I. ASSISTIVE TECHNOLOGY AND ITS APPLICATIONS

As the world's population ages at an unprecedented rate, societies find themselves in a predicament where the communicative power of technology strides ahead, leaving behind an underserved population segment that stands to gain immeasurably from its full and proper adoption. The term 'digital divide' refers to that gap between those people with effective access to digital and information technology and those without access, and reveals just how critical it is to include a growing elderly population in every technological advance made. Europe's i2010 policy framework is one strategy amongst many implemented to foster inclusion and better public services and quality of life for all through the use of information and communication technologies (ICTs).

Assistive technology is a broad term used to describe all assistive, adaptive and rehabilitative devices for older people and for those people with disabilities. While this broad definition encompasses both high- and low-tech devices, this chapter does not include a discussion of the assistive technologies in common use (e.g., wheelchairs, walkers and hearing aids), but focuses rather on those new and emerging assistive technologies that enable older adults to more independently perform activities of daily living and give them an opportunity to participate in society longer and more fully, thereby addressing the problems of the digital divide and fostering e-inclusion. The following is an overview of the assistive technologies that have taken shape over the past several years, as well as those that are just beginning to emerge.

1. EMERGING TECHNOLOGIES

When technologies improve human capabilities, they have the potential to satisfy the needs of the elderly solutions and to promote inclusion. These solutions also offer otherwise elderly 'disabled' bodies the same access to information, technology and services as younger 'abled' bodies and extend the time in which the elderly can remain active in the workforce. The following technologies serve as building blocks for broad applications, which are redefining how the elderly can remain fully engaged in society and independent in their homes. The survey also provides some examples of specific development projects that have been undertaken to advance the technologies or their applications in practical settings.

1.1 Robotics

The science of robotics studies the behaviour of intelligent beings to develop methodologies for machines (i.e., robots) that can interact with the environment through sensors and actuators to accomplish specific tasks. While robotics is a branch

---

[5] This Chapter includes adaptation of some portions of deliverables from the SENIOR Project, including in particular: D1.1: Environmental Scanning Report, D2.1: Ubiquitous Computing, D2.2: Ubiquitous Communication, D2.3: Intelligent User Interfaces, D2.4: AI & Adaptive Software, and D2.5: AT & Robotics.

of engineering, it also incorporates biology, physiology, linguistics, psychology, automation, electronics, physics, informatics, mathematics and mechanics.

The term robot (from the Czech word robota, meaning compulsory labour) refers to any machine (anthropomorphic or not) able to accomplish a given task in substitution for human labor. Robots are devices that assist humans in performing tasks. They do so more or less independently. With the intervention of artificial intelligence, robots can also 'learn' their functions by interacting with the environment and with humans.

The goals of robotic technologies are focused upon improving and supporting a user's capabilities, rather than replacing the need for human assistance entirely. Several different types of robots are emerging. Personal robots are service robots designed to work in the domestic environment, or the work environment, or applied in daily life. Assistive robots, defined as devices that cooperate with a user through physical activity in the user's environment[6], can help the elderly in a number of ways.

Lack of mobility is a key issue amongst the elderly population, whether sudden and short-term (e.g., injury due to a fall), or a slow diminishing of capabilities over time; mobility limitations impact an individual in terms of their ability to perform activities of daily living (ADLs), causing them to lose independence in physical terms, as well as losing opportunities to remain socially engaged within their community and continue as active participants in the workforce.

Robotic technology is being employed to address the needs of the elderly, through intelligent walkers, mobile robotic guides and assistive robotic agents. Intelligent walkers, or i-Walkers, are based on intelligent multi-agent systems technology and are similar to traditional walkers, but also have the ability to communicate with the user and react to their surroundings. They adapt to the specific needs of the individual and can recognise voice commands given by the user. The i-Walker is also used in rehabilitation to modify the amount of support given to the user. For example, the effort made in walking, distance travelled, calories burned, etc. is documented by the i-Walker and subsequently adjusted by a medical professional depending on progress made.[7]

A US project illustrating practical use of robotics focused on the development of an assistive robotic device with specific goals that could be altered based on the needs of the user. The device was intended to keep the user from falling down or hitting anything, as well as to assist in ensuring arrival at their destination.[8] The user always remained in control of this assistive device, unless the walker itself sensed that the user was about to have a collision or collapse. In such cases, the walker took action and attempted to steer the walker elsewhere. If this could not be done without affecting the user's balance, brakes were activated. Similar walkers have also been researched for the elderly blind, along with smart canes.

Other devices in which robotics have been implemented to improve daily life for the elderly include:

---

[6] Meng, Q. and M.H.Lee, 'Design Issues for Assistive Robotics for the Elderly', University of Wales, Wales, UK, 2006.
https://cadair.aber.ac.uk/dspace/bitstream/2160/450/1/AEI06.pdf
[7] Universitat Politècnica de Catalunya, 'Intelligent Walker Designed to Assist the Elderly and People Undergoing Medical Rehabilitation', *ScienceDaily*, 2008. http://www.sciencedaily.com/releases/2008/11/081107072015.htm
[8] Wasson, Glenn, Jim Gunderson, Sean Graves and Robin Felder, 'An Assistive Robotic Agent for Pedestrian Mobility', University of Virginia, 2001, p. 1. http://www.cs.virginia.edu/~gsw2c/research/agents01.pdf

- aids for lifting and transfer
- home adaptation and intelligent user interfaces
- special controls for driving
- limb prostheses
- aids for self-care
- aids for games, exercise, sports, entertainment
- aids for memory
- diagnostic monitoring.

Additionally, when artificial intelligence (as discussed in the following section) is integrated with robotic devices, the robots can be used to look after and monitor elderly patients and even provide some level of perceived nurture. These types of robots have been implemented to assist elderly people suffering from cognitive disorders and physical disabilities. Some specific examples include:

- The Nursebot project incorporated intelligent reminding for those with mild cognitive issues. The robot was programmed with information about the user's daily routines and observed the user, offering reminders when necessary. Such robots are not necessarily needed to monitor everything the user does, but for critical activities, such as taking medications and non-critical, but preferred activities, such as watching a favourite television show, the robot provides reminders if the activities are forgotten. The robot also learned which activities must be monitored daily and which only needed periodic monitoring.[9]
- Robot care bears were introduced in a retirement home in Japan. These bears watched over patients and monitored specific interests of doctors, such as response times and lengths of time spent on specific tasks. They also alerted staff of any changes in these areas. The difference between these robots and many others is their friendly exterior which enables them to act as a companion for many elderly residents.[10]
- Similar to robotic care bears, robot dogs have been introduced to act as companions. Living pets may be difficult for elderly individuals to manage, whether because of physical limitations of the elderly to provide the daily exercise, feeding and grooming routines, or because the elderly person is living in a care facility where animals are not typically allowed. Aibo, a robotic dog with touch sensors, sound, voice and face recognition, the ability to learn from its environment and express emotion, was introduced to elderly patients in St. Louis, Missouri, and results showed that it was just as companionable as a real dog.[11] Animal-assisted therapy is a solution to the loneliness and depression that occur on a regular basis in nursing homes. While Aibo did not have the ability to provide his user with reminders or collect information about the user to help doctors or nursing home staff, he was deemed a great companion by the users.

---

[9] Ramakrishnan, Sailesh, and Martha E. Pollack, 'Intelligent Monitoring in a Robotic Assistant for the Elderly', University of Pittsburgh, 2000, p. 1. http://www.eecs.umich.edu/~pollackm/distrib/aaai00stupos.pdf
[10] Lytle, J Mark, 'Robot Care Bears for the Elderly', BBC News, 21 February 2002.
http://news.bbc.co.uk/1/hi/sci/tech/1829021.stm
[11] Cartledge, Sue, 'Robot Dogs Keep Elderly Company', Helioza, 2008.
http://www.helioza.com/Directory/Science/Technology/Robot-Dogs-Keep-Elderly-Company-7.php

- The LIREC (LIving with Robots and IntEractive Companions) project[12] embraced a multi-faceted theory involving artificial long-term companions that can perform numerous functions, including rehabilitation, fetch and carry, security, dispensing medicine, and cognitive prosthetic tasks. These robots move autonomously and must 'know' certain facts, such as the organisation of items around the house, housekeeping preferences of the user, any special needs the user might have, and interaction styles of the user with both individuals and in social situations involving more than one person.[13]

Robotic technology is increasingly entering hospitals, care centers, dangerous environments, industry and retail settings. According to the International Federation of Robotics, the total value of professional service robots sold by the end of 2008 was about $11 billion. However, the value of service robots for personal and domestic use is only a fraction of that, as they are produced for a mass market with completely different pricing and marketing channels. So far, service robots for personal and domestic use are mainly in the areas of domestic (household) robots, which include vacuum cleaning and lawn-mowing robots, and entertainment and leisure robots, including toy robots, hobby systems, education and training robots. Millions of these low-cost products have already been sold and almost 12 million are forecast to be sold between 2009 and 2012 representing an estimated value of $3 billion.[14]

Taking into account the shifting demographics, many countries continue to invest in development of care robots, with some of the most significant developments taking place in Japan, which has the largest percentage of senior citizens amongst developed nations. Some of the most exciting recent developments regarding robotic technology with elder care benefits include the following:

- General Robotix and the National Institute of Advanced Industrial Science and Technology (AIST) in Japan have developed a 70-centimeter tall robot, named 'Taizo' (a play on the word '*taisou*,' which means 'calisthenics'), with a friendly appearance designed to motivate elderly people to engage in more physical exercise.[15]
- GeckoSystems International, a US-based company, has developed its first robot called CareBot which includes two engines: a self-navigating mobile platform that uses environmental cues and GeckoChat, a language recognition and processing engine.[16]
- Cyberdyne, a Japanese electronics company, has developed a robotic suit, known as the Hybrid Assisted Limb (or HAL), which is designed to boost its wearer's strength by a multiple of 10. Recently, the suit allowed a nursing home patient in Tsurugashima, Japan, to walk for the first time in two years.[17]

---

[12] http://lirec.eu/

[13] Syrdal, Dag Sverre, Dautenhahn, Kristen,Walters, Michael L., and Kheng Lee Koay, 'Long-term Robotic Companionship in the Home', Adaptive Systems Research Group, University of Hertfordshire, 2008. Presentation give at the Future of AI & Self-Adaptive Software, Artificial Intelligence and Adaptive Software Workshop on ICT and Ageing, SENIOR Project, held in Brussels, December 2009. http://seniorproject.eu/resources/5ExpertMeeting/Syrdal.pdf

[14] International Federation of Robotics. http://www.ifr.org/news/ifr-press-release/professional-service-robots-are-establishing-themselves-87/

[15] http://www.generalrobotix.com/product/taizo/index.htm

[16] http://www.geckosystems.com/

[17] http://www.cyberdyne.jp/English/

- InTouch Health, a Santa Barbara Calif.-based robotics company, offers two types of robotic diagnostic stations used by more than 200 hospitals in the US, which enable doctors to interact with hospital patients at a distance.[18]

- Fujitsu Frontech Limited and Fujitsu Laboratories Ltd launched the sale of its service robot, enon(TM), in Japan. Jointly developed by the two companies, enon is an advanced practical-use service robot that can assist in such tasks as providing guidance, escorting guests, transporting objects, and security patrolling.[19]

- Panasonic is developing a new robotic bed that is able to convert into a joystick-controlled wheelchair when the owner commands it to transform.[20]

- The RIKEN-TRI Collaboration Center for Human-Interactive Robot Research (RTC), which was established as a joint collaboration project by RIKEN and Tokai Rubber Industries Ltd (TRI) in Japan, has developed the robot nurse 'Riba', able to lift medical patients who weigh up to 134 pounds, allowing a patient to shift from a wheelchair to a bed. RIBA does this using its very strong human-like arms and by novel tactile guidance methods using high-accuracy tactile sensors.[21]

1.2. Artificial Intelligence

Popular culture has long been fascinated with the intelligent machine, able to replicate the best of man's rational and logical thought and decision-making processes, and improve upon them through the elimination of emotional burdens. Today's artificial intelligent (AI) systems are oriented towards adapting to unpredictable situations, often made unpredictable because of the presence of humans in the environment.

The field of artificial intelligence has been evolving over the past 50 years[22] and a perhaps more tightly-focused, but closely connected area of research – self-adaptive software – has emerged only in the last decade.[23] Self-adaptive software has the

---

[18] http://www.intouchhealth.com/

[19] http://www.frontech.fujitsu.com/en/forjp/robot/servicerobot/

[20] http://www.engadget.com/2009/09/18/panasonics-robotic-bed-makes-sleeping-with-robots-a-reality/

[21] http://rtc.nagoya.riken.jp/RIBA/index-e.html

[22] The term Artificial Intelligence for this area of research is commonly attributed to John McCarthy (Professor Emeritus, Stanford University) in 1956. In his web-published article 'WHAT IS ARTIFICIAL INTELLIGENCE? (rev. 12 November 2007, http://www-formal.stanford.edu/jmc/whatisai/whatisai.html), McCarthy provides extensive background on AI, and its definition as 'the science and engineering of making intelligent machines, especially intelligent computer programs.' He credits the English mathematician Alan Turing as the first researcher in this area: 'He gave a lecture on it in 1947. He also may have been the first to decide that AI was best researched by programming computers rather than by building machines. By the late 1950s, there were many researchers on AI, and most of them were basing their work on programming computers.'

[23] From a DARPA Broad Agency Announcement on Self Adaptive Software (BAA-98-12) in December 1997:

'Self Adaptive Software evaluates its own behavior and changes behavior when the evaluation indicates that it is not accomplishing what the software is intended to do, or when better functionality or performance is possible.

…This implies that the software has multiple ways of accomplishing its purpose, and has enough knowledge of its construction to make effective changes at runtime. Such software should include functionality for evaluating its behavior and performance, as well as the ability to replan and reconfigure its operations in order to improve its operation. Self Adaptive Software should also

capacity to dynamically alter its own behaviour to best satisfy the requirements of its environment. Its environment includes anything the system is able to recognise, any inputs from external hardware devices (sensors) and network instrumentation.

A self-adaptive artificial intelligent solution gathers information from its environment and organises it into themes, such as user context and application requirements. It examines and evaluates the data that has been collected and determines its importance to the system. Then, it makes decisions based on this analysis and adapts to the given situation by making changes in how the system is run. As the system learns more about its environment, its accuracy improves.

Artificial intelligence is commonly one technological component amongst many in an assistive product solution. For example, consider the robotic solutions discussed above that enhance mobility. A number of other applications built upon or integrating AI or adaptive software are emerging and beginning to have an impact on the elderly. In particular, artificial intelligence is also being used in medical diagnosis and to produce new instruments to support medical research and training. Programs such as medical decision-support system and patient-centred health information systems can help medical professionals make care decisions. The system analyses medical history, symptoms, etc., providing diagnoses for the patient's conditions and recommending appropriate treatment alternatives. These systems may also monitor and manage the patient's conditions.[24]

More complex systems can also narrow the number of diagnostic possibilities very quickly, using reasoning techniques to determine which diagnosis would make the most sense, creating models of specific patient's ailments and explaining how they arrived at this conclusion. This allows healthcare professionals to check the logic of the diagnosis and correct any flaws in the system.[25]

Affective computing is another branch of artificial intelligence that deals with the design of systems and devices that can recognise, interpret and process human emotions. Many assistive technologies for the elderly rely on the ability to detect a user's personal capacities and skills, including cognitive and learning deficiencies. Chips, lab-on-chips and physiological sensors track affective cues that accompany the learning effort such as valence, intensity and uncertainty. Cognitive sciences then interpret those data in real time and interface with computers which communicate to the user the appropriate advice. Research on 'affective perception' of technologies, however, is in the early stages of development[26]; in addition, tracking 'emotions'

---

include a set of components for each major function, along with descriptions of the components, so that components of systems can be selected and scheduled at runtime, in response to the evaluators. It also requires the ability to impedance match input/output of sequenced components, and the ability to generate some of this code from specifications. In addition, DARPA seek this new basis of adaptation to be applied at runtime, as opposed to development/design time, or as a maintenance activity.'

[24] Ishak, Wan Hussain Wan, and Fadzilah Siraj, 'Artificial Intelligence in Medical Applications: An Exploration', Universiti Utara Malaysia, 2006. http://www.hi-europe.info/files/2002/9980.htm
[25] Szolovits, Peter, Ramesh S. Patil and William B. Schwartz, 'Artificial Intelligence in Medical Diagnosis', Massachusetts Institute of Technology, 1988. http://groups.csail.mit.edu/medg/ftp/psz/SchwartzAnnals.html
[26]Picard, Rosalind W., 'Affective Computing: Challenges', *International Journal of Human-Computer Studies*, 59, (1-2), July 2003, pp. 55–64.

encroaches (pretending to see not 'what a person is doing' but digging in deeper to determine 'how that person is doing it') on the opacity of *persona(*l) privacy.[27]

Artificial intelligence is also one of the key technologies that contributes to intelligent telemonitoring and smart home development used to enable the elderly to live more independent, healthy and engaged lives in their own homes. These solutions are discussed later in this chapter.

1.3. Sensing and surveillance technology

Sensing technology has been around for decades; however, more recent technological advances have led to a dramatic increase in human-machine intimacy. Sensors are also becoming smaller and cheaper to produce, with limited power consumption, enabling them to be used in a broad range of scenarios, including movement (monitoring when an object is moved or measuring vibrations), light (measuring varying colour and intensity of light, which could include determining whether indoors, outdoors or change in time based upon a change in location of light source), proximity (which could monitor the presence of activity nearby, trigger applications that would otherwise be dormant), audio (level, pitch, etc.), temperature of an object or of the ambient environment, force (which may be used to determine weight of an object, for example, as a vessel is being filled), humidity, acceleration and magnetism. It is possible to use them in novel ways, enabling the objects into which they are placed to become 'smart'.

The development of smaller sensors and wireless sensing networks that enable their effective use for more applications has been significant – most notably, the Smart Dust project sponsored by the US Defense Advanced Research Projects Agency (DARPA)[28], and carried out at the University of California in Berkeley. The project resulted in the development of the TinyOS open source operating system as well as highly miniaturised 'motes' which are part of the sensor network, providing sensor input as well as storage and other functions.

Smaller sensors also provide the opportunity for technology to be used in increasingly novel ways, enabling the objects and environments into which they are placed to become 'smart'. For example:

Sensors are increasingly being embedded into textiles, enabling clothing to measure an individual's physical condition, whether for medical applications, entertainment or for monitoring sports-performance.

Sensors are being used within carpet materials, embedded in canes or in the insole of shoes to measure and recognise an individual's gait. Current research is aiming to identify changes in an individual's gait as a proactive predictor of weakness or loss of balance that may lead to falls.[29]

---

[27] On the conception of privacy as opacity, see De Hert, P. , and S.Gutwirth, *Privacy, data protection and law enforcement. Opacity of the individual and transparency of power,* in E. Claes, A. Duff and S. Gutwirth (eds.), *Privacy and the criminal law,* Intersentia, Antwerpen-Oxford, 2006.

[28] The vision for the original funding of the 'Smart Dust' project by DARPA was to provide a way to sense battlefield conditions, where thousands of sensors might be scattered over an area by plane or helicopter to obtain information about vehicle movement in remote locations or environmental data.

[29] Significant research efforts are focused on this issue, due to the high incidence of falling injuries as both a cause of death or non-fatal injuries resulting in hospital admission for trauma amongst older adults. According to the US Center for Disease Control (CDC), more than one third of adults 65 and older fall each year in the United States (CDC 2006). http://www.cdc.gov/ncipc/factsheets/adultfalls.htm

Vibration sensors are embedded into the environment, able to distinguish between a dropped object and a person falling on the floor.[30]

In assistive systems for the elderly, the sensing components are those technologies that include sensors for movement, physical health parameters, temperature, pictures, etc. When sensors are coupled with other surveillance technologies, a new realm of assistive products becomes possible.

When we think about surveillance technologies, we naturally think about cameras peering at us from every angle as we walk through public places, potentially motivating good behaviour or, at the least, providing a forensic tool in response to the opposite. However, surveillance cameras on every street corner, traffic light and underground station are only the tip of the iceberg when we consider the direction surveillance may take in years to come. New technologies are emerging which enable the environment to be monitored for much more than a physical image.

Surveillance technologies have also become sufficiently low cost to make their way from public and industrial applications to the home environment. Webcams have been deployed by home users for more than a decade, providing for some very limited (both in scope and quality) surveillance capabilities, and more commonly used for enhancing personal communications and entertainment applications. However, with advances in availability and speed of IP connections, more robust monitoring cameras and other devices have become commonplace, monitoring home or pets while on vacation, monitoring children within the home, etc. In the home environment, however, monitoring with cameras introduces significant challenges to privacy. Solutions to these challenges have included systems that blur captured images, or otherwise aim to provide some level of physical privacy to individuals being recorded.

Enabling surveillance and, in point of fact, extending the use of many digital technologies is the continued enhancement and accessibility of underlying communications technologies. Access to high-speed broadband connections has become a necessity to respond to the ever increasing size of applications and shared data files. In urban areas, the speed and reliability of wireline and wireless connections are being enhanced and accessibility levels are quite high (though the price of this and all technologies being discussed here can present a key accessibility barrier for many of the e-excluded). In many rural areas, however, there remains limited access to broadband connections which are generally dependent upon point-to-point wiring. Wireless broadband services complement these services to reach remote users, but the technology is continuing to be developed and deployed. There are strong levels of competition to address the needs of wireless mobile users, more so than for the fixed wireless broadband market in these areas. Initiatives to increase coverage for rural locations are being funded by governments including expansive programs by the US Department of Agriculture to support rural communities[31] and a commitment by the European Union to attain 100% coverage of broadband internet between 2010 and 2013.[32]

---

[30] Alwan, M., P.J. Rajendran, S. Kell, et al., 'A Smart and Passive Floor-Vibration Based Fall Detector for Elderly', *Information and Communication Technologies Medical Automation Research Center (MARC)*, Department of Pathology, University of Virginia, 24-28 April 2006.
[31] 'USDA Rural Development: Bringing Broadband to Rural America', US Department of Agriculture, Rural Development Agency, May 2007. http://www.rurdev.usda.gov/rd/pubs/RDBroadbandRpt.pdf
[32] 'Key Issues Paper 2009 - contribution from the Competitiveness Council to the Spring European Council,' 5-6 March 2009.

Surveillance cameras do not in and of themselves ensure safety of course, but rather they must be coupled with intelligent content analysis programmed to determine whether an alert should be issued (e.g., identifying a possible fall or other unusual event). Another solution provided to the privacy problem is to monitor behaviours rather than live images in the environment. Behaviour monitoring is accomplished through systems comprised of sensors (motion sensors, sensors detecting use of an appliance, detecting physical weight in a chair, in a bed, etc.). Such systems can range from purpose-specific ones (e.g., a monitor in a bed triggers a light to dim up slowly once it is determined that the occupant has arisen) to broader systems that monitor an individual's movement through the residence to analysis for adherence to an established behavioural norm.

Several recent EU-funded projects related to developing sensor-based technology to monitor the elderly include:

- EMERGE: Emergency monitoring and prevention[33] –Led by Fraunhofer IESE of Germany, with eight other partners, the aim of the EMERGE project (Feb 2007 – Oct 2009) was to support elderly people with emergency monitoring and prevention. The project aimed to detect deviations from typical behaviour patterns and acute disorders in their health in case of strokes, falls or similar emergencies. The project used ambient and unobtrusive sensors to monitor activity, location and vital data. Daily routine was tracked in order to detect abnormalities and to create early indicators for potential emergencies. In case an emergency cannot be handled by the senior citizen or friends or caregivers, an integrated emergency medical service (EMS) could be called and informed about the case.

- ENABLE: A wearable system supporting services for the elderly[34] –Led by the Vienna University of Technology, with eight other partners, the project (Jan 2007 – Dec 2009) developed a personal system, with services for senior citizens in or out of the home, to mitigate the effects of any disability and to increase autonomy, mobility, communications, care and safety. The system used a mobile phone and wrist unit as an open platform by means of which third parties could add other services by 'plugging' into defined interfaces. The project addressed problems of everyday living such as using the phone, raising an alarm to get help, monitoring for health conditions, taking medicines, ensuring appliances are turned on and off, etc.

- Netcarity: Networked multi-sensor system for elderly people[35] –Led by the Italian National Research Council, with 14 other partners, Netcarity (Feb 2007 – Jan 2011) fosters the development of a 'light' technological infrastructure, to be integrated in senior citizens' homes, that provides basic support of everyday activities as well as detection of health emergencies, and encourages social and psychological engagement.

- SENSACTION-AAL: SENsing and mobility in Ambient Assisted Living[36] –Led by the University of Bologna (Italy), with seven other partners, the SENSACTION-AAL project (Jan 2007 – June 2009) aimed to assist older

---

[33] http://www.emerge-project.eu/
[34] http://www.enable-project.eu/
[35] http://www.netcarity.org/
[36] http://www.sensaction-aal.eu/

people to remain independent and injury-free by developing sensor-based technology to allow medical professionals to initiate interventions in the home environment. The SENSACTION-AAL project designed and tested wireless on-body systems to monitor ADLs and physical performance using sensory augmentation and biofeedback.

- BiosensorNet: Autonomic Biosensor Networks for Pervasive Healthcare[37] – (funded by the EPSRC[38] Wired and Wireless Intelligent Networked Systems (WINES) Programme from October 2005 to March 2009). This project's emphasis was on sensor-based measurements to provide information from the body including dynamic and quantitative differences between vascular and tissue compartments, enabling clinical decisions.

1.4. Biotechnology

Biotechnology is the science of using living organisms or systems to manufacture products to benefit the human race or other animal species. Biotechnology has long been used in the medical industry to discover the causes of many diseases, and to develop antibiotics and immunisations. It has also been used to enhance the production of food in the farming industry, and is now being used in bio-fuels research. The highly controversial stem cell research falls under the umbrella of biotechnology. In everyday life, one encounters the application of biotechnology in many objects, including biodegradable plastics, detergents and fabrics, amongst others.[39]

During the last decades, understanding of the human brain has increased, prompting the development and use of pharmacological and technological products and devices. Tapping into nerves allows the development of brain-computer interface (BCI) devices. BCIs aim at assisting, augmenting or repairing human cognitive or sensory motor functions. Long term progress is expected in electronic medicine: cyber-drugs and cyber-narcotics to cure cancer or to relieve clinical depression.[40] Today, neural implants are already being used to help regulate certain functions of the brain of Parkinson's patients.

BCIs translate a brain's electrical activity into a signal that controls an artificial component, and thus hold promise in the application of assistive technology to better the lives of the elderly. BCIs are being designed to restore lost motor and sensory functions and to overcome damages in the nervous pathway. Applications for the elderly include stimulation for chronic pain therapy, limb prostheses for anatomical compensation of damaged neural pathways, implantable neuro-stimulation devices, cochlear and retinal implants.[41]

The Ambient Corporation's Audeo is being developed to create a human-computer interface for communication. The approach uses electrical activity

---

[37] http://vip.doc.ic.ac.uk/biosensornet/m432.html
[38] Engineering and Physical Sciences Research Council.
[39] Portions adapted from SENIOR: Intelligent User Interfaces (D2.3).
[40] Cavaliere, Thomas , 'Tapping into nerves', ELE 282 Biomedical Engineering Seminar I, Biomedical engineering, University of Rhode Island, 8 April 2008. http://www.ele.uri.edu/Courses/ele282/S02/Tom_2.pdf
[41] Nsanze, Fabienne, *ICT Implants in the Human Body – a review*, In: Ethical aspects of ICT implants in the human body, European Group on Ethics in Science and New Technologys to the European Commission, 2005. http://bookshop.europa.eu/eubookshop/download.action?fileName=KAAJ050203AC_002.pdf&eubphfUid=155714&catalogNbr=KA-AJ-05-020-3A-C

generated when a person's brain sends instructions through the nervous system, normally intended to stimulate the muscles to produce speech. This electrical activity will be used to simulate speech where disease or disability may prevent the muscle stimulation to be effective.[42]

The technology associated with brain computer interfacing is still in its infancy. Some applications being researched today include aiding long-term memory function by replacing parts of the hippocampus with a mechanical device, decision-making tools for the elderly, an aid to maintain brain plasticity to enable an enduring ability and capacity to learn, aids for well-being and virtual reality gaming to facilitate independent living, thought-controlled prosthetic devices, sensory replacement devices, and the ultimate in brain computing technology – an artificial brain.

Some publicly funded projects related to BCI research include the following:

- The EPSRC Wired and Wireless Intelligent Networked Systems (WINES) Programme has funded a project called Analogue Evolutionary Brain Computer Interfaces[43], which is using new brain computer interface technology as a way of allowing people to control computer access devices via brain waves. The team has developed a prototype BCI mouse capable of full 2-D motion control. Further work is being done to examine the optimal visual presentation conditions that minimise cognitive load, perceptual errors and interference which distracts from the target.
- The European Commission funded the FP7 project BRAIN - BCIs with Rapid Automated Interfaces for Non-experts[44]. This project aims at developing Brain-Computer Interfaces into assistive tools for a range of disabled users, enhancing the ability to interact with people, devices in their environment, and technologies.

Regenerative medicine also falls under the umbrella of biotechnology. This field applies tissue science and tissue engineering, along with other biological and engineering principles to restore damaged tissues and organs. This field encompasses innovative approaches to treatment of disease through the use of therapies that encourage the autonomous regeneration of tissues, directly transplant healthy new tissue and use implants engineered from tissue to promote regeneration[45]: Government initiatives that further the use and application of regenerative medicine include, among others[46]:

- The United States Health and Human Services department (HHS) proposed the Federal Initiative for Regenerative Medicine (FIRM), a biotech program that promises to provide tissues and organs 'on demand' for every American by 2020. It is anticipated that with replaceable tissues and organs available, doctors would be able to prevent more deaths from a broad range of human ailments.
- The Kobe Medical Industry Development Project is investing in a broad range of therapies and infrastructure to raise the standard of living of Japan's elderly, with cell therapy and regenerative medicine research as one element of its work.

---

[42] http://www.theaudeo.com/tech.html
[43] http://gow.epsrc.ac.uk/ViewGrant.aspx?GrantRef=EP/F033818/1
[44] http://www.brain-project.org/
[45] http://www.hhs.gov/reference/newfuture.shtml
[46] Ibid.

- The European Union has established an infrastructure for regenerative medicine. The European Commission's Directorate General Enterprise is responsible for developing and organising regenerative medicine efforts in the EU including establishing the governing regulatory environment.[47]

1.5. Biometrics

Biometric technologies (which use scans of fingerprint, iris, face, palm print, vein, retina, voice, skin, hand geometry, ear shape, etc.) have featured especially in security applications over the past decade, and the advances associated with these technologies have generally served a security agenda. As the total cost of ownership for biometrics continues to drop, their prevalence in the market is becoming more mainstream and in some cases more obligatory (in relation to social service entitlements, immigration and international travel, physical or logical access at one's job).

Even though there are numerous options for identification through biometric technologies (including behavioural means such as keystroke dynamics, gait and signature verification), research continues, bringing ever-more-obscure methods out of the laboratory in search of the highest level of accuracy at the greatest level of efficiency. DNA identification is certainly not new, but continued work in this area has reduced DNA testing cost to the point where it is routinely used by consumers (particularly for paternity testing), and not merely for security applications. With continued work in mapping the human genome, and targets set to bring the mapping process closer to $1,000[48], use of DNA technology to identify not only a person, but any disease to which he or she may be pre-disposed is easy to foresee. This technology, in its most beneficent form, can be used in predictive medicine to target treatments for individuals before the onset of disease, and has the potential to have a significant impact on addressing the needs of our ageing population.

In the US, at the Massachusetts Institute of Technology (MIT) AgeLab, researchers are conducting studies on the application of telemedicine technologies to manage chronic conditions such as congestive heart failure (CHF), diabetes and obesity. AgeLab researchers hope to make a 'check-up-a-day' not only possible, but a reality for everyone. The prevention demands of today's older population and ageing boomers will drive health delivery from the clinic to the home. Working with the Philips Corporation, AgeLab researchers, MIT's Department of Computer Science and Artificial Intelligence and the MIT Department of Mechanical Engineering are developing a system to provide early detection and warning for CHF patients and their families, using a home set of simple, non-invasive commercial medical instruments.[49]

One project funded by the European Union related to developing biometric-based technology to monitor the elderly is called HeartCycle: Compliance and effectiveness in heart failure and chronic heart disease closed-loop management.[50] The HeartCycle project is developing systems for monitoring people with a heart condition at home with the aim of improving disease management through telemonitoring. These

---

[47] Regulation (EC) No 1394/2007 of the European Parliament and of the Council of 13 November 2007 on advanced therapy medicinal products and amending Directive 2001/83/EC and Regulation (EC) No 726/2004.
[48] The goal of reaching the $1,000 genome was set as a goal to achieve within 10-15 years of the original challenge, and which is widely expected to be achieved by the year 2014.
[49] http://web.mit.edu/agelab/projects_wellness.shtml
[50] http://heartcycle.med.auth.gr/

systems will comprise unobtrusive sensors built into the patient's clothing or bed sheets and home appliances such as weight scales and blood pressure monitors and report relevant medical data back to clinicians to monitor therapies and progress.

In-home monitoring via the implementation of biometric technologies has become increasingly important as an effective method for the elderly to maintain their independence. Two key applications in this area are:

- Telecare works through a series of discrete sensors positioned around one's home. These sensors alert either the call centre or the user's caregiver if they detect a problem.[51] Most of this monitoring is focused upon behavioural profiles and exceptions, and while some care systems utilise cameras, for most individuals the use of video-based systems is deemed far too privacy-invasive, and most emerging systems use sensors and enriched devices throughout the home to monitor and ensure the occupant's safety. For example, a smart home can have movement sensors and contact switches to get in touch with medical personnel in case of an emergency. There are many benefits to this technology, including 'increased safety (e.g., by monitoring lifestyle patterns or the latest activities and providing assistance when a potentially harmful situation is developing), comfort (e.g., by adjusting temperature automatically), and economy (e.g., controlling the use of lights)'[52].

- Telemonitoring, on the other hand, is focused on enabling individuals with severe illnesses or disabilities to live and function in their own homes for a longer period of time. Existing telemonitors detect abnormal physiological conditions and typically send an audio-visual alert to a doctor. The doctor must then silence the alarm and tend to the patient. This routine can become burdensome on a doctor who is monitoring numerous patients. Research is being done to incorporate artificial intelligence into these systems, which allow them to self-manage alerts.[53] Telemonitoring would require less management oversight, enabling a medical professional to effectively monitor more patients. These medical devices can also be embedded into clothing, which can then constantly monitor the vital signs of the patient. Also known as self-managed cells, these systems would support self-configuration, self-healing, self-optimisation, self-protection and context-aware adaptation.[54] Doctors can monitor patients at a distance and the smart home can detect if there is a change in the patient's condition and make emergency phone calls, if

---

[51] For example, *Just Checking* is a system designed to enable caregivers to check on the person they care for remotely from work or home and then can plan for visits that are meant to be purely social, rather than simple reassurance about the loved one's condition. From Mort, Maggie, 'Achieving 'good care in sociotechnical networks: ethical frameworks for new care technologies for older people', EFFORTT, Lancaster University, 2008. Based on a presentation at the Future of AI & Self-Adaptive Software, Artificial Intelligence and Adaptive Software Workshop on ICT and Ageing, EU SENIOR Project, Brussels, December 2008.

[52] Augusto, Juan Carlos, and Paul McCullagh, *Ambient Intelligence: Concepts and Applications*, Invited Paper by the International Journal on Computer Science and Information Systems, volume 4, Number 1, pp. 1-28, June 2007, p. 6.

[53] Baxi, Amit, and N. Kodalapura, 'A Self-Managing Framework for Health Monitoring', *Intel Technology Journal*, Intel Corporation, Vol. 10, No. 4, 2006, p. 314. http://download.intel.com/technology/itj/2006/v10i4/v10-i4-art06.pdf

[54] Dulay, N., S. Heeps, E. Lupu, R. Mathur, O. Sharma, M. Sloman and J. Sventek, 'AMUSE: Autonomic Management of Ubiquitous e-Health Systems', Imperial College London, 2005. http://www.dcs.gla.ac.uk/amuse/AHM2005-slomanFinal.pdf

necessary.[55] The overall goal of smart homes is to provide people with a cost-effective, safe, comfortable environment and for the elderly or chronically ill, can incorporate components that can contribute to a programme of healthcare, while enabling the individual to remain in a familiar and safe environment.[56]

1.6. Nanotechnology

The concept of 'nanotechnology' was introduced by Richard P. Feynman, physicist at the Los Alamos National Laboratory and later professor at the California Institute of Technology (Caltech), in a talk titled 'There's Plenty of Room at the Bottom' in 1959.[57] In that talk, Feynman introduced the concept of manipulating and controlling things on a staggeringly small scale. In nanotechnology, 'small scale' means at or around the scale of a nanometer, where one nanometer is a billionth of a meter or about 1/80,000 the width of a human hair.

Today, nanotechnology stretches across the entire spectrum of science and technology – with research and application in physics, chemistry, engineering and electronics, as well as medicine. For example, nanotechnology provides the basis for:

1. Ever smaller data storage devices while at the same time increasing memory capacity;
2. Highly efficient filters for wastewater treatment;
3. Photovoltaic windows;
4. New materials allowing the automotive industry to produce ultra light engines and car body panels;
5. Artificial joints whose nano-surface coatings can be tolerated better by the human body[58].

As of late 2009, the Project of Emerging Nanotechnologies reports over 1,000 nanotechnology-enabled consumer products, reflecting the increase use of tiny particles in everything from conventional products such as non-stick cookware and lighter, stronger tennis racquets to more unique items such as wearable sensors that monitor posture.[59]

Additionally, most smart devices used to aid the elderly in living independently have some type of embedded nanotechnology. In order for the technology to be ubiquitous and unobtrusive, the micro-processing component must be very small. In addition to sensor technology, robotics and biometrics, the smart home innovations discussed earlier in this chapter incorporate the use of nanotechnology to enhance the autonomy and quality of life of the elderly and disabled people by simplifying their interactions with devices at home, improving their living space, enabling their mobility and monitoring their health.

- Nanotechnology is also being used in conjunction with biotechnology (called nanobiotechnology) to construct devices able to go inside the

---

[55] Ramos, Carlos, Augusto, Juan Carlos, and Daniel Shapiro (guest editors), *Special Issue on Ambient Intelligence*, IEEE Intelligent Systems, vol. 23, no. 2, pp. 15-18, Mar/Apr, 2008, p. 4.
[56] Phillips, Becky, 'No Place Like Home -- Student's Sensors May Help Elderly', Washington State University, 2008. http://school.eecs.wsu.edu/node/612
[57] Feynman, Richard P., 'There's Plenty of Room at the Bottom: An Invitation to Enter a New Field of Physics', *Engineering and Science*, Vol. XXIII, No. 5, February 1960.
[58] Wiedemann, Peter M., and Holger Schutz, 'Framing Effects on Risk Perception of Nanotechnology,' *Public Understanding of Science*, Vol. 17, No. 3, 2008, pp. 369-379.
[59] http://www.nanotechproject.org

human body to extend the limitations of biology and ultimately be applied to resolve issues related to the ageing process and disease. Examples of applications of nanobiotechnology research include:The use of intelligent 'nanobots' will provide non-invasive, surgery-free neural implants which can be distributed to millions or even billions of points in the brain. This will lead to expansion of human intelligence, multiplying the natural 100 trillion connections of the brain many times over.[60]

- Nanotechnology theorist Rob Freitas designed a robotic red blood cell, called a respirocyte. The simply designed red blood cell gathers oxygen and lets it out at prescribed times. Primary applications can include transfusable blood substitution; partial treatment for anemia, perinatal/neonatal and lung disorders; enhancement of cardiovascular/ neurovascular procedures, tumour therapies and diagnostics; prevention of asphyxia; artificial breathing; and a variety of sports, veterinary, battlefield and other uses.[61]

- Rob Freitas has also designed a robotic white blood cell, called a microbivore, which downloads software from the Internet to combat specific pathogens. Microbivores constitute a potentially large class of medical nanorobots intended to be deployed in human patients for a wide variety of antimicrobial therapeutic purposes.[62]

1.7. RFID technologies

Radio-frequency identification (RFID) is a technology applied to an item in an effort to identify or track the item using radio waves. RFID tags are most commonly used for supply chain applications to provide unique identification for objects. The recent main advances in RFID have been in the area of miniaturization of the tags, and the ability to produce such tags more economically. With the advent of IPv6 and more easily deployed RFID technology, it is possible to have physical objects assigned unique identification, as part of what has been termed 'the Internet of Things'.

In the assistive technology realm, RFID technology has been implemented in different products and solutions, including:

- RFID is commonly used in wander management applications in care homes where there is a concern for residents suffering from dementia. Wander management applications have also moved past the controlled environment of the senior citizens' residence, and in some cases to law enforcement, as in the case of Project Lifesaver launched by the Sarasota, Florida, Police Department.[63]

---

[60] Quote attributed to Raymond Kurzweil. http://www.auntminnie.com/index.asp?sec=ser&sub=def&pag=dis&ItemID=58359

[61] Freitas, Robert A. Jr., 'A Mechanical Artificial Red Cell: Exploratory Design in Medical Nanotechnology,' 1999.
http://www.foresight.org/Nanomedicine/Respirocytes.html

[62] Freitas, Robert A., 'Microbivores: Artificial Mechanical Phagocytes,' *Institute for Molecular Manufacturing*, Report Number 25, 2001.

[63] http://www.sarasotagov.com/InsideCityGovernment/Content/Police/Lifesaver.htm

- Research is also being done in the use of RFID skin patches, which would allow for post-surgery monitoring by both physicians and patients.[64]
- With far less market uptake to date, VeriChip[65] developed an FDA-approved RFID tag (about the size of a grain of rice) which is meant to be injected under the skin, and which is intended to act as identification should an individual be brought into a medical facility where they are unable to communicate effectively.
- RFID is emerging as an option for tagging frequently lost objects and providing cognitive support to the elderly in the early stages of dementia.

There are many new applications using RFID emerging from the global research community, both academic and industrial, in response to new markets and availability of research funding. As an example, the SESAMONET (Secure and Safe Mobility Network) project, co-funded by the EC, prototyped a path for safe navigation for the visually impaired, through the combination of RFID tags embedded in the ground, along with a smart walking stick, phone and headset, providing recorded messages about location. Interestingly, while the costs of RFID tags are decreasing, this project kept costs at a minimum by using recycled chips which had previously been used for tracking cattle.[66]

Another project funded by the European Commission under FP7 is called CONFIDENCE: Ubiquitous care system to support independent living. Led by the Centro de Estudios e Investigaciones Tecnicas de Guipuzcoa of Spain with nine partners, CONFIDENCE is developing and integrating technologies for the detection of abnormal events (such as falls) or unexpected behaviour, both outdoors and indoors. The user will wear a few tags, whose positions are determined using radio technology. The tags' coordinates will be used to reconstruct the user's posture. This information, together with some environment information, will be analysed to decide whether to trigger an alarm.[67]

In the United States and Canada, Project Lifesaver is a system (since 1999) using RFID technologies. The solution consists of a bracelet with a tracking device to be worn by cognitively impaired persons. The bracelet is a one-ounce, battery-operated, wrist radio transmitter emitting an automatic, individualised tracking signal. If a client is determined to be missing, trained personnel respond to positively locate and identify the individual and ensure their safety.[68]

The Ambient Kitchen[69] project is exploring the use of pervasive computing for assisted living. The kitchen provides a platform for the application of pervasive computing technology in a domestic setting. The Ambient Kitchen uses standard kitchen units and objects with RFID tags and readers, as well as cameras integrated into the walls to support lab-based research in the environment.

As more objects (and locations) are 'tagged' and are given unique numbers and identifiers, one can see a connection between all these objects and how they might each become nodes in the 'Internet of Things'. Complemented by other types of

---

[64] 'RFID Skin Patches For Medical Applications', *Wireless Healthcare*, 17 May 2007. http://www.wirelesshealthcare.co.uk/wh/news/wk20-07-0006.htm
[65] http://www.verichipcorp.com/
[66] European Commission Joint Research Centre, 'SESAMONET- improved mobility of the visually impaired', 19 October 2007. http://ec.europa.eu/dgs/jrc/index.cfm?id=4210&lang=en
[67] http://www.confidence-eu.org/index.html
[68] http://projectlifesaver.org
[69] http://culturelab.ncl.ac.uk/ambientkitchen/

tagging mechanisms (graphical tags, SMS tags, etc.), RFID-tagged objects may be joined in a wireless and self-configuring network to support new and evolving applications impacting daily life. Supporting the emergence of RFID and other tagging mechanisms as unique identifiers of objects (and in some cases, people or animals) is IPv6, with vastly larger addressing capability (addresses under IPv6 are 128 bits in length as compared to 32 bits under IPv4)[70], which provides for approximately 5×10^{28} (roughly 2^{95}) addresses for each of the 6.5 billion (6.5×10^{9}) people alive today.[71]

1.8. GPS technologies

The past decade has witnessed significant advancement in the availability of location-based monitoring, moving GNSS (Global Navigation Satellite System) technology out of the realm of scientific, tracking and surveillance applications, and into mainstream commercial and consumer uses. GPS (the US-based Global Positioning System) is routinely included as part of standard equipment in commercial and non-commercial vehicles alike, providing convenience for drivers and enabling safety systems. Mobile phones also now include GPS receivers, providing the ability to pinpoint an individual's location.

These applications, tied to personal safety and convenience, provide benefits to the user who chooses to make use of them; however, for others, GPS technology may have different implications. There are several assistive products on the market now that make use of RFID tags, GPS and transponders to assist in navigation for disabled people and/or visually challenged seniors to navigate in an indoor or outdoor location. These same technologies are integral to providing alarms to carers or relatives if an elderly person moves beyond a designated area (with respect to wandering for cognitively impaired seniors).

GPS developers are joining with other manufacturers to find new applications for deployment of the technology – for example, GPS embedded into shoes combined with a tracking protocol will issue a Google alert if a loved one (or their shoes, at least) travels outside a predefined perimeter or 'geo-fence'.[72] Similar technology has been embedded into other items, such as bracelets and cell phones, to track elderly users.

The embedded GPS technology not only helps tracks the elderly users, but also gives them the ability to roam further from home than they might otherwise feel comfortable in doing so. For example, an older woman may feel more comfortable going to visit friends when she has her GPS-enabled cell phone, knowing that if her car breaks down her family can more easily determine her location. As a result, she can stay in direct contact with friends and family, and remain an active participant in her social network.

Several projects funded by the European Union related to exploring location-tracking technology for the elderly include:

---

[70] In a summary of its policy regarding support for the deployment of IPv6, the Commission expressed the view that IPv6 is 'an essential technology for implementing ambient intelligence'. http://ec.europa.eu/information_society/policy/ipv6/index_en.htm

[71] Estrin, Deborah (ed.), *Embedded, Everywhere,* Committee on Networked Systems of Embedded Computers of the Computer Science and Telecommunications Board, National Research Council, National Academy Press, Washington, DC, 2001. http://www.nap.edu/openbook.php?isbn=0309075688

[72] 'New GPS Shoes Join in Trend to Help Elderly'. http://www.switched.com/2009/06/16/new-gps-shoes-join-in-trend-to-help-elderly/

- LOCOMOTION: Location-based mobile phones for elderly citizens – Led by the Mobility Solutions Unit of Indra Sistemas of Spain, with eight partners, the LOCOMOTION project (Apr 2002 – Oct 2004) developed a remote and nomadic location monitoring device for use in the telecare of people with dementia and learning difficulties. The aim of the project was to provide individuals with special needs, as well as their carers, with relevant information according to their geographical position via mobile phones equipped with position determination capabilities. These services were aimed at increasing mobility of users, along with enhancing independent living and social inclusion.
- CAALYX[73] (Jan 2007 – Dec 2008) is an extensible health monitoring platform that uses GPS to support health monitoring and emergency handling. It does not continuously track older people, rather location information is only sent in an emergency or when an alarm is raised.[74]
- COGKNOW: Helping people with mild dementia navigate their day[75] – The COGKNOW project (Sept 2006 – Aug 2009) was aimed at development of a service, including a PDA which users could carry in order to enable reminders and detailed information that could be sent to the carers who could decide if the patient was in danger.

1.9. Connectedness: social networking, accessibility, and communications technologies

In addition to the ageing global population, socio-demographic changes taking place across society reveal a disturbing trend toward increased social isolation[76], presenting a significant social problem for the elderly, who increasingly remain living in their own homes but largely devoid of human contact.

The physiological and psychological changes caused by ageing often prevent seniors from participating in the community to the extent they may wish. Visual and hearing impairment and decreased mobility are common among senior citizens, and have the tendency to affect seniors' socialisation. Assistive communication technologies have the potential to allow senior citizens to continue their engagement in specific social settings or communities by providing necessary support and assistance. At the same time, these technologies may create access to new communities, thus either changing or increasing the individual's social network and possibilities of engaging actively in social relations.

Social networking

Social relations and social interaction are changing with the development of new technologies and systems. These technologies are also changing our notions of social interaction and relationships, as well as the notion of community. Online communities have become a reality and they may provide great (online) support for many people,

---

[73] http://caalyx.eu/
[74] Boulos, Maged N Kamel, et al., 'CAALYX: a new generation of location-based services in healthcare', *International Journal of Health Geographics*, Vol. 6, No. 9, 2007. http://caalyx.eu/index.php?option=com_content&task=view&id=13&Itemid=31
[75] http://www.cogknow.eu/
[76] Hawkley, L. C., and J. T Cacioppo, 'Aging and Loneliness,' *Current Directions in Psychological Science,* Vol. 16, No. 4, pp. 187-191, 2007.

e.g., with health problems or recreational/interest groups, and may allow the elderly to remain active or become active in new ways.

But while online social networking systems could provide assistive aid to the elderly, the elderly often do not participate in using the latest technologies. Studies in the US have shown that the share of adult Internet users who participate in an online social network site had more than quadrupled from 8% in 2005 to 35% by the end of 2008. Still, younger online adults are much more likely than their older counterparts to use social networks, with 75% of adults aged 18-24 using these networks, compared to just 7% of adults 65 and older.[77]

Social networking is in large part enabled by the development practices and principles associated with what is known as Web 2.0, which is intended to facilitate interactive information sharing, interoperability, collaboration and user-centric designs. Currently, there are a limited number of social networking websites catering explicitly to the elderly, but more are emerging as commercial interests focus on tapping into the significant market potential represented by this group. Some examples include:

www.aarp.org
www.eons.com
www.rezoom.com
www.silverplanet.com
www.sagazone.co.uk

Accessibility

In addition to offering demographically appropriate information, entertainment and forums, websites for older adults also need to be designed to contend with age-related changes in vision and cognition. Various guidelines have been issued to aid site developers in this, including guidelines from the US National Institute on Aging and the National Library of Medicine[78] which address the needs of the elderly. More broadly, Web Content Accessibility Guidelines (WCAG[79]) provide recommendations for making Web content more accessible to a wider range of people with disabilities, including blindness and low vision, deafness and hearing loss, learning disabilities, cognitive limitations, limited movement, speech disabilities, photosensitivity and combinations of these. The European Commission has indicated that all public websites should comply with WCAG.[80] Similarly, the US requires compliance with Section 508 to ensure all IT systems are accessible.

The exact benefits of the use of any ICT product vary considerably depending on the individual's ability and attitude towards human computer interaction. The ability

[77] Lenhart, A., 'Pew Internet Project Data Memo', *Pew Internet & American Life Project*, 2009.
[78] National Institute on Aging, February 2001 (last revised March 2009). http://www.nia.nih.gov/HealthInformation/Publications/website.htm
[79] http://www.w3.org/TR/2008/REC-WCAG20-20081211/
[80] European Commission, European i2010 initiative on e-Inclusion: 'To be part of the information society', Communication from the Commission to the European Parliament, the Council, the European Economic and Social Committee and the Committee of the Regions, COM(2007) 694 final, Brussels, 8 Nov 2007, p. 4. The EC says that as of the end of 2006 a minority of surveyed public websites were fully compliant with these Guidelines. See also European Commission, 'Commission wants a web that is better enabled for the disabled', Press release, IP/08/1074, Brussels, 2 July 2008.
http://europa.eu/rapid/pressReleasesAction.do?reference=IP/08/1074&format=HTML&aged=0&language=EN&guiLanguage=nl

to understand the application, to access it and trust in the technology is a key condition for its successful adoption and subsequent e-inclusion benefits. But for senior citizens, just being given the opportunity to use the technology can have a positive effect on their quality of life, their independence and on their family and social life, as well as their ability to participate in a work environment.

The social and economic impact of the world's ageing population could be somewhat minimised if senior citizens remained in the labour force longer, if they were able to contribute more to the overall productivity of the economy and if they remained active in society longer. However, to achieve this, various aspects of the digital divide need to be overcome. A telling indicator of the digital divide is that only 10 per cent of senior citizens over the age of 65 used the Internet (in 2005), compared to 68 per cent of those aged 16-24.[81] In the US, according to the Pew Research Center's Internet & American Life Project surveys taken from 2006-2008, the Web continues to be populated largely by younger generations, as over half of the adult internet population is between 18 and 44 years old.[82]

According to the SeniorWatch 2 study, 'among older people who are still working in gainful employment (or self-employment), almost two-thirds (63%) use computers and one-half (47%) use the Internet at work at least occasionally. Comparing this with former workers shows the tremendous increase in ICT use at the workplace, also of older workers, that has taken place. Compared to today's 63%, among those who retired or were last employed before 1991, only 12% used computers at the workplace, and for instance those before 2001 but after 1997 already had a 40% share of computer users. Employment policy in Europe now gives a high importance to increasing employment rates of older workers and encouraging older workers to remain longer in the workforce. Older workers' ICT skills will play a key role in reaching these goals.'[83]

Examples of projects funded by the European Commission related to developing Web-based interfaces and ICT to keep older workers in the labour force longer include the following:

- DIADEM: Adaptable browser for the disabled and elderly[84] – Led by Brunel University (UK), with six other partners, the project (Sept 2006 – Aug 2009) aimed to provide an adaptable Web browser interface to help individuals with reduced cognitive skills remain active and independent both at work and at home. The project developed an 'Expert System', which monitors the user, adapting and personalising the computer interface.

- ICT for ALL: Measuring interaction with ICT –Led by ASM Market Research and Analysis Centre (Poland), with four other partners, the ICT for ALL project (Oct 2006 – Sept 2008) focused upon indicators of the use of ICT by immigrants (including internal migration), the disabled, unemployed and older citizens. Its aim was to establish a framework for measuring the interaction of these populations with ICT and, in particular, broadband Internet, 3G, digital TV and ambient intelligence, as compared to other members of society.

---

[81] Riga Ministerial Declaration made by EU Ministers on eInclusion concerning 'Inclusive eGovernment', 11 June 2006. http://europa.eu.int/information_society/events/ict_riga_2006/index_en.htm

[82] Fox, Susannah, and Sydney Jones, 'PEW Internet & American Life Project', *Generations Online in 2009*, 28 Jan 2009.

[83] 'SeniorWatch 2: Assessment of the Senior Market for ICT, Progress and Developments', Final Study Report, (Deliverable D4 external), European Commission, April 2008.

[84] http://www.project-diadem.eu/

Communications technologies

In addition to the GPS technology embedded into mobile phones which can aid in tracking location, cell phone manufacturers have designed new products to facilitate use by the elderly, and thereby foster communication and enable socialisation. Those cell phone design issues that promote use by the elderly include better font spacing and size, bigger screens, larger device sizes and easy-to-grip surfaces. Many of the devices include hearing aid capabilities for better voice quality and emergency response services. Examples of cell phone manufacturers and their products that cater to the elderly include:

- Jitterbug handset and mobile service provider
- ClarityLife C900
- LG LX150
- Doro HandlePlus 334gsm, PhoneEasy 410, and PhoneEasy 335
- Alcom E110S Elderly Friendly GSM Phone
- Motorola W259
- UTStarcom Coupe 8630

2. AGEING WELL WITH CONVERGING TECHNOLOGIES

With every technological advance, we are challenged to ensure that all segments of society are included as beneficiaries. Emerging technologies must be equally accessible and beneficial to everyone regardless of age or ability. Ambient intelligent solutions, as discussed in this section, have the potential to fulfil this challenge and to assist elderly individuals in living healthy, safe and comfortable lives in an independent environment.

A number of applications built upon or integrating the technologies discussed above are emerging, and are beginning to have an impact on the elderly, if not now, then in the very near future. For example, a wearable device used to monitor the health of an elderly person may make use of affective intelligence to detect the wearer's mood, biotechnology to detect the wearer's blood pressure, sensing technology to detect the wearer's location, and nanotechnology to perform the micro-processing needed to assess the wearer's health. A convergence of various technologies is required to deliver this comprehensive solution which, in this example, may be allowing the elder wearer to go to work or to participate in social activities without worrying about the state of his health or may even intercept in an emergency situation and provide required first aid.

Scientific leaders and policy-makers across a broad range of fields are evaluating the potential impact of converging technologies on improving human capabilities at the microscopic, individual, group and societal levels. A vast potential lies in expanding human cognition and communication, improving human health and physical capabilities, enhancing group and societal outcomes, influencing national security, and unifying science and education.[85]

---

[85] *Converging Technologies for Improving Human Performance: Nanotechnology, Biotechnology, Information Technology and Cognitive Science*, National Science Foundation-sponsored report, June 2002. http://www.wtec.org/ConvergingTechnologies/Report/NBIC_report.pdf

2.1. The foundation: ubiquitous computing

No one can deny the significance that computing technology has had on our world; however, when that technology is unnoticeable and undetectable, the implications for its adoption become unlimited. According to visionary Mark Weiser, 'The most profound technologies are those that disappear. They weave themselves into the fabric of everyday life until they are indistinguishable from it.'[86] Eventually we will be using technology in the course of everyday activities without even realising it. And access to that technology may be everywhere – on your walls, in your furniture, on the packaging of your food, and in your clothes. Weiser referred to this technology as 'ubiquitous computing'.

Ubiquitous computing (UbiComp) is the model of human-computer interaction in which information processing has been thoroughly integrated into everyday objects and activities. As opposed to the desktop paradigm, in which a single user consciously engages a single device for a specialised purpose, someone 'using' ubiquitous computing engages many computational devices and systems simultaneously, in the course of ordinary activities, and may not necessarily even be aware that they are doing so.

Weiser coined the phrase 'ubiquitous computing' during his tenure as Chief Technologist of the Xerox Palo Alto Research Center (PARC). In a 1993 paper, he wrote, 'Ubiquitous computing enhances computer use by making many computers available throughout the physical environment, while making them effectively invisible to the user.'[87]

2.2. Context-aware computing and ambient intelligence

Ubiquitous computing lays the foundation for the technological paradigm called ambient intelligence (AmI). By adding communication abilities to ubiquitous computing devices, a whole new world of services based on 'context awareness' becomes available. These services obtain information about the circumstances under which they are able to operate, and based on rules or an intelligent stimulus, they adapt their behaviour accordingly. These services sense the user's environment while simultaneously accessing remote data repositories and other humans, and exchange information without the user being involved.

While ubiquitous computing means that computing access is unobtrusively all around us, ambient intelligence goes one step further. Not only is the computing all around us, but the electronic environments are responsive to the presence of people. In other words, the systems themselves are both context-aware and responsive.

The concept of context awareness emerged out of ubiquitous computing research at Xerox PARC and elsewhere in the early 1990s. The term was first used by Schilit and Theimer in their 1994 paper 'Disseminating Active Map Information to Mobile Hosts' where they describe a model of computing in which users interact with many different mobile and stationary computers and classify a context-aware system as one

---

[86] Weiser, Mark. 'The Computer for the 21st Century', *Scientific American*, 265, No. 3, Sept 1991, pp. 94-104.
[87] Weiser, Mark, 'Some Computer Issues in Ubiquitous Computing', *Communications of the ACM*, Vol. 36, No. 7, July 1993, pp. 74-84.

that can adapt according to its location of use, the collection of nearby people and objects, as well as the changes to those objects over time.[88]

An ambient intelligent environment uses unobtrusive computing devices to improve the quality of people's lives by acknowledging their needs, requirements and preferences and thus act in some way on their behalf even if the users themselves cannot do so. Using various embedded sensors and devices, an ambient system is able to obtain information about the circumstances under which it is operating (i.e., its context) and adapt its behaviour accordingly on its own. Ambient systems do so by detecting and processing the following four aspects:

1. The first aspect is **location**: Where is the device (and thus the user) currently located? Is the device mobile or fixed? Can its location be determined by the device itself, or must it be inferred from another device (GPS) or from the general layout of the service (hospital or home network)? Hence, accurate location information may thus depend on multiple sensors or inferred knowledge from networks and other services.

2. The second aspect is related to **information about co-events**: What is actually happening around the user? Is it raining? What is the time of the day? Are there other users in the vicinity? What services are available? All this information must be infused from appropriate sensors, devices, services, etc., and made available to some kind of inference mechanism. The inference can be made based on simple pre-defined rules, business process engines or some kind of higher level intelligence with knowledge discovery, semantic resolution and processing.

3. The third aspect is related to the **history of events**: What happened in the past? Did the patient take medication in the morning? How many times did the doorbell sound? What can be seen from video pictures captured in the 10 minutes prior to a break-in? A history of events requires data persistence and storage facilities, either in backend systems (data repositories) or in distributed networks (devices, gateways, network controllers, etc.), which thus poses serious data protection and security concerns.

4. The fourth and final aspect is related to **status monitoring**: What is the present status of the user? Is the house empty? Is the blood pressure stable? Has the user signed up for social services? Status can be inferred directly from devices and repositories or can be inferred from rules or higher-level intelligence. When a status changes unexpectedly, it usually causes an alarm to be invoked.

2.3. Integrated, personalised, adaptive, and anticipatory

In addition to the four aspects defined above used to assess a user's situational context, ambient intelligent systems are also characterised as:

- Integrated – the ambient system is embedded into the environment.
- Personalised – the ambient system can be tailored to a specific user's needs.
- Adaptive – the ambient system changes in response to the user.

[88] Schilit, Bill N., and Marvin M. Theimer, 'Disseminating Active Map Information to Mobile Hosts', *IEEE Network,* September/October 1994, pp. 22 – 32.

- Anticipatory – the ambient system anticipates the user's desires without direct mediation.

Ambient systems aim to improve the quality of peoples' lives by creating and monitoring a desired atmosphere via intelligent, interconnected and personalised systems and services. The ambient system is able to anticipate the user's needs and subsequently adapt to those inputs for future evaluations.

By adapting its behaviour according to the immediate and future needs of the user, ambient intelligent applications become limitless – homes, offices, stores, vehicles, hospitals, schools, sports facilities and many more – and the implications for using the technology to address the needs of the elderly population become evident in terms of both an assistive and e-inclusive strategy.

II.   BARRIERS AND RISKS

Advocates of the benefits of technological change typically see emerging technologies as offering hope for the betterment of the human condition, while critics are quick to warn of the dangers they pose. As with all new technology, the emergence of new assistive products and services includes both benefits and risks, which have been described earlier in this Chapter, as well as elsewhere in this volume. One of the key risks that bears some further examination here are those barriers that currently constrain development and market adoption of these technologies. The assistive technology (AT) market is diverse and fragmented[89], and facing a number of challenges, including:

- **Low awareness by users.** There has been a low level of knowledge among the elderly population about the assistive technology devices which have been commercialised and made available in the market. In a study conducted with Belgian seniors residing in community living[90], it was found that, though the seniors were aware of assistive devices relating to using the toilet, there was a low level of awareness of assistive devices related to mobility, communication and other self-care aspects. Efforts in this area are led by international and national organisations, including EASTIN (European Assistive Technology Information Network) which specifically focuses upon providing information about European products for daily living in terms understandable by end-users and their carers.
- **Lack of effective response to social factors in technology development.** Technology evangelists, in earlier commercialisation efforts, have always focused on developing a product which is accurate and precise, most of the time ignoring the 'social and human factors'[91] involved in its usage. An example of this was seen in the first generation of assistive robots developed to assist elderly at home akin to the industrial robots. The acceptance rate was low since it was missing the 'empathy' factor and was designed to serve narrowly defined health-care problems. While there is a significant effort to enhance design of public spaces and places, as well as objects and artefacts used in the range of human experience,

---

[89] 'Analyzing and federating the European assistive technology ICT industry,' Final Report, March 2009.
[90] Roelands, M., P. Van Oosta, A. Buyssea and A. M. Depoorterb, 'Awareness among community-dwelling elderly of assistive devices for mobility and self-care and attitudes towards their use,' *Social Science & Medicine*, Vol. 54, Issue 9, May 2002.
[91] Meng and Lee.

in Europe, especially as driven by Design For All[92] initiatives, research has indicated that acceptance of assistive technology would be greater with better attention to user preferences than was previously assumed.

- **Cost of assistive technology devices**. Assistive technology is quite costly, especially when devices or products must be purchased in a lump sum (often, as a proportion of the elder's pension, such purchases are out of reach). Reimbursement policies differ around the globe and across Europe. In many cases, adult children of the elder bear the cost of such purchases directly, and are thus involved in purchasing decisions. Difficulty in determining how to pay for AT can constrain users from making purchases, and likewise, constrain manufacturers from entering new markets, if only based upon a lack of knowledge of how best to price and market products in various regions.

- **Difficulty in achieving economies of scale**. For AT developers, being able to generate sufficient levels of uptake of new products, negatively impacts overall market growth, continuing to keep profit margins low and reducing further investment in R&D. Because of the lack of effective product distribution models, absence of strong service models to support deployment, diverse reimbursement schemes and lack of significant investment by large industrial players, AT manufacturers continue to struggle, and fail to build the market. The AAATE (Association for the Advancement of Assistive Technology in Europe) actively supports efforts to increase the uptake of AT within the European market, as do national level organisations.

The adaptation of new technologies always requires different business models and disciplines to converge and cooperate. All industrial concerns that play a role in the future technologies must be willing to make the required investments in order for the technologies to take root. Because ambient technology has the potential to be applied to products and systems that aid the elderly, there is a significant risk if industry and government policy cannot drive the new technology forward. Rather than ease the increasing burden on health and nursing care facilities, the failure of the technology to take root may result in even further demand upon these facilities and the potential neglect of needs of ageing individuals living independently.

As we move towards Kurzweil's Singularity, it is critical that the inclusive society provide the opportunity for all to make use of new technologies as they are developed. These emerging assistive technologies have the opportunity to create significant changes in the life of individuals, and through their ability to promote independent living and foster the development of assistive products and services, they also provide an extraordinary opportunity to close the digital divide.

REFERENCES

Alwan, M., P.J. Rajendran, S. Kell, et al., "A Smart and Passive Floor-Vibration Based Fall Detector for Elderly", *Information and Communication Technologies Medical Automation Research Center* (MARC), Department of Pathology, University of Virginia, 24-28 April 2006.

---

[92] http://www.edean.org

Augusto, Juan Carlos, and Paul McCullagh, *Ambient Intelligence: Concepts and Applications*, Invited Paper by the International Journal on Computer Science and Information Systems, volume 4, Number 1, pp. 1-28, June 2007.

Baxi, Amit, and N. Kodalapura, "A Self-Managing Framework for Health Monitoring", *Intel Technology Journal*, Intel Corporation, Vol. 10, No. 4, 2006, p. 314. http://download.intel.com/technology/itj/2006/v10i4/v10-i4-art06.pdf

Boulos, Maged N Kamel, et al., "CAALYX: a new generation of location-based services in healthcare", *International Journal of Health Geographics*, Vol. 6, No. 9, 2007.

Cartledge, Sue, *Robot Dogs Keep Elderly Company*, Helioza, 2008. http://www.helioza.com/Directory/Science/Technology/Robot-Dogs-Keep-Elderly-Company-7.php

Cavaliere, Thomas , "Tapping into nerves", ELE 282 Biomedical Engineering Seminar I, *Biomedical engineering*, University of Rhode Island, 8 April 2008. http://www.ele.uri.edu/Courses/ele282/S02/Tom_2.pdf

Converging Technologies for Improving Human Performance: Nanotechnology, Biotechnology, Information Technology and Cognitive Science, National Science Foundation-sponsored report, June 2002. http://www.wtec.org/ConvergingTechnologies/Report/NBIC_report.pdf

De Hert, P. , and S.Gutwirth, Privacy, data protection and law enforcement. Opacity of the individual and transparency of power, in E. Claes, A. Duff and S. Gutwirth (eds.), *Privacy and the criminal law*, Intersentia, Antwerpen-Oxford, 2006.

Dulay, N., S. Heeps, E. Lupu, R. Mathur, O. Sharma, M. Sloman and J. Sventek, "AMUSE: Autonomic Management of Ubiquitous e-Health Systems", *Imperial College London*, 2005. http://www.dcs.gla.ac.uk/amuse/AHM2005-slomanFinal.pdf

Estrin, Deborah (ed.), Embedded, Everywhere, Committee on Networked Systems of Embedded Computers of the Computer Science and Telecommunications Board, National Research Council, *National Academy Press*, Washington, DC, 2001. http://www.nap.edu/openbook.php?isbn=0309075688

European Commission Joint Research Centre, "SESAMONET- improved mobility of the visually impaired", 19 October 2007. http://ec.europa.eu/dgs/jrc/index.cfm?id=4210&lang=en

Feynman, Richard P., "There's Plenty of Room at the Bottom: An Invitation to Enter a New Field of Physics", *Engineering and Science*, Vol. XXIII, No. 5, February 1960.

Fox, Susannah, and Sydney Jones, "PEW Internet & American Life Project", *Generations Online* in 2009, 28 Jan 2009.

Freitas, Robert A. Jr., "A Mechanical Artificial Red Cell: Exploratory Design in Medical Nanotechnology," 1999.

Freitas, Robert A., "Microbivores: Artificial Mechanical Phagocytes," *Institute for Molecular Manufacturing*, Report Number 25, 2001.

Hawkley, L. C., and J. T Cacioppo, "Aging and Loneliness," *Current Directions in Psychological Science*, Vol. 16, No. 4, pp. 187-191, 2007.

Ishak, Wan Hussain Wan, and Fadzilah Siraj, "Artificial Intelligence in Medical Applications: An Exploration", *University Utara Malaysi*a, 2006.

Kurzweil, Raymond. "The Law of Accelerating Returns", KurzweilAI.net, 7 Mar 2001. http://www.kurzweilai.net/articles/art0134.html

Lenhart, A., "Pew Internet Project Data Memo", Pew Internet & American Life Project, 2009.

McCarthy, J., (Professor Emeritus, Stanford University), 'What is Artificial Intelligence? (rev. 12 November 2007, http://www-formal.stanford.edu/jmc/whatisai/whatisai.html

Meng, Q. and M.H.Lee, "Design Issues for Assistive Robotics for the Elderly", University of Wales, Wales, UK, 2006.

Mort, Maggie, *"Achieving 'good care in sociotechnical networks: ethical frameworks for new care technologies for older people"*, EFFORTT, Lancaster University, 2008. Based on a presentation at the Future of AI & Self-Adaptive Software, Artificial Intelligence and Adaptive Software Workshop on ICT and Ageing, EU SENIOR Project, Brussels, December 2008.

Nsanze, Fabienne, ICT Implants in the Human Body – a review, In: Ethical aspects of ICT implants in the human body, European Group on Ethics in Science and New Technologies to the European Commission, 2005. http://bookshop.europa.eu/eubookshop/download.action?fileName=KAAJ050203AC_002.pdf &eubphfUid=155714&catalogNbr=KA-AJ-05-020-3A-C

Phillips, Becky, "No Place Like Home -- Student's Sensors May Help Elderly", Washington State University, 2008. http://school.eecs.wsu.edu/node/612

Picard, Rosalind W., "Affective Computing: Challenges", *International Journal of Human-Computer Studies*, 59, (1-2), July 2003, pp. 55–64.

Ramakrishnan, Sailesh, and Martha E. Pollack, *Intelligent Monitoring in a Robotic Assistant for the Elderly*, University of Pittsburgh, 2000. http://www.eecs.umich.edu/ ~pollackm/distrib/aaai00stupos.pdf.

Ramos, Carlos, Juan Augusto, and Daniel Shapiro (guest editors), *Special Issue on Ambient Intelligence*, IEEE Intelligent Systems, vol. 23, no. 2, pp. 15-18, Mar/Apr, 2008.

Reding, Viviane, "Why the Internet must be open, global and multilingual", *Opening speech at the Internet Governance Forum Sharm El Sheikh*, 15 November 2009.

Roelands, M., P. Van Oosta, A. Buyssea and A. M. Depoorterb, "Awareness among community-dwelling elderly of assistive devices for mobility and self-care and attitudes towards their use," *Social Science & Medicine*, Vol. 54, Issue 9, May 2002.

Schilit, Bill N., and Marvin M. Theimer, "Disseminating Active Map Information to Mobile Hosts", *IEEE Network*, September/October 1994, pp. 22 – 32.

SeniorWatch 2: Assessment of the Senior Market for ICT, Progress and Developments", *Final Study Report*, (Deliverable D4 external), European Commission, April 2008.

Syrdal, Dag Sverre, Dautenhahn, Kristen,Walters, Michael L., and Kheng Lee Koay, "Long-term Robotic Companionship in the Home", Adaptive Systems Research Group, University of Hertfordshire, 2008. Presentation give at the Future of AI & Self-Adaptive Software, Artificial Intelligence and Adaptive Software Workshop on ICT and Ageing, SENIOR Project, held in Brussels, December 2009. http://seniorproject.eu/resources/ 5ExpertMeeting/Syrdal.pdf

Szolovits, Peter, Ramesh S. Patil and William B. Schwartz, "Artificial Intelligence in Medical Diagnosis", *Massachusetts Institute of Technology*, 1988. http://groups.csail.mit.edu/ medg/ftp/psz/SchwartzAnnals.html

US Center for Disease Control (CDC) http://www.cdc.gov/ncipc/factsheets/adultfalls.htm

USDA Rural Development: Bringing Broadband to Rural America", US Department of Agriculture, Rural Development Agency, May 2007. http://www.rurdev.usda.gov/ rd/pubs/RDBroadbandRpt.pdf

Wasson, Glenn, Jim Gunderson, Sean Graves and Robin Felder, *An Assistive Robotic Agent for Pedestrian Mobility*, University of Virginia, 2001. http://www.cs.virginia.edu/ ~gsw2c/research/agents01.pdf

Weiser, Mark, "Some Computer Issues in Ubiquitous Computing", *Communications of the ACM*, Vol. 36, No. 7, July 1993, pp. 74-84.

Weiser, Mark. "The Computer for the 21st Century", *Scientific American*, 265, No. 3, Sept 1991, pp. 94-104.

Wiedemann, Peter M., and Holger Schutz, "Framing Effects on Risk Perception of Nanotechnology," *Public Understanding of Science*, Vol. 17, No. 3, 2008, pp. 369-379.

Regulation (EC) No 1394/2007 of the European Parliament and of the Council of 13 November 2007 on advanced therapy medicinal products and amending Directive 2001/83/EC and Regulation (EC) No 726/2004.

European Commission, European i2010 initiative on e-Inclusion: "To be part of the information society", Communication from the Commission to the European Parliament, the Council, the European Economic and Social Committee and the Committee of the Regions, COM(2007) 694 final, Brussels, 8 Nov 2007, p. 4. The EC says that as of the end of 2006 a minority of surveyed public websites were fully compliant with these Guidelines. See also

European Commission, "Commission wants a web that is better enabled for the disabled", Press release, IP/08/1074, Brussels, 2 July 2008.

Riga Ministerial Declaration made by EU Ministers on eInclusion concerning "Inclusive eGovernment", 11 June 2006. http://europa.eu.int/information_society/events/ict_riga_2006/index_en.htm

SENIOR project, D1.1: Environmental Scanning Report, D2.1: Ubiquitous Computing, D2.2: Ubiquitous Communication, D2.3: Intelligent User Interfaces, D2.4: AI & Adaptive Software, and D2.5: AT & Robotics.

Science Daily, Universitat Politècnica de Catalunya, "Intelligent Walker Designed to Assist the Elderly and People Undergoing Medical Rehabilitation", ScienceDaily, 2008. http://www.sciencedaily.com/releases/2008/11/081107072015.htm

BBC News, Lytle, J Mark, "Robot Care Bears for the Elderly", BBC News, 21 February 2002.

   http://news.bbc.co.uk/1/hi/sci/tech/1829021.stm

Swithed.com, "New   GPS   Shoes   Join   in   Trend   to   Help   Elderly". http://www.switched.com/2009/06/16/new-gps-shoes-join-in-trend-to-help-elderly/

CHAPTER SEVEN. GOOD PRACTICES IN E-INCLUSION

By David Wright and Kush Wadhwa

INTRODUCTION

Addressing the challenges of e-inclusion and ageing requires actions on several fronts – policy, legal, regulatory, technology. A key element in the strategy is good practice, practical examples that can be cited and shown as helping to overcome social exclusion. For this reason, good practice became an important focus in the SENIOR project and for the European Commission, so much so that this book would be incomplete without a discussion of what constitutes good practice and a few examples. In 2009, with the support of the SENIOR consortium, the European Commission invited experts from across Europe to three workshops in Brussels to consider these issues: What is good practice in e-inclusion? What criteria should good practice meet? How should good practices be selected? In addition to the more theoretical conceptualisations, the Commission asked SENIOR to identify actual examples of good practice, preferably from different quarters of Europe, from different domains and involving different stakeholders. Actual instances of good practice in e-inclusion provides a useful complement to analysis – the latter can identify problems and issues and propose solutions, while good practice cases can give weight or body to analysis grounded in reality, can show solutions, which is the main point of promoting good practice. This chapter draws on the experience and findings that arose from the work done in support of the Commission and its three workshops.

By way of introduction to this chapter, we invite the reader to note that Member States, the European Commission, industry and NGOs representing users have undertaken several actions to advance e-inclusion. A milestone was the 2006 Ministerial Riga Declaration on ICT for an inclusive Information Society, by means of which Member States committed themselves to concrete targets for Internet usage and availability, digital literacy, and accessibility of ICT by 2010. In the context of the Riga Declaration, the European Commission identified six themes which it uses to foster e-inclusion. The six themes and their overall objectives are the following[1]:

- *E-accessibility*. Make ICT accessible to all, meeting a wide spectrum of people's needs, in particular any special needs.
- *Ageing*. Empower older people to fully participate in the economy and society, continue independent lifestyles and enhance their quality of life.
- *E-competences*. Equip citizens with the knowledge, skills and lifelong learning approach needed to increase social inclusion, employability and enrich their lives.
- *Socio-cultural e-inclusion*. Enable minorities, migrants and marginalised young people to fully integrate into communities and participate in society by using ICT.
- *Geographical e-inclusion*. Increase the social and economic well being of people in rural, remote and economically disadvantaged areas with the help of ICT.

---

[1] See Chapter 1 where we introduced the six thematic issues of e-inclusion

- *Inclusive e-government*. Deliver better, more diverse public services for all using ICT while encouraging increased public participation in democracy.

In 2007, the European Commission launched its i2010 e-Inclusion Initiative to raise political awareness of e-inclusion, encourage replication of e-inclusion success stories throughout the EU, and pave the way for future actions.

An important element in the e-inclusion strategies has been the identification and promotion of good practices.

Good practice e-inclusion awards were a highlight of the European Ministerial Conference on e-Inclusion held in Vienna in late 2008 which was attended by more than 1,000 participants.

In the following sections, we consider what good practices are, note the increasing emphasis on good practices as a matter of e-inclusion strategy, the perceived value of good practices and the criteria for selecting them. The success in using good practices as a matter of strategy and policy is critically dependent on how they are selected and by whom and how well they are promoted (or disseminated). In a last section, three examples of good practices are discussed in more detail.

I. WHAT ARE GOOD PRACTICES?

1. GENERAL

The term 'good practice' suggests something that has worked in a particular situation and that may offer lessons for others. A defining characteristic of good practice is that it must be transferable or applicable to others, at least in part. A good practice implies a practice that can be improved, not one that has finality from which one must not deviate.

There are various definitions of good practice. Often these definitions are contextually based. As our interest is in good practices in e-inclusion, it is instructive to consider the definition of good practice used in the largest online library of good practices in e-inclusion, that collected by the European Commission on its ePractice.eu portal.[2] ePractice.eu describes itself as 'the one stop place for the exchange of advice, experiences and events on practices of eGovernment, eHealth and eInclusion, offering the most complete information and exchange opportunities for these areas in Europe'. As of mid-2009, the portal had more than 1,100 good practice case studies. It describes these cases as

> written summaries of real-life projects or business solutions developed by public administrations, entrepreneurs and corporations. Case studies included in our portal are based on actual experiences, and reading them provides a picture of the challenges and dilemmas faced by the professionals working in eGovernment, eHealth and eInclusion... The use of ICT leading towards the reorganisation of eGovernment, eInclusion or eHealth processes must be a basic factor in all the cases published in the portal.'

---

[2] http://www.epractice.eu/en/einclusion

The Commission goes on to say that 'Research projects or events are not considered cases. In order to be included in the database, a case must be a real-life project, already executed and developed in a particular context.'[3]

This definition seems a bit severe in that one can envisage a good practice that does not necessarily involve a reorganisation of e-government, e-inclusion or e-health processes. Similarly, one can envisage a good practice in a research project that merits being used by other research projects. For example, the MAPPED project, a project funded by the European Commission under its Sixth Framework Programme (FP6), certified on its website that it complied with ethical guidelines. We think this is a good practice which merits replication by other research projects. In our view, even a policy could be a good practice. For example, the Commission's policy on e-inclusion merits replication by the Member States. So far, e-inclusion is a 'soft' policy, i.e., it is not the subject of a directive or regulation which obliges Member States to implement it. Nevertheless, the wisdom and good sense of the Commission's policy on e-inclusion has found favour with the Member States, as evidenced by the Riga Declaration by means of which Member States committed themselves to introducing various measures to overcome exclusion of digitally disadvantaged persons and bringing them into the mainstream of Europe's Information Society.

In spite of the rigidity of the ePractice criteria for good practice case studies, one could agree that a good practice should have some measurable results in order to evaluate whether it is good practice or not. Without real-world application, where is the proof of its goodness? A good practice should reach beyond theory to real-world application in some context, where its impact can be observed or measured in some way.

The authors of a report on good practices in e-health observe that a good practice comes from real life and should offer a learning experience and recognisable benefits. They say that

> What is judged as 'best' will always depend on the national, cultural, structural context and subjective assessments. What might be judged by some as best in one context may not be applicable at all in another, even similar context or not 'work' for other reasons like legal requirements or habits and attitudes of citizens. On the other hand, good practice cases ... – in spite of reflecting unique experiences – can provide useful insights for others, likely to stimulate creativity, self-reflection and the transfer or adaptation of good ideas.[4]

The authors also noted that of the good practice cases they collected 'Project managers and users from various backgrounds described the success of their eHealth solutions mostly in ... 'how' the respective solution was implemented and did not relate success much to 'what' was implemented'.

A good practice should not imply that others must follow it rigidly, as one might be expected to do in the case of a standard. A good practice is one that offers lessons from which one can learn and possibly apply in a similar or even different situation or context. But it may not be possible to completely transfer the practice, simply because there are cultural or environmental or other contextual factors that are different. Thus, careful evaluation is needed before adopting any so-called good practice. One

---

[3] http://www.epractice.eu/info/cases

[4] Stroetmann, Karl A., Reinhard Hammerschmidt,Veli N. Stroetmann, Ingrid Moldenaers, eHealth in Action: Good Practice in European Countries, Good eHealth Report, Office for Official Publications of the European Communities, Luxembourg, January 2009, p. 6. See also p. 9.

person's good practice is not necessarily the best for another person, company or country. Applying a good practice unquestioningly might have a negative impact in a different context.

The Tavistock Institute in its report on e-inclusion good practices presented some examples of good practice and commented that

> What all these examples have in common is that they have chosen an approach which combines the 'primary task' of addressing the particular needs of the eInclusion dimension (e.g. providing access to ICTs by making available PCs or high-speed Internet access) with measures that embed these activities within the wider socio-economic context of the target groups that are being addressed. This ensures that some of the inherent barriers to the take-up of ICTs are being addressed and at best overcome. Looking back at the possible strategies for tackling social exclusion, this means that what the selected examples... have in common is an underlying preventative approach / vision for tackling issues of digital exclusion.[5]

A good practice is inherently a case study. It must be capable of being described and transmitted, or promoted, to others. In some fashion, it must offer guidance for others.

Taking account of the foregoing, but perhaps adopting a more inclusive approach to what constitutes a good practice than the ePractice.eu portal, we envisage good practices in e-inclusion being of three main types, i.e., projects, guidances, and policies and programmes.

2. PROJECTS

By projects, we include research projects such as those funded by the EC under its Framework Programmes and their equivalent in the Member States which are typically of fixed duration (from a year or so up to several years in the case of Integrated Projects and Networks of Excellence). We also include projects of an operational or ongoing nature.

3. GUIDANCES

Some projects or organisations or associations, agencies or other entities have published guidances which could be considered as good practices. In some cases, the guidance has been prepared by a consortium for the guidance of its partners. In other cases, the guidance has been prepared for others. For example, the UK Information Commissioner's Office (ICO) has prepared guidance on good practice in security of personal information.[6]

---

[5] Cullen, Joe, Kari Hadjivassiliou and Kerstin Junge, *Status of eInclusion measurement, analysis and approaches for improvement*, Topic Report 4: Recommendations for future action, Final Report, Tavistock Institute, February 2007, p. 53.
[6] For this and many other good practice notes from ICO, see
http://www.ico.gov.uk/tools_and_resources/document_library/data_protection.aspx

4. POLICIES AND PROGRAMMES

The EC and Member States have adopted policies and programmes on e-inclusion which could be considered as good practices. For example, the Commission and various Member States have adopted policies and programmes the aim of which is to make broadband access to the Internet available to all citizens.

II. VALUE OF GOOD PRACTICES

Good practice cases have strategic value, i.e., as an element in strategies aimed at overcoming e-exclusion, but they may also have value as examples of ways of responding to ethical challenges. Collecting and disseminating good practices is a way of supporting stakeholders in their efforts to address common challenges, to facilitate implementation of e-inclusion strategies and to promote the benefits that flow from the e-inclusion of all citizens. Good practice cases can be an important resource for decision-makers, who require reliable evidence of the benefits of e-inclusion ethics.[7]

Well disseminated good practices have an economic value too, in avoiding duplication of effort or avoiding the cost of reinventing the wheel. A UK study found that 'lack of evaluation can lead to a poor appreciation of the benefits of ICT for social inclusion, poor replication of good practice, or duplication of effort where the experience of past initiatives is not drawn upon.'[8]

Good practice cases are intended to influence others engaged in similar activities. The rationale for an e-learning manual is described thusly: 'This Manual provides examples of good practice collected from different European countries in the field of e-inclusion and e-learning for people with psychological disabilities. Its purpose is to provide all actors involved in the fight against the digital divide with ideas and successful paths that could be included within their own activities'.[9]

Good practices may make the difference between e-excluded groups joining or not joining mainstream digital society, as found:

> Various social pressures were non-conducive to maintaining participants' engagement with the Internet, with some participants feeling stigmatized when they joined the project. In any residential environment that planned to introduce Internet facilities, a clear and obvious commitment from the management and care staff would be helpful, and an opinion leader could be encouraged to be part of the project. The introduction of computers to groups who already share some common activities, even if not much more than a friendly cooperative arrangement, would improve the chances for success when combined with patient, readily-available support.[10]

Thus, in this case, good practice would ensure a supportive, rather than stigmatising social context, even in a relatively small social context such as that of an

---

[7] Stroetmann et al., op. cit., p. 10.

[8] Social Exclusion Unit (SEU). Inclusion Through Innovation: Tackling Social Exclusion Through New Technologies. Final Report. Office of the Deputy Prime Minister, London, November 2005, p. 62.

[9] e-ability project, *Good Practice Manual: Promotion of digital literacy in people with psychological disabilities: Some European Initiatives*, European Commission Directorate-General for Education and Culture, Brussels, [no date], p. 8.
www.elearningeuropa.info/out/?doc_id=8577&rsr_id=9950

[10] Mellor, David, Lucy Firth and Kathleen Moore, 'Can the Internet Improve the Well-being of the Elderly?', *Ageing International*, Vol. 35, 2008, pp. 25-42 [p. 41].

individual assisted living facility. The case described by Mellor et al. shows that even bad or poor practice can have value in pointing out what to avoid.

One might assume that good practice cases do influence other practices and policy-making, based on circumstantial evidence. The, for example, has said that the EU has to innovate in the way it sets policy frameworks, in its legislation, in bringing people together in the exchange of best practice and in catalysing new approaches.[11] Similarly, the UK government says its recent *Digital Britain* report 'allows the Government to assess the excellent work already achieved, and to suggest a step change in the ways to help the digitally disconnected, *building on the best practice to date*, and on the knowledge and understanding we now have about the barriers and the ways to overcome them' [Italics added].[12]

While one might assume that good practice cases do influence other practices and policy-making in e-domains, notably e-inclusion, so far there appears to be limited empirical evidence to support that assumption.

III. SELECTING GOOD PRACTICES

Good practices are selected in different ways. They may be designated as a good practice by the organisation that follows the practice or by the authors of a report or by a committee of independent experts.

The European Commission has a good practice portal (ePractice.eu) where individuals can lodge what they take to be a good practice, at least to some extent. The portal does have an Editorial Board which seems to exercise some judgement in what is accepted for publication on the website.[13] As of mid-2009, the portal has accumulated and published more than 1,100 good practice cases since its launch in June 2007, which, it says, proves 'the growing interest of European professionals in sharing practices and being informed about the latest developments in the eGovernment, eInclusion and eHealth domains'.[14]

Under contract to the European Commission, the German consultancy Empirica produced two reports on good practices in e-health and e-inclusion, but in neither case is an explanation offered on how the good practice case studies were selected or by whom they were selected.

Some good practices or the best of good practices are designated as such as a result of their selection by a jury of independent experts. The European Commission invited the submission of e-inclusion good practices in 2008. It received 469 cases from which it selected five for each of seven categories, and of those it selected one from each of the seven categories as the winners of its e-inclusion awards.

---

[11] European Commission. Renewed social agenda: Opportunities, access and solidarity in 21st century Europe. Communication from the Commission to the European Parliament, the Council, the European Economic and Social Committee and the Committee of the Regions. COM(2008) 412 final. Brussels, 2 July 2008.

[12] UK Department for Culture, Media and Sport and Department for Business, Innovation and Skills, *Digital Britain*, Final Report, The Stationery Office, Norwich, June 2009, p. 34. www.tsoshop.co.uk.

[13] The portal says that 'ePractice.eu publishes, in good faith, all cases correctly submitted, although in some circumstances the Editorial Board reserves the right to question suitability and remove a contribution. In these occasions, ePractice.eu may contact the author and work with him/her to clarify the situation. Cases are occasionally withdrawn at the request of the author or an institution.' http://www.epractice.eu/info/cases

[14] http://www.epractice.eu/case1000

The criteria used by the judges in selecting the best of the good practices were the following:

- Impact on the community – What positive impact did the project make on the community it serves and how was that impact measured?
- Innovative use of technology – How was the project innovative? Was it the technology used, route to market, method of engagement or another element?
- Embracing all users – How has the project encouraged greater accessibility or improved the user friendliness of digital technology for the community it serves?
- Working with others – How has the project created partnerships with other organisations to improve the experience for all those involved and what were the benefits?
- Sharing the learning and knowledge – How have the lessons learnt and knowledge gained been shared with other organisations to benefit the communities served?
- Long term sustainability – What was the duration of the project, and how did the funding model meet those commitments and obligations?
- WOW factor – Why was the project amazing? Could it be the way it came together, the people involved, the outcomes it achieved, or something else?[15]

In the case of the 2009 e-government awards, the European Commission says the best of good practices will be evaluated and selected by a panel of independent experts. 'The experts will be drawn from across Europe from a variety of backgrounds to ensure the widest possible coverage in terms of specialist knowledge and geographical balance. The panel of experts will be suggested by the European eGovernment Awards Consortium and endorsed by the European Commission services. Experts are bound to confidentiality rules and will have to confirm that they are not involved in conflicts of interest regarding their deliberations.'[16]

Selection criteria for the e-government awards are relevance, impact, innovation, potential for sharing good practice, management approach, and communication and dissemination.

Perhaps somewhat more distant from e-inclusion and e-domains, the European Occupational Safety and Health Agency (OSHA), based in Bilbao, has been conducting good practice competitions for several years. Its experience with selecting good practices for awards makes its selection criteria useful as a point of reference. They are as follows:

Relevance	Is the information directly relevant to Good Practice to eliminate or reduce risks at work?
Focus	Is the example from the workplace or involving interventions aimed at work?
Tackling risks at source	How well does the example eliminate or prevent risks at source through good management practice, and the effective use of risk assessment and implementation of its findings? Are interventions such as training part of an overall approach aimed at eliminating or preventing risks at source?
Implementation	How well have these measures been successfully implemented in practice?
Improvements	How well does the example demonstrate real improvement?

---

[15] http://www.citizensonline.org.uk/e-inclusionawards/judging
[16] European Commission, Teaming Up for the eUnion: European eGovernment Awards 2009. Guidance Notes For Submission, not dated.

Participation	Does the example demonstrate effective participation, including the involvement of employees / workers and their representatives?
Consultation	Where appropriate, how well does the example show evidence of good consultation between management and trade unions / workers?
Sustainability	Will the example be sustainable over time?
Legislation	How far do the measures comply with the relevant legislative requirements of the Member State, and preferably go beyond minimum requirements?
Transferability	How well the information could be used in other situations (e.g. Member States, industry sectors, other workplaces)?
Innovative	Is the example current - i.e. recent and relevant to existing work practices in the EU? Preferably, it should 'add value' to existing practices in the Member State providing the example.
Detail of coverage of information	Does the information provided give sufficient detail?
Design and aesthetics (for the Web)	Is the example clearly and simply described?
Consensus	Is the example acceptable to all National Network partners?

From the above examples, we can see there are different ways of selecting good practices (including self-nomination) and different criteria applied in selecting them, which suggests that there might be room for improving the value of good practice case studies through greater harmonisation of selection criteria.

IV. DISSEMINATING GOOD PRACTICES

The critical success factor for extracting value from good practices is their dissemination, i.e., how they are promoted. A UK study said that evidence suggests that innovations to tackle social exclusion are seldom evaluated, often marginalised and have low visibility. 'Few people know about the successful projects already delivering. A focal point is needed to bring together good practice and initiatives worthy of wider roll out. This report proposes an independent unit to consolidate and promote evidence of highly effective and efficient practices, and raise the political profile of the opportunities.'[17]

Good practices in e-inclusion have been and are being promoted in Europe in several different ways, among which are the following (with examples of each):

1. GOOD PRACTICE AWARDS

The European Commission established the e-Inclusion Awards to raise awareness, encourage participation and recognise excellence and good practice in using ICT and digital technology to tackle social and digital exclusion across Europe. The scheme ran for the first time in 2008 and was open to organisations from Europe from all sectors: government and public, business and private, non-governmental and

---

[17] SEU, op. cit.

voluntary. 469 organisations entered in total.[18] 35 finalists (five per each of the seven categories – see below for details) were invited to exhibit their project at the Ministerial Conference on e-Inclusion in Vienna on 30 November - 2 December 2008 and were presented with a medal for their achievements.

The seven categories and seven winners were the following:

- Ageing Well: London Borough of Newham (United Kingdom)
- Geographic Inclusion: Kyyjarven Mediamyllarit ry (Finland)
- Digital Literacy: Association 'Langas i ateiti' (Lithuania)
- Cultural Diversity: Milton Keynes Council (United Kingdom)
- Marginalised Young People: A-Clinic Foundation (Finland)
- e-Accessibility: Synscenter Refsnæs (Denmark)
- Inclusive Public Services: Sotiria Hospital (Greece).

The European Commission's 2009 call for good practice cases in the field of e-government received a total of 259 submissions which are competing in four categories for the European eGovernment Awards title.[19] Selected finalists will receive invitations to exhibit at the 5th Ministerial eGovernment Conference, to be held from 19 to 20 November 2009 in Malmö, Sweden. According to the Commission, the awards, organised every two years, support the implementation of its e-government policy and action plans. In addition to the four winners selected by the jury, a public prize will be awarded to the case among the 52 short-listed finalists that receives the most votes by ePractice.eu members.

2. PROSYLETISING, GOOD PRACTICE 'MISSIONARIES'

Here are two examples of good practice missionaries:
IDABC is the European Commission programme that promotes the delivery of e-government services in the European Union. IDABC stands for Interoperable Delivery of European eGovernment Services to public Administrations, Businesses and Citizens. It promotes the delivery of cross-border public services to citizens and enterprises in Europe. Its mission is to improve efficiency and collaboration between European public administrations.[20] The IDABC programme is based in the Directorate General Informatics. Among its other activities, it produces and updates twice a year e-government fact sheets for each of the Member States.

In June 2009, the UK government appointed Martha Lane Fox to a two-year assignment as 'champion for digital inclusion'. The idea of appointing a champion emerged in 2008 in the UK's first national strategy for ending the digital divide. The lastminute.com founder, a dotcom pioneer, Lane Fox is supported by a taskforce of experts. As the government's digital champion, Lane Fox says her main strength will be an ability to 'give digital inclusion projects a voice in places where they might not otherwise be heard'. A consultation on the strategy found that the champion 'must have the power and authority to enforce any changes that are necessary to ensure digital inclusion of the most vulnerable groups is delivered'.[21]

---

[18] http://ec.europa.eu/information_society/events/e-inclusion/2008/exhibition/awards/index_en.htm
[19] http://www.epractice.eu/en/news/292104
[20] http://ec.europa.eu/idabc
[21] Cross, Michael, 'Lane Fox to become UK's first digital champion', *The Guardian*, 17 June 2009. http://www.guardian.co.uk/technology/2009/jun/17/martha-lane-fox-digital-inclusion

3. PUBLICATIONS

The European Commission sponsors the *European Journal of e-Practice*, a digital publication which promotes the sharing of good practices in e-government, e-health and e-inclusion.[22]

The Commission's Directorate General for Information Society publishes an e-inclusion newsletter and an e-health newsletter, both of which are delivered via e-mail.

4. GOOD PRACTICE LIBRARIES AND PORTALS

A high-level workshop on ethics and e-inclusion, held in Bled, Slovenia, in May 2008, recommended that stakeholders 'Develop and maintain a good/bad practice case study library which illustrates the ethical dimension of ICT services and products used to promote social inclusion and improved quality of service to those in most need'.[23]

In fact, there are already libraries of good practice now. The EC's ePractice.eu has what it describes as a 'constantly increasing knowledge base of good practice', containing hundreds of e-government, e-inclusion and e-health cases submitted by members of its community. Registered users of ePractice.eu can submit their own projects to the portal and contact the authors of cases already described there. As of mid-2009, 48 countries were participating in this portal with 15,000 members and more than 1,100 descriptions of various projects.[24]

5. SPECIAL EVENTS

Age Concern England encourages and helps older people to get online.[25] It estimates that more than nine million people over the age of 55 in the UK are excluded from using technologies. It promotes events such as myfriends online week (16-20 March 2009) to highlight the opportunities for older people to make new friends and keep in touch with family at home and abroad.

In June 2009, the European Commission published a call for proposals for the organisation of a major awareness-raising campaign associated with EU e-Skills Week in March 2010.[26]

6. CONFERENCES AND WORKSHOPS

The Commission and others have organised numerous conferences and workshops devoted to e-inclusion. Several of the most significant have already been mentioned

---

[22] http://www.epracticejournal.eu

[23] Rogerson, Simon, *Ethics and e-Inclusion: Exploration of issues and guidance on Ethics and e-Inclusion*, Contribution to the European e-Inclusion Initiative. Report of the High-Level workshop held in Bled, Slovenia, 12 May 2008, [published] September 2008, p. 6.
http://ec.europa.eu/information_society/activities/einclusion/events/workshop_ethics/workshop/index_en.htm

[24] http://www.epractice.eu/en/cases/

[25] www.ageconcern.org.uk/myfriendsonline.

[26] http://ec.europa.eu/enterprise/newsroom/cf/itemlongdetail.cfm?item_id=3160&lang=en

above, namely the Ministerial meeting which led to the Riga Declaration in June 2006, the workshop on ethics and e-inclusion held in Bled, Slovenia, in May 2008, and the Ministerial conference on e-inclusion held in Vienna, 30 Nov – 2 Dec 2008.

V. LINKING STRATEGIES AND GOOD PRACTICES

A Belgian project provides a good example of how good practice, e-inclusion strategy, ethics and dissemination activities can be integrated successfully and brought to the attention of policy-makers. The project, entitled 'Colourful Flanders turns to Grey', was designed, initiated and managed by the Flemish Institution for Science and Technology Assessment (viWTA, a parliamentary institution for technology assessment), and conducted by the Centre for Audience Research (Catholic University of Leuven). The ultimate aim of the study was to formulate short-term and long-term policy recommendations with regard to the elderly and ICT.[27] The project set tough, but realistic measures of success for itself: 'The usefulness of the project (and its methodology) will not surface until the framework is reflected in actual policy plans. The project will only be assessable when policy objectives that have been inspired by this study, gradually start to be linked with legislative, policy, service, or budgetary measures.'[28] Among the actions it took was to present the project results directly to the Flemish Parliament.

While individual projects, such as this Belgian example, can link good practice, strategy and policy, higher level co-ordination is also necessary, at the macro level as it were. The European Commission makes this point when it says that action is required across a number of policy areas to deal with Europe's ageing population and that coordination at European level can facilitate the exchange of best practices, develop synergies and reduce negative spill-overs.[29] Co-ordination is a way of improving the efficiency and effectiveness of social spending. The European Commission collaborates with Member States through the so-called open method of coordination (OMC) on social protection and social inclusion. Tangible evidence of this co-ordination on e-inclusion exists beyond the words contained in the Riga Declaration. The i2010 e-Inclusion Subgroup National Reports (Dec 2007) contain a wealth of information, including contact details, examples of e-inclusion good practices and policies.[30]

---

[27] Eggermont, Steven, Heidi Vandebosch and Stef Steyaert, 'Towards the desired future of the elderly and ICT: policy recommendations based on a dialogue with senior citizens', *Poiesis & Praxis*, Vol. 4, No. 3, Sept. 2006, pp. 199-217.

[28] Eggermont et al., p. 215.

[29] European Commission, Dealing with the impact of an ageing population in the EU (2009 Ageing Report), Communication from the Commission to the European Parliament, the Council, the European Economic and Social Committee and the Committee of the Regions, COM(2009) 180/4, Brussels, 29 Apr 2009, p. 10.

[30] http://www.epractice.eu/files/download/i2010_eInclusion_Reports.pdf

VI. SOME EXAMPLES OF GOOD PRACTICE

1. SENIORNETT – TRAINING IN ICT AND E-INCLUSION FOR ELDERLY PEOPLE IN NORWAY

Seniornett Norge[31] is a non-government organisation working towards e-inclusion for elderly people. The organisation has two tiers: the first is the annual 'Senior-surf day', an open house event held at libraries and community centres nationwide for the elderly to learn about ICT. The second tier is a 'club' or training centre established at a local site where senior citizens can continue their learning and become proficient ICT users.

Seniornett Norway is 12 years old, and has grown 'stone by stone', said Seniornett managing director Tore Langemyr Larsen in an interview. 'Its aim is to get all senior citizens over 55 to use computers and use the Internet. There are 1.2 million inhabitants in Norway over 55, about 25 per cent of the total population. Only half of those are using the Internet or have used a computer. Norway is a high-cost country. The government and private enterprise need to reduce costs, so, for example, they are concentrating on net-banking and delivering tax returns via the Internet. It's a big problem if those over 55 can't use the Internet.'

In addition to the economic incentives, familiarity with the Internet has social benefits, for example, in one's being able to contact friends and family whenever one wants. 'Facebook is popular for a reason,' said Larsen. 'Some seniors are beginning to use social networks, but they are behind young people. We started with the motivation phase, to explain that the Internet is not just for youngsters. It's why we started the senior surf day where seniors could get their first taste, to whet their appetite. We have had more than 50,000 seniors going to their libraries to get their first taste of the Internet. We publish adverts encouraging them to try the Internet, but this is not enough. Seniors need training, as in clubs, where they can learn from each other, share experience, genealogy research, photos. We started these clubs and now have about 100 all over Norway. We train the instructors for these training centres. To reach out to 600,000 seniors not on the Internet, our strategy is to train the trainers who can train more instructors which creates a pyramid effect. It's been quite successful. It's why we were a finalist for the EC e-inclusion awards.

'We have had contact with other countries, such as the UK, Japan and the US, but they don't train the trainers and don't have clubs like we do. Our approach is different because we train the trainers. We think we are more efficient. We rely on the pyramid effect. We are proud of it. In Norway last year [2008], more than 100,000 seniors over 65 went on the Internet for first time. We'd like to take some of the credit for that.'

Seniornett has a small core of permanent employees, but it has about 1,000 volunteer instructors who work in the senior citizen clubs providing training and guidance. Seniornett helps the clubs with broadband lines and some equipment.

Seniornett Norway gets funding from government grants and private donations. 'Telenor, the Norwegian telecoms carrier, and the Bill and Melinda Gates Foundation have given us free licences. We get support from banks because they want seniors to use their net-banking services. About 50 per cent of our funding comes from government grants, with the rest coming from the private sector.'

Volunteers can in principle be anybody, but they are mostly senior citizens from all walks of life, said Larsen 'Some are retired, some are not, some are from the IT

---

[31] http://www.seniornett.no/

industry and others not. We have a wide spectrum of volunteers, and most stay with us for a long time. It's a labour of love. It's very inspiring to get seniors on the Internet. Once they get over the fear of the mouse and keyboard or doing something that they think might break it, they become like children in their enthusiasm.'

Oslo is the hub of the network, but the clubs are spread all over Norway. 'Seniors don't want to travel long distances to get to a club. That's why we need clubs as close to the senior citizens as possible We have a very good geographic distribution. Our aim is to have about 300 clubs in the next three or four years, and after that our concentration will shift to the running of the clubs, to make them more efficient and training people to use new software. For example, seniors have had a big problem in going from XP to Vista. We talk to Microsoft quite often about the usability of its software, its user-friendliness, to make it easier to use.'

Telenor was the first mid-wife of Seniornett when it gave a computer to a library about 12 years ago. The library asked what they could do with it. It became obvious that training was needed if the computer was going to be used. 'Telenor has a commercial interest in what we do because it will help them sell more broadband service. Our program is sustainable because it is a win-win situation, everyone benefits from getting seniors on the Net.'

Regarding lessons learned, Larsen cited several. He said that 'to get seniors on the Internet, they need to understand why they should spend the time and money to do so. The biggest obstacle is motivation, is responding to their question: 'Why should I?' We emphasise the new life they can have on the Internet. We concentrate not on the technology, but on the uses. A lot of repetition is needed in training. Also, the train-the-trainer model is quite successful. Even so, getting funding is not easy, even when everybody thinks it's a good idea. I spend about 75 per cent of my time looking for donors. I would tell anyone planning to do what we do not to underestimate the effort needed to get funding.

'Our model of training the trainers is valid for other countries. So is the concept of the club. Our trainers give senior citizens a course of about 24 hours, but the seniors need to practise after that. Their new skills will disappear very quickly if they don't practise. A lot of practice is very important. Clubs are better than training centres or traditional classrooms. The clubs are in libraries, in senior citizen centres, some in social organisations like the Kiwanis and Rotary clubs, some are in volunteer centres. The clubs don't have to pay rent, they get free space. Sometimes they get free broadband connections. Costs are low. I think it's a sustainable project. Once we get up to 300 clubs, we might need to double the number of people we have in the NGO (from four to eight).'

Regarding criteria for good practice in e-inclusion, Larsen said 'a good practice should tailor the training around seniors. They are good learners, but they need a different training from that given to an 18-year-old. There's a long list of things important for seniors, but not for 18-year-olds. Practices and exercises are very important in training. If you use too many technical terms, they get hazy-eyed. It's important to use non-technological terms. Most software and hardware developers have a long way to go to address senior citizen needs. As just one example, the comma and full-stop on a keyboard could be made bigger. We work with government as they develop software and applications for citizens to use. We tell them not to make fonts too small, to make functions appear at the same place from one webpage to the next, to be consistent in the use of terms. Seniors need to understand what happens if they strike a key. There are many things that go into a good practice. It is helpful to have trainers from the same age group, so there is the prospect of good rapport with those to be trained. Senior citizens also need to have a lot of breaks. It's important to accept that there are no stupid questions.'

Larsen said Seniornett has not really encountered any serious ethical issues so far. 'We have, however, prepared some brief guidelines for seniors. For example, if you go on Facebook, remember that the things you post there will be there forever. We tell seniors to be careful with their private information. When it comes to banking, they have to be careful with their PIN codes, never give to give them out.

'Our last senior surf day was in early October, and we received a lot of media attention. We have had many interviews, talking about our work. We are interested in meeting others in Europe to tell them what we are doing. We think we have a good model, perhaps the best in Europe, in getting senior citizens on to the Internet.'

When asked how he learned about the European e-inclusion good practice competition, he said Seniornett's sponsors in the Norwegian government, the people working on e-inclusion, suggested that they should apply for one of the European e-inclusion awards. 'So we did.' It was not the first time Seniornett was in a good practice competition. Before Seniornett was recognised as an e-inclusion good practice at the Ministerial conference in Vienna, 'We won the Rosing prize, an ICT prize, the biggest in Norway, two years ago, for good practice. We were proud of that.'

2. ETHICAL GUIDANCE ON USE OF WANDERING TECHNOLOGIES IN SCOTLAND

Restraints are still a common way to deal with wandering. In order to prevent their residents from getting lost, many care establishments lock doors or use barriers such as keypads or handle arrangements that require skills to open. Not only do these arrangements prevent the free movement of those who are at risk of wandering but also that of all the other residents. Coming up against a locked door can cause frustration or anger for a person with dementia.

To help determine those cases in which wandering technologies can be appropriate, the Mental Welfare Commission of Scotland produced a document, entitled *Safe to wander?*[32]. It sets out ethical principles and guidance on good practice in the use of wandering technologies in support of individuals with dementia who are residents in care homes or hospitals. The technologies include tagging and tracking devices used to alert a care-giver when a person leaves a given area and to help locate a person who has gotten lost. Wandering technology involves the attachment of an electronic device to a person or their clothing, so that if they pass across a particular boundary, an alarm goes off, and staff are alerted. Wandering technology can also involve tracking devices which can locate the wearer if he or she becomes lost or fails to return.

The Mental Welfare Commission has provided both general principles and a checklist. Regarding the use of new technologies, it recommends that

- an intervention must provide a benefit that cannot otherwise be achieved;
- the intervention must be the least restrictive in relation to the person's freedom in order to achieve the desired benefit;
- the past and present wishes of the person must be taken into account;

---

[32] http://www.mwcscot.org.uk/web/FILES/Publications/Safe_to_Wander.pdf

- the views of relevant others should be taken into account; and
- the intervention should encourage the person to use existing skills and develop new ones.

Those considering the use of wandering technologies should take into account the causes of the individual's behaviour, risks to the individual, alternatives to the technology, ethical implications of the system, the views of the individual, relatives, care team, etc. as well as the legal implications. The use of wandering technology devices must be enabling to the wearer, not limiting. If not, the technology could be seen as an unwarranted invasion of personal liberty. If wandering technology is found to be necessary for certain individuals, it should be discreetly applied, so that the resident is not 'labelled'. Furthermore, to be effective, the device should be small, comfortable and unobtrusive for the benefit of the person themselves. A visible, uncomfortable device is likely to be undignified, stigmatising and rejected.

Because individuals with dementia are particularly vulnerable, not in a good position to defend their rights and at risk of getting lost (and being hurt) if left without adequate care, it is important that those who make decisions about their well-being are well aware of the ethical dimensions that are at play in using wandering technologies.

The *Safe to Wander?* guidance says, 'The use of technology, including wandering technology, in care homes and hospitals is not in itself a good or a bad thing. Where technology is used, this should be as a tailored and appropriate response to the identified risks faced by an individual. How technology is applied can make the difference between providing restrictive and inflexible care, or a freedom-enhancing setting.'

Dr Donald Lyons, director of the Mental Welfare Commission (MWC) and co-author of the guidance, said the guidelines were produced in response to the queries the MWC was receiving in response to concerns expressed by stakeholders about practical or ethical difficulties in the application of recent mental health and incapacity legislation. He and co-author Alison Thomson sent the draft guidance for comment to stakeholders including carers, professional and charitable organisations, hospitals, government and care homes as well as specific groups such as the Dementia and Development Centre at the University of Stirling, Alzheimer's Scotland, the Association of Directors of Social Work, the Care Commission, the Royal College of Psychiatrists, the Royal College of Nursing and West Lothian Council. He singled out valuable input received from the Glasgow Dementia Working Group (which has evolved into the Scotland Dementia Working Group), which is composed of people with dementia.

Wandering is not necessarily the best word, he said in an interview. Some people with dementia have a desire to walk, to go somewhere. They are not necessarily wandering aimlessly. He and Ms Thomson contributed a chapter based on the guidance to a book entitled *Walking not Wandering*[33], which makes exactly this point.

The principal technologies used in dementia cases are passive sensors, which transmit an alarm to alert carers or the police if someone is exiting an assisted living facility or their own home. Other technologies include sensor pads (beds, chair, floor), nurse/carer call systems, panic buttons, fall and movement sensors, electronic tagging and tracking systems, CCTV or video surveillance and intruder alerts. So far, GPS-embedded bracelets or necklaces are not in use for tracking people with dementia.

---

[33] Mary Marshall and Kate Allan (eds.), *Dementia: Walking Not Wandering - Fresh Approaches to Understanding and Practice*, Hawker Publications, London, 2006.

Although tracking devices are not much used in UK care homes, the technology is becoming increasingly easily available and financially affordable. Tracking devices with GPS are being used in Spain for some patients with Alzheimer's disease. Even if such devices are used, there will still be a need to ensure the person's safety once he or she has left an assisted living facility.

Dr Lyons cited Scotland's West Lothian Council as an example of an authority implementing passive sensors. He said using such technologies is safer than locking a person in the house, which could expose them to significant risks such as fire. In a care home, some people are able to come and go safely, others are not. If doors are locked, all residents may be deprived of their liberty. It is also demeaning of a person's dignity if they have to ask permission to go out. There are ways of stopping people from accidentally going out and coming to harm, for example, by making the assisted living facility more interesting. Care homes with enclosed gardens, allow people to walk around to their heart's content. However, many care homes are badly designed and not designed with dementia in mind. If someone with dementia does go out, it is very demeaning and inappropriate if a carer has to go out after them and pull them back into the home. Before thinking about technology, said Dr Lyons, one has to think about the circumstances in which it is used. Scottish legislation requires that interventions be the least restrictive to individuals' freedom. Indeed, the legislation was a driver in the production of the guidance, which is intended to increase personal freedom.

The *Safe to Wander?* guidance was produced in early 2007 and is used throughout Scotland. Some entities in England have expressed interest in the guidelines too, but Dr Lyons said that although they reference Scottish legislation, they could be used virtually anywhere.

As an example of a lesson learned since production of the guidelines, Dr Lyons said the MWC is engaging stakeholders at an even earlier stage in the production of other guidance documents. Calls for advice and discussions with stakeholders help the MWC to identify those areas of practice where people are finding it difficult to understand how to work within the law and associated ethical principles. Now when the MWC decides to produce a set of guidelines, it invites experienced representatives from all relevant stakeholder groups to form a group to discuss key issues and to share ideas and examples of good practice. The MWC brings stakeholders together and gives them some anonymised scenarios drawn from real cases and asks them what they would do in the depicted situations. 'We get stakeholders to think through the ethical implications, so that in this way they become more involved in the actual drafting of guidelines.'

The guidelines produced by the MWC represent good practice, in his view, because they involve stakeholders from the outset, including people who have used MWC services, advocates, lawyers, mental health service managers, occupational therapists and others. The MWC, he says, is very well rooted in the community and consults widely. Guidelines are seen as practical, rather something produced in an ivory tower.

Among criteria for good practices, he said compatibility with legislation was paramount. Relevant Scottish legislation includes the Mental Health and Care and Treatment Act, the Adults with Incapacity Act and the Human Rights Act. Good practice has to be based on principles, but applicable to real-life situations that practitioners encounter on a daily basis. MWC guidance documents use anonymised case examples to show how the guidelines can be implemented. Good practice also must have stakeholder buy-in to ensure their relevance and utility; indeed, all key stakeholders should be involved in the production of such guidelines.

In addition to the production of ethical guidelines, the MWC also contributes to professional development activities and gives general advice aimed at helping care providers to incorporate awareness of rights and the law into training and education programmes. It also supports the Principles into Practice Network, which acts as a forum for anyone in Scotland with an interest in discussing and developing good practices based on ethical principles.

The Mental Welfare Commission is funded by the Scottish government, but is an independent organisation working to safeguard the rights and welfare of everyone with a mental illness, learning disability or other mental disorder.

3. DIGITAL STORY-TELLING IN SWEDEN AS A TOOL FOR E-INCLUSION

A challenge for e-inclusion is getting media attention focused on the e-excluded. Fair media portrayal should increase the possibilities for people with disabilities to be included in society and to find employment. A Swedish project, called MediAbility[34], found a novel way of meeting this challenge – it empowered the e-excluded by giving them the tools to make their own digital video stories which generated sufficient interest that they were used by leading media companies.

'Our project was about people with disabilities not being present in mainstream media. We wanted to change that,' said project spokesperson Mia Ahlgren in an interview. 'We worked with public service TV, to make them aware of this injustice. We wanted people to take control of communications tools in their own right.'

The MediAbility project collaborated with mainstream media companies for more and fairer portrayal of people with disabilities. The project was initiated by the Swedish Disability Federation, a Swedish umbrella organisation, representing 43 national disability organisations and 460,000 individual members. The Federation obtained funding for the project from the Swedish Inheritance Fund. The project started in February 2006 and concluded with a final report in June 2009.

The idea of digital storytelling was developed in California about 15 years ago, but the MediAbility project took it a step further by making it easy and inexpensive for the e-excluded to make short videos which were published on the website of UR, the Swedish Educational Broadcasting Company, one of the project partners.[35] The project has also been an active partner in a European networking project.[36]

'We co-operated with Swedish public broadcasting companies. We worked with the educational broadcasting company. They had a Web project, where they were already working with digital TV story-telling, so we grafted our project on to theirs. They helped us with the first workshop. They provided a distribution medium. We also co-operated with the Swedish public TV broadcaster on the study. We collaborated with different educational institutions, which were doing work on the digital divide, and we had some conferences with them.'

'Our project had two parallel actions, a research study on how people with disabilities were portrayed and workshops on what people wanted to convey. The workshops grew. We conducted them in different parts of Sweden. We had small

---

[34] http://mediability.wordpress.com/
[35] http://www.ur.se/rfb/index.php?t=1&tt=9
[36] http://www.mediaanddisability.org

groups of eight people in each workshop. We adapted a method developed in California, using simple technologies. The main thing would be the story. In our project, we started at quite a high level, telling people they should make a video. We had people who didn't know about computers. In a way, we 'tricked' them into using technologies. Developing a story was the motive for using computers. Once people got used to the technology, they became curious and some participants went on to use computers for other purposes.'

'We asked journalists with disabilities to do some stories on what we were doing. Our first workshops were at a school for people with disabilities. Then we ran an advert across our 43 member organisations. We did workshops for them. We also did workshops with educational institutions. Most of the workshops were held where there were already groups. The only criterion was: do you have a story to tell? We didn't say anything about computer skills. I wouldn't say it was easy, but the reward was great.

'For young people, the MediAbility project was just another way of telling story. For some older people, it really changed their lives. But regardless of age, they all felt proud of themselves. They produced a film in two days that would be put on the website of a public broadcaster. We've done our best to show people how easy it is to get going. It's not expensive. You just need a tutor. You also need proselytisers, somebody who can champion and promote this method.

'Our method can be used for different groups of people. We had very mixed groups. We had both young and old people. We had people with cognitive disabilities and mental illnesses, such as schizophrenia, participating in our workshops. We only had one person who was totally blind.

The workshops were two days long. 'Our workshops started with a short introduction where we showed participants some examples of digital stories as a way to build enthusiam and to stimulate their own ideas. We asked them to think a bit before the workshop, for example, about a place that meant a lot to them. We asked participants not to talk about their disabilities. Instead, we encouraged them to prepare stories about something that interested them. It makes people really happy to do a video on what interests them.

'Some workshop leaders used a theme, for example, on human rights, to stimulate ideas, but the participants always decided themselves what story to tell. Their videos were based on their own ideas. For example, the theme of human rights was translated to 'What makes you feel good?' in a group with participants with intellectual disabilities. But one of the participants made a story about the war in Kosovo.

'We started workshops with oral story-telling. We put people in small groups, where there would be some peer-to-peer discussion. People could see they have some things in common. We told them their stories should end with something they have learned.

'In logical and structured steps, and with coaching in story-telling and technology, the participants first worked out a story-line and then made storyboards to determine what kind of images they would need. Then they were given a digital camera. The participants would 'act' to make a good picture. Workshop leaders helped them to use software programs such as MovieMaker for PCs or iMovie for Macs to make their videos. The workshop leaders served as intermediaries to participants to remove barriers in digital communication. The participants' videos were typically two minutes long. The participants' showed each other the videos they made. People could continue to explore digital communication without any extra cost, and sometimes they invented their own ways to make content accessible.

'It's been quite eye-opening, asking people what they wanted to do. Everyone has a story to tell. Their stories are so different. A challenge for some participants was to make a short story. One of the older participants had a brain damage 40 years ago. He wanted to tell a story about how he had recovered. He made a six-minute video. After the workshop, he sent us an e-mail with a one-minute video about how he appreciated the workshop.'

The MediAbility website gives an example of empowerment digital video story-telling as follows:

Barbara is 59 years old and lives in a small community in the countryside. She had hardly used computers when she took part in a MediAbility digital storytelling workshop in August 2006.

She was not really interested in digital communication but she felt she had 'a story to tell'. She made her first two-minute film and made new friends in the workshop. A few weeks later, she decided to join a course to learn how to produce documentary films. Barbara made a digitally edited documentary about a person she had met in the workshop.

Barbara joined another MediAbility workshop on how to start your own blog. Recently, she passed our course for training future workshop leaders. Two years after entering the digital society, she initiated a course on digital storytelling in her local community, where she will be the tutor. Today, she uses a computer for information search and e-mails and she pays her bills electronically. For Barbara, learning about digital storytelling has become a story of empowerment by narration.

'We had about 160 participants in total,' said Ahlgren. 'We thought it would be expensive to do these workshops, but it wasn't. We used other people's computers and meeting places, so we could do a lot more workshops. We did about 25 workshops in different places in Sweden. We had an organising person, who would help identify what was needed. We were facilitators. We made the best solution for each workshop. In some workshops, we used the educational broadcasters.'

Of lessons learned from the project, Ahlgren said, 'When you work with people with disabilities, many people think you need special preparations, but we learned that you could mix different people. You can use the same method even if you have people with different disabilities. The mixed groups were the biggest value. With this method, you learn about things you have in common with other people.' She said their method should work anywhere for people who haven't been heard very much.

She also expressed the hope that technologies and software for people with disabilities will improve. As it was, her project used software that was relatively simple and easy to use.

In response to a question about what makes a good practice, she said 'Good practice depends on the purpose. It should be out of the box, sustainable, inquiring. Sometimes you need to find new ideas, to do something in a different way. It's important that you start from the user point of view. That's been very strong in our project. Good practices should be user-oriented. You need to bring in users from the beginning. You start with users, not the technology. Presentation is an important issue in good practice. Also important is how questions are asked, especially of elderly people. When you talk about elderly people, people with disabilities, there are often prejudices, but they are like the rest of us.'

On ethical issues, she said, 'We talked a lot at the beginning about the difference between private and personal. We tried to discourage workshop participants from talking about their disabilities. If they wanted to do a private story, we would ask them not to show it on the Internet. We had one woman do a beautiful film about the two sons who were taken away from her. We always tried, especially with people with mental illness, to have someone present who knew them. If you are working in these areas, it's important to have contacts with people who know the participants. Another ethical issue for us was to let people be free to do their own stories.

'We also had a contract. Anyone who wanted to spread their films had to sign a contract to allow their films to be shown. We contacted people to ask them if it was okay for their films to be reused in educational broadcasting. We had a couple of girls who put their videos on the Internet, and then wanted them back. We took the film off our website, where we controlled the film, but they understood that people could have downloaded their video. We also didn't want to do films with children.'

The MediAbility project was a finalist in the e-inclusion good practice awards at the Ministerial e-inclusion conference in Vienna in early December 2008. Other recognition came when Ahlgren was asked by the Swedish broadcasting company to be a juror in a competition organised by NHK, the Japanese broadcaster, called the Japan Prize. 'I was probably asked because of our work. The competition was about selecting educational content from TV and the Web. There were a lot of people from different countries. We even met the Crown Prince!'

Digital storytelling was one part of the Mediability project, but the project also included other activities to encourage participation in digital media. In addition to digital story-telling, the MediAbility project organised workshops about blogging and networking on the Web to encourage people to use free-of-charge blog tools. 'All workshop participants started their own blogs, and some have continued blogging regularly.'

VII. THE VALUE OF GOOD PRACTICE CASE STUDIES FOR INCLUSION

From our research in support of the European Commission's workshops on e-inclusion and good practice, we draw several conclusions, as follows.

First, as a matter of definition, a good practice must be from real life; a good practice case study should have some measurable results to enable others to evaluate whether it is good practice or not. A good practice should reach beyond theory to real-world application in some context, where its impact can be observed or measured in some way.

Second, 'good practice' is a better term of usage than 'best practice'; it is more user-friendly. A good practice (as distinct from so-called 'best' practice) implies a practice that can be improved, not one that has finality from which one must not deviate. A good practice should not imply that others must follow it rigidly, as one might be expected to do in the case of a standard. A good practice is one that offers lessons from which one can learn and possibly apply in a similar or even different situation or context.

Third, it may not be possible to completely transfer a good practice, simply because there are cultural or environmental or other contextual factors that are different. Thus, careful evaluation is needed before adopting any good practice. As stated earlier in this chapter, one person's good practice is not necessarily the best for another person, company or country. Applying a good practice unquestioningly might have a negative impact in a different context.

Fourth, while one might assume that good practice cases do influence other practices and policy-making, so far there appears to be limited empirical evidence to support that assumption. Further research is needed to provide this empirical base.

Fifth, there is increasing emphasis on good practice as a matter of e-inclusion strategy, and other related e-domains, such as e-health, e-learning, e-government and e-participation. However, the perceived value of good practices and the prospects for success in using good practices as a matter of strategy and policy is critically dependent on how they are selected and by whom and how well they are promoted (or disseminated). In this regard, the Commission's ePractice.eu portal and its e-inclusion good practice competitions, such as that highlight of the Ministerial conference on e-inclusion held in Vienna in early December 2008, are good initiatives.

Sixth, good practices cases are selected in different ways with different selection criteria, which suggests that there might be room for improving the value of good practice case studies through greater harmonisation of selection criteria.

Finally, we believe good practice case studies constitute an important instrument in e-inclusion policy-making and strategy, just as important as the development of e-accessibility guidelines, assistive technology and anti-discrimination regulation. Indeed, good practice case studies provide the evidence as to whether regulation and technology are achieving results.

REFERENCES

Cullen, Joe, Kari Hadjivassiliou and Kerstin Junge, Status of eInclusion measurement, analysis and approaches for improvement, Topic Report 4: Recommendations for future action, Final Report, Tavistock Institute, February 2007.

E-ability project, Good Practice Manual: Promotion of digital literacy in people with psychological disabilities: *Some European Initiatives*, European Commission Directorate-General for Education and Culture, Brussels, [no date].

Eggermont, Steven, Heidi Vandebosch and Stef Steyaert, "Towards the desired future of the elderly and ICT: policy recommendations based on a dialogue with senior citizens", *Poiesis & Praxis*, Vol. 4, No. 3, Sept. 2006, pp. 199-217.
http://ec.europa.eu/information_society/activities/einclusion/events/workshop_ethics/work shop/index_en.htm

Marshall, Mary, and Kate Allan (eds.), *Dementia: Walking Not Wandering - Fresh Approaches to Understanding and Practice*, Hawker Publications, London, 2006.

Mellor, David, Lucy Firth and Kathleen Moore, "Can the Internet Improve the Well-being of the Elderly?", *Ageing International*, Vol. 35, 2008, pp. 25-42.

Rogerson, Simon, Ethics and e-Inclusion: Exploration of issues and guidance on Ethics and e-Inclusion, Contribution to the European e-Inclusion Initiative. Report of the High-Level workshop held in Bled, Slovenia, 12 May 2008, [published] September 2008.

Stroetmann, Karl A., Reinhard Hammerschmidt, Veli N. Stroetmann, Ingrid Moldenaers, eHealth in Action: Good Practice in European Countries, *Good eHealth Report*, Office for Official Publications of the European Communities, Luxembourg, January 2009.
www.elearningeuropa.info/out/?doc_id=8577&rsr_id=9950

European Commission. Renewed social agenda: Opportunities, access and solidarity in 21st century Europe. Communication from the Commission to the European Parliament, the Council, the European Economic and Social Committee and the Committee of the Regions. COM(2008) 412 final. Brussels, 2 July 2008.

European Commission, Dealing with the impact of an ageing population in the EU (2009 Ageing Report), Communication from the Commission to the European Parliament, the Council, the European Economic and Social Committee and the Committee of the Regions, COM(2009) 180/4, Brussels, 29 Apr 2009.

European Commission, Teaming Up for the eUnion: European eGovernment Awards 2009. Guidance Notes For Submission, not dated.

UK Department for Culture, Media and Sport and Department for Business, *Innovation and Skills, Digital Britain*, Final Report, The Stationery Office, Norwich, June 2009, p. 34.
www.tsoshop.co.uk.
http://www.citizensonline.org.uk/e-inclusionawards/judging

Social Exclusion Unit (SEU). *Inclusion Through Innovation: Tackling Social Exclusion Through New Technologies*. Final Report. Office of the Deputy Prime Minister, London, November 2005, p. 62.

The Guardian, "Lane Fox to become UK's first digital champion", by Cross, Michael, 17 June 2009.
http://www.guardian.co.uk/technology/2009/jun/17/martha-lane-fox-digital-inclusion

CHAPTER EIGHT. ETHICAL RECOMMENDATIONS

By Emilio Mordini

INTRODUCTION

The overall theoretical horizon of these ethical recommendations is the tension between power and frailty. By assuming this tension as constitutive, we make two further assumptions, say, that technology epitomizes human aspirations to power, and that old age is the ideal example of human frailty. So in its essence technology for ageing turns out to be an oxymoron, which includes in itself two of the main sources of moral narratives in the West, the will of power and the ephemeral nature of any living being. *"By curing all kinds of fatal, infectious, and short-term illnesses, medicine has provided us with the gift of much greater longevity. But the price for that gift is a long stretch of time of life lived with chronic and incurable diseases. The elderly are healthy and vigorous as no elderly people have been before. And yet, 40 percent of us will die after a period of protracted debility and feeble dementia stretching on average for some seven to 10 years. The price to be paid for our great medical triumphs is, in fact, a protracted period of considerable misery. In addition, thanks to medicine's success in curing disease and forestalling death, it is not clear that we haven't produced a culture in which death is even more unacceptable and more feared than ever before. We may have increased the demand for new remedies without being properly grateful for the remedies that we have already received. This is a perfect example of the ever-expanding character of human desire, in which we are now doing better but feeling worse".*[1]

The tension between power and frailty is further articulated as tension between the individual and the community, where it becomes increasingly difficult to distinguish between the desire of liberty and the pleasure entailed by dependence. The complex dynamic between the individual (his or her character, selfhood, exceptionality) and the community (its commonality, purpose, unity, momentum) is one of the main specific features of any human society. In order to survive, humans must live together and from infanthood, human beings face the acute awareness of their dependence on other human beings. Such a dependence is destined to last quite a long time beyond the standard mother-newborn dependence in other species.[2] Dependence – in the sense of having one's want correctly anticipated and met – may be a pleasant state for a short period of life, but sooner or later, frustrations and obligations entailed by dependence become too burdensome. Humans develop awareness of the conflict between their dependence needs and the individual nature of their personal desires, which require a certain degree of liberty and autonomy to be fulfilled. In fact, the most prominent aspect of human society is the way in which individuals deal with social obligations and the unavoidable charge of resentment and frustration carried out by these obligations. Even in the least structured human groups, it is possible to

---

[1] Kass LR,, 2004, Human Frailty and Human Dignity, *The New Atlantis*, 7, 110-118
[2] Anthropologists call *neoteny* the tendency of mammals to remain dependant on other individuals and to exhibit juvenile characteristics. Human beings present a higher level of neoteny.

see traces of the tension between the "pleasure" of being dependent and the "desire" to be autonomous[3] and to be left alone.

Since the time of the Greek philosophers, ethics have been evoked to mitigate the tension between individuals and community.[4] However, social bonds can be justified without resorting to ethical categories. For instance, according to Thomas Scheff[5], individualist societies have institutionalised two major defences against the loss of social bonds. One, he says, is the "*myth of individualism, and the denial and repression of the emotions*", and the second follows from this: a simplification of human nature and social order by the exclusion of social feelings, solidarity, for instance, and, in general, emotions. One should include individuals in the society chiefly because they can contribute to the common wealth and can receive from this common wealth accordingly. We should also open up the market to previously marginalised sectors of the society in order to enlarge markets. In the extreme version of this theory, only people who can remain active, either as producers or consumers, are worth being included. Although an echo of a pure economic theory can be traced in EU policies on e-Inclusion (e.g., the emphasis accorded to the need to promote "active" living), it is indisputable that the EU approach to e-Inclusion is based on a different vision. Ethics are an integral part of the EU concept of e-Inclusion: "*e-Inclusion is necessary for social justice, ensuring equity in the knowledge society*"[6].

Finally the tension between power and frailty is articulated with the aim to provide a vision of a decent society in which ICT is used "*for social justice, ensuring equity*". We will adopt –as in much contemporary moral and political theory – a Rawlsian approach. For the purposes of these ethical recommendations there is no need to discuss in detail Rawl's principles or his justificatory strategy, it is enough that we assume that the moral outlook of these recommendations include four main features, 1) recommendations for the allocation of basic rights, liberties, and duties; 2) recommendations for the allocation of resources, notably ICT resources; 3) recommendations for creating binding relationships; 4) recommendations for choosing the right action. Recommendations (1) and (2) will serve to outline an acceptable approach to ICT for ageing and are enforceable at European level, through the implementation of specific policies. Recommendations in (3) are still enforceable by European institutions but concern the way in which stakeholders could move from the status quo to new states of affairs, they are the core of a strategic agenda Recommendations in (4) demand a more direct engagement of the civil society in order to be enforced, they are the basic elements for an action plan.

I. AGEING AS A SOCIAL FACT

While ageing is a biological process, the condition of old age is a social fact that reflects the multifaceted nature of the older-person role, rather than an "objective" category. Social scientists have long been intrigued by the definition of social facts,

---

[3] E.g., Moore, B., Jr, *Privacy: Studies in Social and Cultural History*, Pantheon Books, 1984.
[4] E.g., most virtues listed by Aristotle are actually attitudes such as friendship, honesty, trustfulness, solidarity, etc., which are essential to overcome the conflict between the individual and the community.
[5] Scheff, Thomas, *Microsociology: Discourse, Emotion and Social Structure*, University of Chicago Press, 1990.
[6] European Commission, European i2010 initiative on e-Inclusion: "To be part of the information society", Communication from the Commission to the European Parliament, the Council, the European Economic and Social Committee and the Committee of the Regions, COM(2007) 694 final, Brussels, 8 Nov 2007.

ever since Durkheim wrote about them.[7] Social facts are occurrences produced by social, collective, dynamics. They are real events distinct from psychological, economic, and biological facts because they are direct expression of social interactions, in given social contexts. Questions about social facts have been raised by XX century leading scholars, like the legal philosopher Herbert L.A.Hart[8], who argued that legal validity is a function of certain social facts, and the American philosopher John Searle[9], who defines social facts as collective intentional facts, say, facts directed at something and agreed upon by a large number of people. Social facts include both material and non-material facts. Material social facts are social structures, say, political institutions, economic organizations, the legal, educational and communication systems, and so on. Nonmaterial social facts consist in a web of meanings shared by each group and by larger communities. They include beliefs, values, customs, behaviours, rituals, narratives, ceremonies, roles and norms. Nonmaterial social facts are often "internalized", in the sense that as strange, bizarre, irrational, they may appear to outsiders, they are taken for granted by people within that society. Social facts order human collective action and, through the collective, they also norm individual's existence. The normative role of the collective, both conscious and unconscious, has been recently explored by social scientists[10,11,12] and psychoanalysts.[13,14,15]

As a social fact, ageing includes both material elements (e.g., the overall apparatus for handling older people, which embraces the pension system and various retirement plans, legislation about older citizens, the so-called "grey economy", social and health care for the elderly, nursing homes, assistive technologies, etc.) and non-material elements (e.g., narratives about ageing, rites of passages, implicit and explicit definitions of ageing, elderly role descriptions, age-related values, etc.). An important non-material element that contributes to shaping old age conditions is the dynamic between social inclusion and exclusion. Although biological, economical, technological, psychological, factors may also play an important role, the polarity of inclusion/exclusion has essentially to do with social interactions. Inclusive and exclusive processes do not follow the all-or-none law. They are nuanced, and fluctuating, since all individuals are contemporarily included and excluded to different degrees, in the multiple groups to which they belong through birth, assimilation, or achievement. In other words, the couple inclusion/exclusion reflects multifaceted power relations between individuals and their social environments.

Understanding power relations that affect the aged person is essential in order to understand ageing processes and their chief ethical implications. Ageing always implies – at least to a certain extent and from certain viewpoints – a form of weakening of the individual. With age, abilities diminish, one loses physical strength, visual and hearing acuity, memory and learning capacities, dexterity, sexual appeal, reproductive capacity, and so. These changes produce different effects in urban or

---

[7] Durkheim E, (1938) *The Rules of Sociological Method*, New York, The Free Press

[8] Hart H.L.A. (1983), *Essays in Jurisprudence and Philosophy*, Oxford: Clarendon Press

[9] Searle, J. (1995) *The Construction of Social Reality*. New York: The Free Press

[10] Jameson, F. (1981), *The Political Unconscious: Narrative as a Socially Symbolic Act*, Ithaca, N.Y.: Cornell UP

[11] Taylor, C. (1989), 'Modern social imaginaries', *Public Culture* 14(1), 91-124

[12] Maffesoli, M. (1993), 'The imaginary and the sacred in Durkheim's sociology', *Current Sociology*, 41(2), 1-5

[13] Castoriadis, C. (1987), *The imaginary institution of society*, Cambridge, MA: *MIT*

[14] Mordini, E. (1996), 'L'Inconscio Sociale', *Rivista di Teologia Morale*, 110, 58-75

[15] Hopper, E. (2003), *The Social Unconscious: Selected Papers*, London: Jessica Kingsley

rural environments, in pre-industrial, industrial, and post-industrial societies, in diverse social groups. Roles and social contexts can either mitigate or emphasise age related impairment, which may result in major or in minor losses of social power. For instance, the increasing dependence from other people, which is often a consequence of ageing processes, has very different outcomes in societies with strong community ties, or in societies, which highly value independent living and the lonely search for the meaning of life. This holds true not only in terms of social interactions, but also in psychological terms, as people used to considering isolation as a sign of liberty and autonomous power, will probably feel age-related dependence as a humiliating and degrading experience.

Recommendation no. 1: Ageing society is a chiefly social phenomenon, which implies a shift within different age groups in a society towards the older ones. At the individual level, ageing is about people living chronologically longer. The effect of ageing on people has more to do with the social context than with medical conditions. An ethical scrutiny of policies which address ageing should be based on a thoughtful distinction between biological and social facts.

II. POWER AND POWER RELATIONS

Generally speaking, power is the ability to overcome obstacles in order to achieve some ends, say, power is a will directed to specific purposes. Power can be classified on the basis of the means used to achieve the ends. According to the classical theory (e.g., Aristotle, Aquinas, Machiavelli, Hobbes, Sun Tzu, Marx) power embraces both the ability to deliver goods (*power of disposition*) and to threaten damage (*power of coercion*). Recent political philosophers (e.g., Gramsci, Foucault, Derrida, Luhmann) have focused on other forms of power as the ability to accumulate knowledge and information, the ability to influence the public opinion, and to shape the cultural milieu. From a more operational point of view[16], power can be described as 1) *Power Over*: ability to influence and coerce; 2) *Power To*: organise and change existing hierarchies; 3) *Power With*: increased power from collective action; 4) *Power from Within*: increased individual consciousness.

Power is not an inherent quality of the person (no one is powerful per se), it is rather a possession, which can be present at different degrees, and can decrease or increase according to several variables, age included. Power always operates *in relation with* something or somebody, say, power is by definition relational. The notion of *power relation* is used to describe the balance of power between different parties which compete to achieve the same ends, in a particular context. It is important to emphasise that, given the fluid nature of power, power relations are always relative to a specific situation. Any attempt to crystallize power relations into stable, rigid, schemes unavoidably ends up misrepresenting the reality.

The notion of *power relation* implies a theory about the nature and the dynamic of power. Overall, one can distinguish between distributive and generative theories. According to distributive theories, power in any specific society tends to remain constant. This means that, at the end of the day, any power conflict is a zero sum game, where one participant's gains result only from another's equivalent losses.

---

[16] Rowlands, J. (1997) Questioning Empowerment: Working with Women in Honduras. Oxford, UK: Oxfam.

Ultimately this perspective understands power relations as non-negotiable conflicts, in the sense that they will imply winners and losers (of course mediation is possible, but it will be a compromise, rather than a true mediation). Distributive theories of power include prominent thinkers like Hobbes, Locke and Rousseau, who, though from different perspectives, looked at human beings as sets of single individuals, only aiming to fulfill their individual ends. For these thinkers there is no "common good" on which one could ground an alliance between parties, at most there is a "common convenience", which could only justify a temporary compromise. Also the so called "theorists of suspicion" - according to Ricoeur's definition of Marx, Freud and Nietzsche – conceive human beings as driven only by self-interest. Economic, libidinal, and selfish links allow humans to establish groups and larger communities, but not to overcome their fundamental, irreducible, "wilderness", which could explode with fury in any moment.

On the contrary, generative theories of power argue that power can be increased without any detrimental effect on any other actor. Say, power is understood as resulting from processes of competition and collaboration rather than from non negotiable conflicts. Competition and collaboration are complementary strategies and very often – as the theory contends - one can compete more effectively if one also collaborates when it is time to collaborate. In principle, competition does not aim to exclude other parties, or to deprive them of their rights, on the contrary is a process through which individuals search for new opportunities, which, after being discovered, can be used also by others. According to generative theories of power, individuals are bound together not only by immediate interests (who are not excluded), but by true bonds of solidarity. Here the idea of power is ultimately justified by the concept of "common good" (e.g., Aristotle, Aquinas), which is a good shared by a collectivity that cannot be disaggregated.

Recommendation no. 2: Ageing always implies a certain weakening of the aged persons, and consequently modifies the power relations which affect them. An ethical analysis should consider the tension between individuals and the collective, and should address the change of power relations among actors.

Finally power can be also investigated from its sources. One possible categorisation is based on a simple distinction between power generated by the ability to exchange, or share, objects, activities, ideas (*power of exchange)*, and power generated by the ability to links humans to each other (*power of coordination).*

Power of exchange consists in the possession of goods, properties, and skills (including scientific and technical knowledge) that can be advantageously exchanged with other goods, properties and skills. The more one possesses exchangeable commodities, the more one is powerful. Obviously the concept of "exchangeable" commodity - say, the relative value of various goods, skills, and knowledge - varies between and within societies. In contemporary society technical knowledge, and data ownership, are among the most "valued" commodities, and this explains why contemporary society is often defined an "information society". In the contemporary world knowledge and information are a primary source of power.

Power of coordination consists in the ability to create networks and to promote common values and inclusive communities. Power of coordination is the typical power of the "network society"[17] and can take on two main aspects. First power of

---

[17] Castells M, 1996, *The Rise of the Network Society*, Blackwell

coordination is the ability to determine the aims of a network or, at least, to influence decisions within the network. Second, power of coordination consists in the ability to switch. Switchers are bridges between networks. Isolated networks are fragile, whereas being connected is a form of power. Yet coordination demands a still more basic element, say, time. Flows between nodes and hubs, interconnectivity between networks, as well as simpler human interactions, cannot be defined without reference to time, and demand time to become effective. Time is then the other primary source of power together with knowledge and information. Without knowledge and time, there is no power, at least in a human sense, because power necessarily implies will and future. Aeschylus, the ancient Greek tragedian, arrived to a similar conclusion.

In the "Prometheus Bound"[18], Aeschylus tells why Prometheus, the titan, was punished. As Zeus, the king of gods, took the power, "*he began to allocate to each god their various responsibilities and powers. But for the wretched mortals he showed no interest at all; in fact he wanted to destroy the whole human race and replace it with another, a new one*" (230). Prometheus decided then to oppose Zeus and to save humans, the "*ephemeral creatures*" (240). He blinded humans with hopes, and gave them the gift of fire. So thanks to hopes, humans "*cannot foresee their own death*" (250), and thanks to fire they "*learned many crafts*" (250). Here the myth achieves a sublime blend of insight and pessimism, irony and philosophical reflection. Thanks to Prometheus (whose name means "prescient"), humans got mental time (say, the time that allows hopes to deploy themselves) and knowledge (say, the ability to see and manipulate the world, since fire is both an instrument for enlightening and for forging). Yet hopes are misleading (actually time is already over for each one of us) and knowledge is only crafts (which means technique, but also trickery). In its essence, human power is then illusory, since human beings are - and remain – frail, powerless, "ephemeral creatures": "*Who of you by worrying can add a single hour to his life ? Since you cannot do this very little thing, why do you worry about the rest?*" (Luke 12, 25-26).

Recommendation no. 3: The main sources of power are capacity for exchange and for coordination, which can be further turned into possession of time and possession of knowledge. Although largely illusory, time and knowledge are the most precious goods that human beings can ever possess, because they save humans from annihilation. It is an ethical tenet to avoid that any social dynamics create people that, for any reason, perceive themselves without time and knowledge.

III. KNOWLEDGE, TIME, AND AGEING

Power can therefore be described according to several accounts, but, ultimately, is grounded on knowledge and time - will and future, hopes and technique - which are the enabling elements that allow the parties to be empowered. Yet the paradox inherent to any kind of human power is precisely that knowledge and time are always on the verge of fading away, of revealing their illusory nature: "*The cloud-capp'd towers, the gorgeous palaces, the solemn temples, the great globe itself, Yea, all which it inherit, shall dissolve, and, like this insubstantial pageant faded, leave not a rack behind. We are such stuff as dreams are made on; and our little life is rounded*

---

[18] Griffith, Mark (1983), *Aeschylus' Prometheus Bound*, Cambridge: Cambridge UP

with sleep. Sir, I am wex'd; bear with my weakness; my old brain is troubled." (*The Tempest*, IV, i, 153-159) Prospero is one of the greatest Shakespearean old men.[19] His time is over, his world fades into thin air. As all old men, he doesn't have much time and his power is now vanishing. Old men cannot make projects, because their time is too short; they cannot hope because their hopes don't have time to be deployed.

The deception is subtle, who could deny indeed that Prospero, and with him all old men, is right? But are we sure that these statements describe only old men's condition or would we do better to realize that they speak of the *human* condition? Who could claim to know how much time they still have? *"The land of a rich man produced plentifully, and he thought to himself, 'What shall I do, for I have nowhere to store my crops?' And he said, 'I will do this: I will tear down my barns and build larger ones, and there I will store all my grain and my goods. And I will say to my soul, Soul, you have ample goods laid up for many years; relax, eat, drink, be merry.' But God said to him, 'Fool! This night your soul is required of you"* (Luke 12, 16-20)

Yet, although we are all "ephemeral creatures", only older people are "forced"[20] to realise that their time is limited, and this is probably the first, and deeper, reason of their social weakness.[21] This holds particularly true in contemporary society, where a continuous acceleration of technological, economic and social processes is eroding any regular temporal sequence. The terrific social pressure towards rejuvenating technologies, cosmetic surgery, and medications would not be comprehensible without understanding that the illusion of eternal youthness, of an endless life span, is today the key to power.

Lack of "social time" is, however, only the first element that contributes to the processes of exclusion and victimisation of aged people. The second, critical, element concerns knowledge and information. In pre-industrial societies, mechanisms for knowledge transmission chiefly relied on human abilities. The older individual was physically weaker, but, insofar as he conserved mental capacities, he was the precious medium used by societies for the transmission of knowledge through human generations. Such a role was paramount in pre-literate societies where humans had no other means to transmit cultural contents other than the memories held by their elders, who were consequently regarded with religious awe and reverence and constituted a very powerful social group, notwithstanding their physical limitations.[22]

Older people's social functions started weakening with the first literate societies, although handwritten documents could not easily replace the elders (furthermore in the so called "literate societies" of the past only a minority of people were actually literate). Only with the "print revolution", did literacy start to deprive elders of their social functions. Book diffusion made it increasingly inadequate to rely on a "living repository of information", and with the industrial revolution, older people became more and more powerless, at least when they belonged to the lowest social classes (Marx's famous, and vivid, description of workers' life in XIX century London,

---

[19] *The Tempest* was Shakespeare's last play, and one might like to imagine that Prospero's words resonate Shakespeare's feelings as well.

[20] It is not only a matter of subliminal messages and social pressures, the social obligation to consider old man's time over is made up by material facts, like the impossibility to get a loan, or to purchase an insurance, or to sign a mortgage.

[21] Admittingly the feeling that the time is over could in principle also create a sense of liberty and independency from material constraints. Yet this reaction is rare, at least in the Western, secularised, civilisation.

[22] However it is to note that when the elderly was not able to fulfil his role of "collective memory", he rapidly lost power also in pre-literate societies. The dementing older (the "old idiot") was hardly respected in societies which highly evaluated the "wise elder".

showed well the degraded living conditions of older workers). To be sure, mid and high income people conserved their relative power when they became aged, but such a power was no longer due to their alleged knowledge or wisdom, but to their wealth. In early industrial societies, wealth accumulation among ordinary people was mainly due to savings. As a consequence, old people were – all other conditions equal – usually wealthier than the young, since they had time to accumulate cash and property. This explains why the "old bourgeois", who was no longer perceived deserving a special moral respect (think for instance of Balzac's novels), was still reverenced and feared.

With the XX century, any pretention that older people had a moral superiority definitely faded away, and old persons also lost their relative economic advantage. In the industrial, capitalistic, society richness is incremental, rather than cumulative, and it is strictly related to production. Once persons have removed themselves from active employment, they are likely to become gradually poorer or, at least, not to increase any longer their wealth. Trends in family structures (e.g., declining birth rates, tendency towards families with fewer members, single-parent families, and childless, rather than extended families, etc.) and trends in work mobility, which increase physical distance between generations of a family, have finally resulted in weakening family ties and making less and less relevant (if any) grandparent's role in the family. Little by little, older people have ended up being perceived only as "retired" persons, destined, once they become too frail and weak to live alone, to be confined in retirement communities or in nursing homes: "*Admission to an old people's home usually means not only the final severing of old affective ties, but also means living together with people with whom the individual has had no positive affective relationships. Physical care by doctors and nursing personnel may be excellent. But at the same time the separation of the old people from normal life, and their congregation with strangers, means loneliness for the individual [...] Many old people's homes are therefore deserts of loneliness*" (p.74)[23]

There is no social role for aged persons in the post-industrial society. As long as they succeed in remaining "young enough", they are included in the wider societal context, but when they give in to the passage of time, their social power rapidly evaporate and they are progressively expulsed and excluded. Economic power – as much it is - is insufficient to compensate the fading away of a temporal perspective in which they can place themselves (for the sake of clarity, I would like to repeat and emphasise that such a temporal perspective has little to do with any insurance-like calculation of individual's life expectancy: I'm referring here to the social perception and construction of time, as rigorously defined by Norbert Elias[24]), and the loss of informational power (not only are older people no longer a repository of collective memory, but also their individual knowledge tends to become obsolete because of the rapid pace of technological innovation). Without *a-time-for-living* and an appropriate knowledge, without a specific social function, older persons either succeed in denying their ageing[25] (interestingly enough, empirical studies have reported that people increasingly describe their experience of growing older by drawing on the idea that

---

[23] Elias N, 1985, *The Loneliness of the Dying*, Blackwell: Oxford
[24] Elias N, 1992, *Time: an Essay*, Blackwell: Oxford
[25] Jones RL, 2006, 'Older people' talking as if they are not older people: Positioning theory as an explanation
Journal of Aging Studies, 20, 1: 79-91

they remain the same person but a mask of an older person appears on their face[26]) or they are going to become the new outcasts.

Recommendation no. 4: In contemporary society, old people are increasingly people without time and knowledge. This makes it an ethical imperative to address their social role and functions, and to understand how they can be empowered.

The parable started with the elders of the pre-literate village could be now closed with Willy Loman, the tragic character of Arthur Miller's play "*Death of a Salesman*". After being a traveling salesman for the Wagner Company for thirty-four years, the 63yo Willy Loman starts perceiving himself ageing, he sees his impeding weaknesses and incoming frailty. He - who had always bet only on appearance and personal attractiveness - now feels his life getting out of hand. Little by little Willy realizes how senseless has been a life spent by striving for being the "*number-one man*". He wanted to be the best of salesmen, and he pretended that he was. Now he realizes that he was not, and decides to commit suicide as the only way to prove that he was not a failure. Yet Willy fails also in death as he failed in life. No one shows up at his funeral, and his life insurance doesn't cover suicide. His story is not only an American tragedy, but it is our, standard, ridiculous, human tragedy, because we are all Willy Loman, when we pretend to be the "*number-one man*".

"*Everything in the world is a jest* – sings *Falstaff* in the final fugue of Verdi's last opera - *We always fool ourselves*". *Falstaff* is an opera that tells the humorous story of an old, fat, man who still pretends being a great seducer and is made a fool of by his companions. The highest dramatic moment is in the final fugue, when the music stops for a few seconds, and the singer who plays Falstaff points to the audience and laughing at them says "*We always make fool ourselves, you too… you too*". Then, after a short pause, the second theme of the fugue explodes and the opera rapidly ends. *Falstaff* - written in Verdi's ninth decade of life, when all music critics thought he was only an old, out of fashion, Italian *maestro* - was probably his supreme opera, universally recognised as an absolute masterpiece. Is *Falstaff* an old man's music composition? Is there ever any sign which might allow us to understand an artist's age from his works? Art (be music, painting, poetry, or sculpture) does not "know" author's age. There is probably a lesson to be learned here.

Recommendation no. 5: Human flourishing and excellence have little to do with power fantasies. Technologies for human augmentation, including anti-ageing and rejuvenating technologies, cosmetic surgery, and medications, are ethically questionable inasmuch as they pretend to offer what they cannot deliver.

IV. AGEING IN THE INFORMATION SOCIETY

"*Europeans are living longer than ever thanks to economic growth and advances in health care. Average life expectancy is now over 80, and by 2020 around 25% of the population will be over 65. Fortunately, the Information Society offers older people the chance to live independently and continue to enjoy a high quality of life.*

---

[26] Featherstone M., Hepworth M., 1991,The mask of ageing and the postmodern life course. In M. Featherstone, M. Hepworth, & B. S. Turner (Eds.), *The body: Social process and cultural theory*, Sage, London: 371–389

Currently, however, a number of barriers prevent the older generation from fully embracing Information and Communication Technologies (ICT). In response, the European Commission is developing actions to improve ICT uptake amongst the elderly."[27] It would be difficult to summarise better, and more concisely, the overall strategy of the European Commission (EC) on inclusion of older people into the Information Society. The recent *Overview of the European strategy in ICT for Ageing Well* also provides a sound rationale for such a strategy *"The number of people over 50 will rise by 35% between 2005 and 2050. The number of people over 85 will triple by 2050. Recent OECD analyses forecast escalating costs as a result of ageing populations in Japan, the US and Europe. As fertility rates are also declining, the ratio between people at work and remaining population will change from 4-1 today to 2-1 by 2050 in average in Europe!! Without a higher level of participation of the elder population in employment, and without better tailored and more effective health and social care services, these trends will put serious pressure on Europe's social models and public finances."*[28]

The argument states that i) society is rapidly ageing because of both a reduction in the fertility rate and an increase in life expectancy; ii) ageing implies increasing economic and social costs; iii) economic costs are chiefly related to the growing imbalance between active and retired populations, and also include health care costs; iv) social costs chiefly concern the risk of creating a larger and larger segment of disengaged and disaffected citizens, which are only marginally included in the societal mainstream; v) ICT has the potential for mitigating both categories of risks and costs; vi) barriers which oppose ICT uptake among the elderly should be removed; vii) drivers which could promote ICT uptake among the elderly should be implemented.

The first cause of societal ageing (decreased fertility rate) depends on many complex, and badly understood, factors. Increasing the fertility rate in western countries – provided that it would be a sensible answer – is anything but easy. The second cause of societal ageing, the increased lifespan, could hardly be considered a target because it is evidently welcome to most. Ageing is still the best alternative to dying, if one had to chose, and provided that ageing is not too burdensome. Old age is not itself a disease and, although one is expected to become physically weaker and suffer from minor short memory impairments, overall health conditions are expected to remain more than acceptable until at least the ninth decade of life. Yet, while the onset of the most severe disabilities is coming later and later in life, most people in the West are still starting their old people's career at 65, when they retire. From that moment on, they start counting the days until they have to enter a nursing home. This increasing mass of people removed from active employment and destitute of any social function but being consumers, is a source of social pressure. Most assumptions about the financial impact of ageing overestimated health spending. Recent figures[29] show that the final two years before death consume about one-quarter of an individual's lifetime healthcare costs, no matter whether this comes at 9 years or 90. This means that health care costs are only marginally increased by societal ageing (costs are mainly a function of the number of people who have access to health care) and when statistics show that health expenditure rises in over-65s, it is chiefly because

[27] http://ec.europa.eu/information_society/activities/einclusion/policy/ageing/index_en.htm
[28] http://ec.europa.eu/information_society/activities/einclusion/docs/ageing/overview.pdf
[29] Herwartz H, Theilen B, 2009, The determinants of healthcare expenditure: new results from semiparametric estimation", *Health Economics*, Published Online: 7 Aug 2009 http://dx.doi.org/10.1002/hec.1540

most people die in this age group. Actually the financial and social burden of old people suffering from various chronic conditions, or affected by mild disability is not as great as is often assumed.[30]

There are two real financial and social issues related to ageing. The first issue concerns the increasing population of old people who are merely frail. They are not counted among either sick or disabled persons. While the sick and the disabled receive help according to different social-health care systems, those who have become so infirm that they cannot live alone any longer, must go into a care home and pay for it (unless they are particularly poor, no social care system in Europe provides a totally free of charge nursing home system). In these cases, the income of all old people - from pensions, savings, benefits and other sources, like the sale of their house if they own one - go towards paying the care home fees. This system is hardly tenable for many reasons, not least because it is not economically sustainable and it is not ethically tolerable. The second financial and social issue related to ageing is the decrease in the proportion of people in the workforce. This means that the impact of the ageing population is taking place in a context of fiscal constraint, and this unavoidably limits what societies can to do for older citizens.

What can ICT do for mitigating these impacts? ICT could both increase the proportion of people in the workforce, and reduce the need for frail old people to move to care homes. In a nutshell, this is the EC Action Plan for "*Ageing Well in the Information Society*"[31], which assumes that ICT has the potential to enable "*older people to stay active and productive for longer; to continue to engage in society with more accessible online services; and to enjoy a healthier and higher quality of life for longer*". In social science terms, what the action plan aims to do is to modify the social fact called "ageing". Both material elements of ageing (e.g., the pension system and various retirement plans, legislation about older citizens, the "grey economy", social and health care for the elderly, nursing homes, assistive technologies, etc.) and non-material elements (e.g., narratives about ageing, implicit and explicit definitions of ageing, elderly role descriptions, age-related values, etc.) are expected to be modified by the massive use of ICT. In particular, the dynamic between social inclusion and exclusion is one of the main targets of the "*Ageing Well in the Information Society*" strategy, which is part of the larger e-Inclusion policy that means both inclusive ICT and the use of ICT to achieve social inclusion. The Action Plan for "*Ageing Well in the Information Society*" is thus essentially a plan for empowering old people.

Recommendation no. 6: ICT can effectively address the two main issues related to ageing, say, the increasing population of frail old people, and the decrease in the proportion of people in the workforce. Reducing the social and economic burden of these two social trends is ethically tenable if it is part of larger strategy, which aims to reshape the old persons role and empower old people.

---

[30] White C, 2007, Health Care Spending Growth: How Different Is the United States From the Rest of the OECD, *Health Affairs*, 26(1): 154-161

[31] COM(2007) 332 final

V. EMPOWERING OLD PEOPLE BY ADDRESSING THE OLD-PERSON-ROLE

As we have seen (section 4), old people are characterized by a twofold vulnerability. First, they all suffer – sooner or later - from some physical weakening, which also includes a reduction of memory and learning capacities. Second, they all suffer – sooner or later – from some form of social exclusion. Both sources of vulnerability can be postponed and mitigated but not completely avoided because they are generated by biological processes and by the lack of a positive social function for older age in post-industrial societies, where collective memories are effectively stored in, and communicated by, a wide range of electronic media, so making obsolete the need for the "wise elder". Postponing and mitigating these vulnerabilities means anything but aiming to dissolve the social fact of ageing as human societies have understood it for centuries, say, since humans have started to record their history and their stories and to transmit cultural contents through generations by using old peoples' memories. This is what makes the "Ageing Well" strategy much more politically ambitious, and ethically challenging, than it is often assumed.

Starting from the seminal work of Philippe Ariès, much work has been devoted to the birth of childhood in the West, and there is now a general agreement among scholars that childhood– say, a period in which the young human learns cultural norms and begins to reflect them – grew into existence in the European upper classes in the 16th and 17th centuries, solidified itself in the 18th century, and finally flourished in the 20th century. The birth of childhood was a by-product of the great social, political, philosophical and scientific turmoil, which characterized the passage to the industrial society. In the same way the invention of adolescence – a period of time between childhood and adulthood, a sort of "extended puberty" in which a sexually mature person is treated as a "growing child", and remains under parental supervision - was a result of the late industrial revolution, which required a longer educational and training period before entering in the workforce. Adolescence has been described as a particular stage of life with precise age parameters, developmental possibilities and social requirements, yet it is by no means an "objective" fact, rather it is a pure social construction. No one should be surprised then to discover that we are now looking at similar radical changes in the social construction of older ages. The elder - someone who should rely on the family, the tribe, or the enlarged community, to survive, but who is still able to contribute to social life through knowledge and practical wisdom accumulated during his life - does not exist any longer, he dissolved *"like this insubstantial pageant faded"*, leaving *"not a rack behind"*. What remains is the 'elderly', and the sole ethically legitimate goal of any policy addressing ageing should be "to abolish" the 'elderly' as it exists today. Age periods can come into existence - as happened with childhood and adolescence - and can disappear, and this should now be the destiny of old age. To be sure, aged persons will always exist, but the old-person role could disappear.

Recommendation no. 7: From an ethical perspective reshaping the old person role means cancelling it altogether, because it no longer confers any kind of advantage to those who play it.

VI. EMPOWERING THE 'EXTENDED MIDDLE AGE' GROUP

ICT can allow *"older people to stay active and productive for longer"*. This means that ICT can deeply modify the most important rite of passage between adulthood and old age, which is retirement, both by postponing it and by making it futile. By changing the meaning of retirement ICT can also change one of the main factors which determine the weakening of old people, say, what we called the "lack of social time" (section 3). Retirement is indeed the signal for most people that their social function is over and that their time, in which they can project themselves and cultivate hopes, is almost terminated as well. If we want to empower old people, and give them the possibility of escaping their role, we need to reshape their concept of time. ICT is by definition a technology which modifies the perception of time and space, and it can allow us to expand the social time of people who are chronologically old. In other words, ICT could give people more subjective time (say, time could be dilated by filling it with meaning and events) and also more "objective" time (say, ICT could be used to find practical solutions to overcoming barriers like the impossibility to get a loan, or to purchase insurance, or to sign a mortgage because of age limits).

ICT is already contributing to creating a new age category, the so called "extended middle age" group, which is an age group between current retirement age (around 65 years) and the start of age related, severe, physical and mental illnesses and disabilities. These people are currently forced to remove themselves from active employment, yet their physical and mental abilities are almost unaltered, and ICT could easily compensate any minor physical and mental impairments, they could show. This would also address one of the main causes of societal ageing, which is the decrease of active people in the workforce. A vast array of everyday electronic devices (e.g., computers, mobile phones, the internet) could allow people belonging to the "extended middle age" class to remain in the workforce, to participate in social and political life, and to overcome barriers, mainly normative and concerning retirement legislations, which tend to force them into the old-person role.

Recommendation no. 8: A new age category, the so called "extended middle age" group, is emerging, also in connection with the wider usage of ICT. Promoting their inclusion in the information society should be a pillar of the Ageing Well strategy.

As much as empowerment is a social process, it is generated by policies which address existing power relations. Technology can be an important element of these policies, but it can never substitute them. The goal to allow *"older people to stay active and productive for longer"* is a policy goal, which requires policy perspectives.

The first policy issue to be addressed concerns older people's vulnerability. We have told (section 5) that their vulnerability is twofold, say, a physical weakening (which includes both bodily and mentally weakening) and a social weakening (which is due to retirement and a lack of social function for retired people). Vulnerability refers to a condition in which a person finds himself or herself particularly susceptible to injury or harm. Old people who belong to the "extended middle age" group are mainly more susceptible to social harm rather than to physical harm. They lose both *power of disposition* and *coercion* (section 2) when they retire. The loss of these two types of power implies a loss of *exchange* and *coordination powers* (section 2) as well. Old people find themselves increasingly excluded by social networks and they have less and less "value" to exchange with others. Their main sources of power remain their wealth and, sometimes, a surrogate parental role (not to be confused with the traditional grandparent role) in the case of the failure of their sons and daughters' families. In practice they can still exchange only their consumers' capacity and their spare time, and they have a minor role to play in social networks.

Some have proposed that old people could increase their social value by devoting time and resources to voluntary work and charitable activities. This is not only insulting (as though there were two categories of people, those whose work must be paid; and those whose work can be given for free), but it is also hardly effective. Voluntary work and charitable activities rarely give volunteers any individual power. Usually these activities give a sort of collective power to the overall organisation, and bestow only the leaders with individual power. Old persons are vulnerable because they are less able to assert claims to rights that they possess as far as citizens, and this cannot be solved by "fictitious", and ad hoc invented, social roles (of course voluntary work is laudable, but it cannot be thought as an easy fix for the lack of social role of older citizens). There is no loophole, the main instrument to empower old people remains the adoption of appropriate legislative, and administrative, measures to modify or abolish all existing laws, regulations, customs and practices in the working place that constitute discrimination against persons on the basis of their chronological age. People should conserve the right to retire after a certain age threshold, but they should never be obliged to retire, unless they become manifestly unable to perform their work and they cannot be differently employed. ICT should be used to allow people to perform their duties at work, safely, securely, and effectively, in particular in case they start suffering from any minor physical or mental impairment.

Recommendation no. 9: All citizens should enjoy full social and economic rights independently from their age. People who belong to the "extended middle age" group should enjoy just and favourable conditions of work. Discriminatory practices on grounds of old age should be banned and ICT should be used to facilitate inclusive processes at work.

Here one meets the issue of e-Accessibility. ICT itself can become a barrier to entering into the "extended middle age" group. If people are computer illiterate, if they are unable to use a keyboard, or unable to see a monitor, if they cannot access the Internet, or are confused by things like flashing banners, pop-up windows and small font sizes, their business perspectives may be limited. If the buttons on a mobile phone are too small for people with dexterity problems, their communication options are limited. If people do not know how to surf the net, they are limited in terms of their ability to access goods and services available solely on line. These limitations are disabilities in today's world. As such, we can say that as much as technology can help to dissolve the old-person role, it can also dramatically reinforce it. This is the great ambiguity of ICT, which – like Prometheus' gift - could turn into an offer or into a sentence (section 2). On the one hand ICT can allow people to participate in society but, on the other hand, it can also become one of the strongest barriers to participation within society.

In order to avoid ICT becoming a barrier it is important that some basic requirements are met. They include

- Most information and communications technologies and systems, including the Internet, should be available at reasonable cost.
- ICT should be designed keeping in mind specific minor disabilities (notably concerning sensory perceptions, and dexterity) that could prevent their usage. Older

persons should be actively involved in ICT production and should incorporate their own perspectives in technology design.
- ICT should adopt different forms of language such as use of sign languages, Braille, augmentative and alternative communication, and all other accessible means, modes and formats of communication.

Participatory practices involving people who belong to the "extended middle age" group could be also justified in view of designing personalized or user centred technology. The risk is that such gatherings never challenge entrenched assumptions, interests, power-structures and imaginations, and end up manipulating their publics or imposing top-down conditions and framings.[32]

Recommendation no. 10: Lack of accessibility can become a serious barrier to the uptake of ICT in people belonging to the "extended middle age" group. An ethical approach to e-accessibility should be based on the preliminary fulfillment of a few basic requirements.

Yet it would be misleading to believe that the main barriers to the uptake of ICT among people of the "extended middle age" group concern either economic or educational factors, or accessibility elements, which are more important in other vulnerable groups. A critical aspect of power relations is the way in which they can be internalised: power can operate through consent as well as coercion. The main effect of ageism and disempowerment is that they prevent people from even considering that there can be an alternative to the situation they are in. As people internalise ageism, their own reactions to any form of ICT training are problematic, because they can easily assume that they are unable to learn and that age prevents them from changing. An important element to focus on is self-respect. "Extended middle age" people need to become self confident and to develop a sense of agency before they can effectively face the challenge of learning any new technology. In other words, technology innovation can be effectively incorporated into a social practice only if the relevant actors have a sufficient sense of self-esteem that allows them to put up with education, and organizational transformation.

Most people belonging to the "extended middle age" group paradoxically have their rights violated because of a formal or informal label of 'old, vulnerable, person' being applied to them. It is important not to judge these persons as being vulnerable in such a way that they become stigmatised or subject to greater risk of discrimination. It is not a person who is vulnerable, but rather some aspect of their circumstances that makes them vulnerable, that is (a) at a particular time; (b) in a particular respect; and (c) vis-à-vis a particular harm or harms. A person of the "extended middle age" group can move in and out of being vulnerable, and the nature and extent of their particular vulnerability can change. It is important to recognise that the vulnerability of a person changes over time and can have multiple and/or varying sources. Many private companies, whose organisation of work relies almost exclusively on information and communication technologies, are wary of hiring older persons because they fear old age is a barrier to picking up ICT skills. Experience shows that when properly trained or assisted in the early stages, older persons are capable of learning to use the few applications that usually run in an enterprise. Non discrimination directives, in particular Council Directive 2000/78/EC of 27 November 2000 establishing a general

---

[32] Cooke, B. and U. Kothari, "Participation: The New Tyranny?", London: Zed., 2002.

framework for equal treatment in employment and occupation, could be updated to take into account the specific issue of ICT and the elderly. The actual version of article 6 of the Directive is arguably not clear enough about discriminating against the elderly because of their presumed lack of ICT skills.

The source of the vulnerability of the "extended middle age" group is chiefly a result of their position with respect to others, in the sense that they are either retired people or about to retire. Other important co-factors, which can contribute to determining their degree of social vulnerability include; gender, ethnicity, education, social conditions, migrant conditions, and disabilities. It is important to consider the full range of potential sources of a particular person's vulnerabilities and strengths to ensure that both the ethical and practical issues are fully considered and properly addressed. Explicit attention to the vulnerability of people encourages better practical and ethical engagement with them. On the other hand it is important to avoid the opposite mistake, say, to assume that a person is weak just because he is older, which is definitely false. People of the "extended middle age" group share the common vulnerability of being old according to most social norms, but usually they are still empowered according to their socio-economic status, gender, ethnic group, etc. When in an age group there are significant power differentials, as it is in this case, awareness of vulnerabilities and strengths avoids unwarranted assumptions being made.

Recommendation no. 11: Self exclusion and social victimization are likely to be the most dangerous factors which may lead to a failure in e-Inclusion processes. The symbolic value of retirement should not be underestimated. In principle ICT should be used to turn retirement into an effective right, enjoyed by each person according to his own will and needs, instead of some pre-fixed schemes.

VII. EMPOWERING THE 'FRAIL OLD PERSON' GROUP

Technology allows people to live longer and longer, but it cannot revert the arrow of time. Although ICT can effectively contribute to dissolving the old-person role into the new "extended middle age" role, there are little doubts that some people are destined to enter into a still more vulnerable and weaker group, the frail people. Frailty is not really a disease but rather a combination of a variety of medical and social problems. Medical doctors[33] define frailty as a condition in which at least three of the following factors are met: 1) unintentional weight loss (five kg or more in a year), 2) general feeling of exhaustion, 3) physical weakness (as measured by grip strength), 4) slow walking speed, 5) low levels of physical activity. As we have seen (section 4) most health costs are expected to occur during the last two years of life of any age group. Modern medicine can make people survive by "freezing" them at the threshold of dying for a certain length of time. The frail people group then includes· people who have entered in their last period of life because of any major disease (most of them are over 65 but they are not frail because of their age but because of the illness), and individuals in their late eighties and nineties, who start showing substantial losses in physical mobility and cognitive functioning. Technology (bio and info) could probably still push ahead the average age of this group of older old, and frailty could start at a hundred years or even more, but this would not change the

---

[33] Fried LP., Tangen CM, Walston J et al., 2001, Frailty in Older Adults: Evidence for a Phenotype, *Journal of Gerontology: Medical Sciences*, 56a, 3: 146-157.

features of the problem because there will be always a group of very frail older people.

The "*Ageing Well in the Information Society*" strategy addresses this group of people when the plan mentions that ICT should help older people "*to enjoy a healthier and higher quality of life for longer*", which is briefly expressed by the nice slogan "*Ageing well at home*". There is no doubt that ICT may improve living conditions of these people in various manners. Memory assistance, robotics, neuro-ICT interfacing, navigation systems, speech, sign and movement recognition, alternative communication environments and virtual worlds, are all examples of ICT which could contribute to contrast frailty and make it possible to postpone, or even to avoid, placement in a care home. Families living in situations of poverty with elderly dependents are particularly exposed and in particular need of assistance: adequate training, counselling, financial assistance and respite care.[34] New technologies could transform the way care is delivered and supported within families and communities. Yet, it is clear that technology cannot renovate frail persons, although it can play an essential role in empowering them.

Recommendation no. 12: Frail, old, people are probably destined to exist notwithstanding any technological innovation. ICT can however play an essential role in empowering them and improving their quality of life. It is then paramount to invest resources and promote research in this field.

First, technology can contribute to prevent elder abuse, which is probably one of the most important public health and societal problems, and a significant reason for the disempowerment of old, frail, people. Elder abuse is indeed facilitated by the disempowerment of old frail people and it is in its turn a cause of further disempowerment. Frail people often need other people who take care of them, notably of their body. In these situations the border between care and intrusion tends to become very subtle. Physical boundaries are also boundaries of personal integrity. The word integrity literally means "the quality or state of being complete or undivided". Physical and mental integrity thus refers to the inviolability of a person's body and mind, say, it refers to the right against being touched (in physical and metaphorical senses) without consent.

Historically, the notion of body integrity comes from the legal conception of *Habeas Corpus* (Latin: you shall have the body), originally the legal action through which a person can seek protection against an unlawful detention. The *Habeas Corpus* affirms the right not to be imprisoned arbitrarily and to not have the body violated in any other way (e.g., physical inspection, torture, abusive treatments, and so on). Body integrity is threatened by physical pain, injuries, sexual assaults, rape, physical inspections, and the like. Mental integrity is violated any time when emotional and cognitive processes are brutally invaded, abused and/or disrupted. We all have an interest in protecting our integrity. This is clearly expressed by the *Universal Declaration of Human Rights* (art.3) which states that everyone has a right to the inviolability of his or her person, and by the *Convention on Human Rights and*

---

[34] According to Madeleine Starr of Carers UK, those providing heavy end care are "twice as likely than the general population to be in poor health themselves, as a result of caring…[they also experience] significant financial disadvantages; very frequently people have to give up work and therefore give up their income…this affects not only their working lives but it also affects their ability to put into the pension system…[thereby] creating a situation where carers themselves might go into poverty in their own retirement." SENIOR, D.1.5 WP 1 Report Final, p. 97.

Biomedicine[35] (art.1), which states that "Parties to this Convention shall protect the dignity and identity of all human beings and guarantee everyone, without discrimination, respect for their integrity and other rights and fundamental freedoms with regard to the application of biology and medicine".

The principle of body integrity does not concern only violations of the body resulting in suffering or in adverse health conditions, but it also deals with intrusions without harmful effects. This leads to an additional issue, say, does a bodily or psychological intrusion constitute a violation of integrity only if it is perceived as such by the victim? Or, on the contrary, are there objective criteria to establish when there is a violation of personal integrity? The principle of the "inviolability of the body" includes two cognate, but different[36], concepts: 1) the view "that the body is a 'sacredness' in the biological order"[37]; and 2) the view of the body as personal property, whose borders cannot be trespassed without the owner's consent. There are then two different perspectives about body integrity, the former contends that the right to integrity is inherently part of the notion of human dignity[38], the latter maintains that personal integrity is the right of every human being to protect his physical privacy[39]. Yet elder abuse, as much as it involves physical intrusion and offence to modesty feelings, unavoidably also implies a sense of physical degradation, and humiliation, and threatens the sense of self-esteem, and self-respect, which are constitutive elements of the notion of dignity. The supreme dignity of the frail person dwells in his frailty, that must be honored as such (to be sure, respecting frailty does not imply accepting it, but it implies consideration of the frail human as completely human, say, frailty does not diminish in any manner the human condition).

The definition of elder abuse adopted by the World Health Organization – "a single, or repeated act, or lack of appropriate action, occurring within any relationship where there is an expectation of trust which causes harm or distress to an older person" [40]– emphasises the breach of trust relations, and opens the notion of abuse also to the issue of data protection.

---

[35] The concept of body integrity has important applications in the biomedical sphere, where inter alia it requires that invasive actions cannot be lifted without the informed consent of the patient.

[36] Actually, together with Giorgio Agamben, one could argue that these two concepts are anything but the two sides of the same coin, being the notion of sacred body only the other side of the notion of body as a property. In his analysis of the *habeas corpus*, Agamben argues that "the root of modern democracy's secret biopolitical calling lies here: he who will appear later as the bearer of rights and, according to a curious oxymoron, as the new sovereign subject (*subiectus superaneus*, in other words, what is below and, at the same time, most elevated) can only be constituted as such through the repetition of the sovereign exception and the isolation of *corpus*, bare life, in himself. If it is true that law needs a body in order to be in force, and if one can speak, in this sense, of "law's desire to have a body," democracy responds to this desire by compelling law to assume the care of this body. This ambiguous (or polar) character of democracy appears even more clearly in the *habeas corpus* if one considers the fact that the same legal procedure that was originally intended to assure the presence of the accused at the trial and, therefore, to keep the accused from avoiding judgment, turns -- in its new and definitive form -- into grounds for the sheriff to detain and exhibit the body of the accused. *Corpus is a two-faced being, the bearer both of subjection to sovereign power and of individual liberties"* (*Agamben G, 1988,* Homo Sacer: Sovereign Power and Bare Life. Stanford UP, Stanford, CA. P 124-125)

[37] Murray TH, (1987), On the Human Body as Property: the Meaning of Embodiment, Markets, and The Need of Strangers, *Journal of Law Reform* 20, 4:1055-1089

[38] See for instance, Maschke KJ, (2003), Proxy Research Consent and the Decisionally Impaired: Science, the Common Good, and Bodily Integrity, *Journal of Disability Policy Studies* 13, 4

[39] Schloendorff v. Society of New York Hospital, 1914, quoted by Maschke KJ, (2003).

[40] http://www.who.int/ageing/projects/elder_abuse/en/

Concerning the protection of private life, the challenge is to create trust in the ageing information society while avoiding the risk of undue social categorization. Some older persons, for instance those living in institutions or conditions of vulnerability and unbalanced power relations, may have reduced capacity to resist anti-ageing practices and attitudes. However, the protection of privacy must be carefully balanced with or sometimes against the need of sharing the burdens, joys, troubles, concerns, and life decisions with others. Privacy in ICT for the elderly should, in our view, factor in the "collective" dimension of old age when social contacts, help, assistance become of paramount importance. Thus, on the one hand, the duty to respect private life, on the other the duty to intervene, *as appropriate*, in order to assist, offer help, provide reasonable accommodation. Consideration could be given to the designation of persons or bodies for the purpose of authorising interventions of different types, including ICT systems, in contexts such as family, living institutions, workplace or health care.[41] Our proposal is to promote new thinking about having, in different social settings, a 'concierge' which can assist individuals when they are in need.

In the field of data protection, building trust between operators, data controllers, and data processors suggests that privacy by design principle (PbD) be binding both for technology designers and producers as well as for data controllers who have to decide on the acquisition and use of ICT. Privacy enhancing technologies (PETs) should become a default setting of ICT products and services. The legal framework should also create a level of transparency and accountability. To this end, it is advisable to convert the currently punctual requirements into a broader and consistent principle of privacy by design. [42] The requirements are well established data protection principles, *viz.* **data minimization;** the processing of personal data should, by design, be engineered towards the minimization of the amount of data which need to be processed; **controllability**: an IT system should provide the data subjects with effective means of control concerning their personal data. The possibilities regarding consent and objection could be supported by technological settings; **transparency**: both developers and operators of IT systems have to ensure that the data subjects are sufficiently informed about the means of operation of the systems; **user friendly systems**: user interfaces can play a valuable role in assisting occasional users or non expert users, such as many senior citizens, navigating the risks posed by aggressive spam, malware, phishing, requests for personal data against free services etc.; **data confidentiality**: by design only authorised entities have access to personal data in IT systems; **data quality**: data controllers should support data quality by technical means; **use limitation**: IT systems which can be used for different purposes; data run through connected systems, such as data warehouses, cloud computing, digital identifiers. IT systems should guarantee that data and processes serving different tasks or purposes can be segregated from each other in a secure way.

Privacy by design principle should be binding both for technology designers and producers as well as for data controllers who have to decide on the acquisition and use of ICT. Privacy enhancing technologies (PETs) should become a default setting of ICT products and services. The legal framework should create a ground level of transparency and accountability.

---

[41] Recommendation 99 (4) of the Council of Europe on the legal protection of incapable adults, 23 February 1999.

[42] Article 29 Data Protection Working Party, *The Future of Privacy. Joint contribution to the Consultation of the European Commission on the legal framework for the fundamental right to protection of personal data*, Adopted on 01 December 2009, 02356/09/EN, WP 168, paragraph 46.

Recommendation 13: ICT for the elderly highlights the importance of creating trust. The breach of trust relations in the field of data protection is an offence to personal integrity and ultimately a form of elder abuse. Creating trust may require both new thinking in the area of private life/privacy and regulatory measures in terms of data protection.

Technology can contribute towards protecting from abuse in two major ways. First ICT can allow the frail person to communicate with the "external world", say, with the world outside the care setting. Communication is a basic empowerment tool, because it allows people to get in contact with other people and to establish alliances. Communication technology can also allow frail people to appeal to formal rules and structures, institutions and procedures, and to have access to tools such as lobbying, media and litigation. Finally communication may allow frail persons to participate in decision making at various institutional levels, which can directly affect their life, and not to be excluded from the wider societal and political life (e.g., e-democracy and e-governance).

Technology can also be used to protect personal spaces and people's intimacy. By providing some practical services (e.g., making it easier to wash themselves, allowing people to feed without assistance, allowing people to take medication autonomously, etc.) assistive technologies can soften the burden of dependence and partly restore some autonomy in frail people. To be sure, one could still prefer to be washed by a human fellow, if he feels it warmer and more devoted, but in case he is not completely happy with the way in which the caregiver handles his body, or if there is a risk to be neglected, technology may offer an alternative.

Recommendation no. 14: Respect for personal integrity is the first ethical tenet when ICT is applied for improving older peoples quality of life at home. Assistive technology for ageing should allow people to live better and to prevent any form of degradation and humiliation.

There is a risk in using technology to substitute the human caregiver. Frail people could become socially invisible (and this is a process which has already started). There is something psychologically unbearable in the sight of the frail person (be they aged or younger) who is losing his mental and physical abilities, until the point of not being able to take care of himself any longer. No one can easily tolerate to look at his own frailty, mirrored by another human being. Only a compassionate gaze, which is able to take on itself the weakness of the other and it is not scared by it, could put up with the view of human frailty, when it becomes so extreme. Only such a compassionate gaze could empower from outside the frail person, who would become included in the human community by being perceived as a member of this community by the caregiver. Yet such a compassionate gaze is not a matter of "good feelings", or a special moral disposition, but it is a consequence of a sort of "philosophical" training developed by living side by side with frail people. Today very few formal and informal caregivers have had in their life such an existential training to human frailty. Human frailty is denied and hidden. Maybe this makes contemporary life easier and "rosier", but it certainly makes us ill-prepared to deal with human frailty when there is no alternative but to face it. The great ethical challenge raised by ICT for ageing is then that technology – which cannot always succeed in overcoming frailty –can more easily succeed in hiding frail people.

Out of sight, out of mind tells an old saying, which is particularly true in this case. During the Edo period in Japan, older people used to end their life by going to the mountains where they died for starvation. Japanese poets made tender, melancholic, poems of this collective suicide. Legends told dreadful stories of witches (mountain women, *yamamba*) who would come down to raid the towns for food and vengeance. The story was actually simpler and more trivial. In that period, people were very poor and faced hard times with limited resources. To survive, citizens banished the unproductive elderly, who were sent to die where no one could see them, where they could disappear without bothering. Modern ICT threatens to do the same. Technology could be used to create a dispersed, decentralized, system of "individual nursing homes" where frail people are destined to spend their last years of life, segregated by the human community, isolated into a technological prison made up by electronic bracelets, wireless sensors, networked communication, automatic supervisors, and robotic companions.

Free and informed consent requires as a precondition the possibility to make a choice between two or more options. Frail persons often live in contexts, and suffer from conditions, which make it impossible to take free and informed decisions, such as that of wearing a bracelet for monitoring movements or not, or to accept a robotic companion which is covertly monitoring health parameters. The possibility to choose fails when there is no other possibility. As happens in the medical field, the need for informed consent should never relieve decision takers from their moral and legal responsibility.

Recommendation no. 15: Independence, self-sufficiency, and autonomy of the frail person should never be turned into isolation and social invisibility. Investments in technology should not prevent promoting effective training of professionals and staff working with older persons and providing better assistance and services. Informed consent cannot be used as an alibi to avoid facing moral and legal responsibilities.

VIII. RECOMMENDATIONS

1. RECOMMENDATIONS FOR THE ALLOCATION OF BASIC RIGHTS, LIBERTIES, AND DUTIES

Recommendation no. 1 (from section 1): Ageing society is a chiefly social phenomenon, which implies a shift within different age groups in a society towards the older ones. At the individual level, ageing is about people living chronologically longer. The effect of ageing on people has more to do with the social context than with medical conditions. An ethical scrutiny of policies which address ageing should be based on a thoughtful distinction between biological and social facts.

Recommendation no. 2 (from section 2): Ageing always implies a certain weakening of the aged persons, and consequently modifies the power relations which affect them. An ethical analysis should consider the tension between individuals and the collective, and should address the change of power relations among actors.

Recommendation no. 3 (from section 2): The main sources of power are capacity for exchange and for coordination, which can be further turned into possession of time and possession of knowledge. Although largely illusory, time and knowledge are the most precious goods that human beings can ever possess, because they save humans from annihilation. It is an ethical tenet to avoid that any social dynamics create people that, for any reason, perceive themselves without time and knowledge.

Recommendation no. 4 (from section 3): In contemporary society, old people are increasingly people without time and knowledge. This makes it an ethical imperative to address their social role and functions, and to understand how they can be empowered.

2. RECOMMENDATIONS FOR THE ALLOCATION OF RESOURCES, NOTABLY ICT RESOURCES

Recommendation no. 5 (from section 3): Human flourishing and excellence have little to do with power fantasies. Technologies for human augmentation, including anti-ageing and rejuvenating technologies, cosmetic surgery, and medications, are ethically questionable inasmuch as they pretend to offer what they cannot deliver.

Recommendation no. 6 (from section 4): ICT can effectively address the two main issues related to ageing, say, the increasing population of frail old people, and the decrease in the proportion of people in the workforce. Reducing the social and economic burden carried by these two social trends is ethically tenable if it is part of larger strategy, which aims to reshape the old persons role and empower old people.

3. RECOMMENDATIONS FOR CREATING BINDING RELATIONSHIPS

Recommendation no. 7 (from section 5): From an ethical perspective reshaping the old person role means cancelling it altogether, because it no longer confers any kind of advantage to those who play it.

Recommendation no. 8 (from section 6): A new age category, the so called "extended middle age" group, is emerging, also in connection with the wider usage of ICT. Promoting their inclusion in the information society should be a pillar of the Ageing Well strategy.

Recommendation no. 9 (from section 6): All citizens should enjoy full social and economic rights independently from their age. People who belong to the "extended middle age" group should enjoy just and favourable conditions of work. Discriminatory practices on grounds of old age should be banned and ICT should be used to facilitate inclusive processes at work.

4. RECOMMENDATIONS FOR CHOOSING THE RIGHT ACTION

Recommendation no. 10 (from section 6): Lack of accessibility can become a serious barrier to the uptake of ICT in people belonging to the "extended middle age" group. An ethical approach to e-accessibility should be based on the preliminary fulfillment of a few basic requirements.

Recommendation no. 11 (from section 6): Self exclusion and social victimization are likely to be the most dangerous factors which may lead to a failure in e-Inclusion processes. The symbolic value of retirement should not be underestimated. In principle ICT should be used to turn retirement into an effective right, enjoyed by each person according to his own will and needs, instead of some pre-fixed schemes.

Recommendation no. 12 (from section 7): Frail, old, people are probably destined to exist notwithstanding any technological innovation. ICT can however play an essential role in empowering them and improving their quality of life. It is then paramount to invest resources and promote research in this field.

Recommendation 13 (from section 7): ICT for the elderly highlights the importance of creating trust. The breach of trust relations in the field of data protection is an offence to personal integrity and ultimately a form of elder abuse. Creating trust may require both new thinking in the area of private life/privacy and regulatory measures in terms of data protection.

Recommendation no. 14 (from section 7): Respect for personal integrity is the first ethical tenet when ICT is applied for improving older peoples quality of life at home. Assistive technology for ageing should allow people to live better and to prevent any form of degradation and humiliation.

Recommendation no. 15 (from section 7): Independence, self-sufficiency, and autonomy of the frail person should never be turned into isolation and social invisibility. Investments in technology should not prevent promoting effective training of professionals and staff working with older persons and providing better assistance and services. Informed consent cannot be used as an alibi to avoid facing moral and legal responsibilities.

REFERENCES

Agamben G, *Homo Sacer: Sovereign Power and Bare Life*, Stanford UP, Stanford, CA., 1988

Castells M, , *The Rise of the Network Society*, Blackwell, 1996,

Castoriadis, C., *The imaginary institution of society*, Cambridge, MA: *MIT* , 1987.

Cooke, B. and U. Kothari, 'Participation: The New Tyranny?', London: Zed., 2002.

Durkheim E, *The Rules of Sociological Method*, New York, The Free Press, 1938

Elias N, , *Time: an Essay*, Blackwell: Oxford, 1992.

Elias N, , *The Loneliness of the Dying*, Blackwell: Oxford, 1985.

Featherstone M., Hepworth M., ,The mask of ageing and the postmodern life course. In M. Featherstone, M. Hepworth, & B. S. Turner (Eds.), *The body: Social process and cultural theory*, Sage, London: 371–389, 1991

Fried LP., Tangen CM,   Walston J et al., , Frailty in Older Adults: Evidence for a Phenotype, *Journal of Gerontology: Medical Sciences*, 56a, 3: 146-157., 2001

Griffith, Mark, *Aeschylus' Prometheus Bound*, Cambridge: Cambridge UP, 1983.

Hart H.L.A., *Essays in Jurisprudence and Philosophy*, Oxford: Clarendon Press, 1983.

Herwartz H, Theilen B, 'The determinants of healthcare expenditure: new results from semiparametric estimation', *Health Economics*, Published Online: 7 Aug 2009 http://dx.doi.org/10.1002/hec.1540

Hopper, E., *The Social Unconscious: Selected Papers*, London: Jessica Kingsley, 2003.

Jameson, F., *The Political Unconscious: Narrative as a Socially Symbolic Act*, Ithaca, N.Y.: Cornell UP, 1981.

Jones RL, , 'Older people' talking as if they are not older people: Positioning theory as an explanation
Journal of Aging Studies, 20, 1: 79-91, 2006

Kass LR, Human Frailty and Human Dignity, *The New Atlantis*, 7, 110-118, 2004.

Maffesoli, M., 'The imaginary and the sacred in Durkheim's sociology', *Current Sociology,* 41(2), 1-5, 1993.

Maschke KJ, ,   Proxy Research Consent and the Decisionally Impaired: Science, the Common Good, and Bodily Integrity, *Journal of Disability Policy Studies* 13, 4, 2003.

Moore, B., Jr, *Privacy: Studies in Social and Cultural History*, Pantheon Books, 1984.

Mordini, E., 'L'Inconscio Sociale', *Rivista di Teologia Morale*, 110, 58-75, 1996.

Murray TH, , On the Human Body as Property: the Meaning of Embodiment, Markets, and The Need of Strangers, *Journal of Law Reform* 20, 4:1055-1089, 1987.

Rowlands, J. Questioning Empowerment: Working with Women in Honduras. Oxford, UK: Oxfam, 1997.

Scheff, Thomas, *Microsociology: Discourse, Emotion and Social Structure*, University of Chicago Press, 1990.

Schloendorff v. Society of New York Hospital, 1914, quoted by Maschke KJ, 2003.

Searle, J. *The Construction of Social Reality*. New York: The Free Press, 1995.

Taylor, C., 'Modern social imaginaries', *Public Culture* 14(1), 91-124, 1989.

White C, , Health Care Spending Growth: How Different Is the United States From the Rest of the OECD, *Health Affairs*, 26(1): 154-161, 2007.

European Commission, European i2010 initiative on e-Inclusion: 'To be part of the information society', Communication from the Commission to the European Parliament, the Council, the European Economic and Social Committee and the Committee of the Regions, COM(2007) 694 final, Brussels, 8 Nov 2007.

CONCLUSION: MAKING VISIBLE THE FRAIL AMONGST THE AGED

The book *Ageing and Invisibility* endeavoured to outline the salient ethical, social and legal issues raised and emerging in the European Union's Information Society strategy for the inclusion of older persons. Built on the research work carried out under the aegis of the FP7 support action *SENIOR project*, the book illustrated the genesis and the main policy references leading up and underpinning the EU e-inclusion strategy for the elderly (chapter I); it pondered critically on the meaning of getting old in highly technological societies (chapter II); it presented the legal references relevant for the governance of e-ageing in chapter III and leaned on the key notions of private life and consent (chapters IV and V, respectively); the book offered an overview of R&TD (chapter VI); discussed some good practices cases and assessed the value of good practices for e-inclusion (chapter VII); it eventually proposed a set of recommendations designed to help regulators navigate the development and implementation of ICT for the elderly (chapter VIII).

In guise of conclusion the authors would like to put forth a final reflection. In sum, it appears to us that political, social, and technological factors and developments concoct to remove the social role and the category of old age from society, because it no longer confers any kind of advantage to those who play it.[1] Such a removal takes place through replacement. Social, and technological factors already are contributing to creating a new age category, the so called "extended middle age" group, which is an age group between current retirement age (around 65 years) and the start of age related, severe, physical and mental illnesses and disabilities.[2]

Simply put, extended middle age effaces old age by trying to expand the boundaries of adult active life to the biological limits of senescence. Where extended middle age provides for the social form of older age life today, active ageing instils it with content. Basically, the meaning active ageing narratives, policies and initiatives offer is twofold. First, they encourage older or middle age citizens to carry on working, consuming, and also participating in cultural and social life as *if* they were active adult citizens and, second, they tend to eschew the norm of senescence, which by nature implies increased frailty and, to differing degrees, loss of social power. Active ageing narratives populate societies where the number of old and very old persons rapidly increase as a proportion of the whole population and are nourished and buttressed by networks of micro-politics operators, which include scientists, academic researchers, politicians, technology developers, psychologists, media gurus, personal coaches, publicists, film directors, medical doctors and so on.[3]

This book underlines the ambiguities of the concept of active ageing and the call for technology supporting it. On the one hand, active ageing policies and technologies may offer the extended middle age group the possibility to pick up new roles and embark on new jobs which will be necessary to sustain our longer – extended – lives, or to attend after ourselves without having to rely exclusively on external support. On the other hand, however, one ought to keep in mind that extending the boundaries of active life is hardly a neutral enterprise. Cultivated by public and private operators with vested interests or stuffed with benevolent intentions, the image of active life

---

[1] See recommendation n. 7, Chapter VIII.
[2] See recommendation n. 8, Ibid.
[3] See Chapter II.

very easily fall to the fallacy of youth at all costs and free of fetters. The other coin of rosy active ageing is bias toward natural ageing, and devalues of graying fading beauties, illness, lowliness and frailty. In the process, old age, its moral endurance and social role are lost.

In our view, active ageing should resist the fallacy which considers it positive, just as such, the conservation of active life. It should instead concentrate on helping those who, within society's older cohort, are most frail and in need of assistance. Crucially, the determination of who is frail and who is vulnerable, and the identification and allocation of the resources necessary to live the last years of one's life in dignity, will not come automatically. It is a matter of taking decisions which impinge on the private/public spheres of ageing: one's plans for later life are in fact affected by existing social and legal arrangements and by the accommodation a society is willing to lend to those who are frailer than the others.

The fallacy of staying young or adult for ever should be rejected as any practices or rules that normalise the experience of getting old by means of removal and though benevolent falsification. Least, failing to remain young is going to become a source of guilt and exclusion for a generation of misfit, unhappy senior citizens who, having tried all means to conceal ageing, and notwithstanding the availability of the technology, will become older.

In conclusion, the really frail are the focus of inclusion. Frailty is not only a condition that *calls for* moral action; it is also generating ethical *value*. First of all, frailty has an ethical dimension because it calls for protection, for help. In other words, it implies the ethics of reciprocity, in its simplest form as the golden rule: "*do to others what you would like to be done to you*". To be sure, there is no guarantee that such a call will be ever responded by someone. Yet it is the mere existence of a call for help, for justice, for protection, which poses the basic ethical issues of reciprocity, altruism, and mercy. In fact, as legal scholar Marta Nussbaum points out, 'usual human life cycle brings with it periods of extreme dependency, in which our functioning is very similar to that experienced by people with mental or physical disabilities throughout their lives.[4] Our own morality and rationality are themselves thoroughly material and animal. 'Disease, old age, and accident can impede the moral and rational functions, just as much as the other animal functions.'[5]

We agree with Nussbaum when she commends recognition of the "diverse frailties of humankind." Being frail and vulnerable is not an exceptional state for human beings (say, when they are older or ill). On the contrary humans are constitutively fragile, easily broken according to the etymology of the word "frail". There is a kind of frailty that is connected to the human essential structure, the awareness that they have of their finitude. Ancient Greeks called humans "mortals", in order to differentiate them from gods (the immortals) and beasts (living beings which are not aware to be mortal). One could say that to Greeks there were two kinds of immortality, the former concerned with an endless existence (gods) and the latter concerned with the lack of awareness of the unavoidability of the death (animals). Humans are then the sole "true" mortal beings, because they know to be mortal. The self consciousness of such a original frailty confers a special value to human beings, because it obliges them to deal with their finitude.[6] Frailty is therefore the true

---

[4] Martha C. Nussbaum, *Frontiers of Justice. Disability, Nationality, Species membership*, The Belknap Press of Harvard University Press, Cambridge (Mass), 2007, p.132-3.
[5] Ibid.
[6] This is also one of the main arguments developed by the ethics of proximity (e.g., Levinas) and feminist ethics of care.

hallmark of the human species, and can be considered as a true source of the somewhat controversial notion of "human dignity", a concept challenged by some as carrier of substantive assumptions.

From a legal perspective, we notice that the notion of dignity has earned approbation and praise since it was codified as the mother right in Article 1 of the 2000 Charter of Fundamental Rights of the European Union.[7] Before the Charter was promulgated the status of human dignity within human rights law was much less explicit. The concept was and still is absent in almost all Member State constitutions, except for the German one.[8] Also in the 1950 European Convention of Human Rights, which is a very straightforward human rights declaration devoid of metaphysical references, there is no general recognition of dignity or of a right to the protection of human dignity.

The difficulty to enforce rights and duties that are not properly internalised by legal subjects concerns also "dignity" when it surfaces in provisions such as article 25 of the EU Charter, "The rights of the elderly", which states that *The Union recognises and respects the rights of the elderly to lead a life of dignity and independence and to participate in social and cultural life.* It is unclear what leading a life of dignity means.

Better guidance can be gained reading article 25 together with article 7 and 8 of the Charter on privacy and data protection. These fundamental rights and the principles elaborated upon them by the European judge can be used to build a strong case to advocate, a) the development of initiatives and technology which are inclusive and accessible to older persons and, b) to protect against solutions and technology that is too intrusive, disciplinarian, and paternalistic.

Indeed, we have a moral and legal duty to reasonably assist, to provide access, and to accommodate problems such as care for children, for elderly people, and people with mental and physical disabilities, from the beginning, in the design of the basic institutional structure, as Nussbaum contends, as well as in the development of technology.

While doing so and when taking decisions, policy makers, law makers and in general all stakeholders and operators should refrain and resist paternalistic and infantilizing initiatives or technological developments which invade the intimate sphere of men and women and offend their dignity.

The proposals and recommendations about ageing and ICT contained in this book were conceived with these thoughts in mind.

---

[7] Article 1: Human dignity is inviolable. It must be respected and protected. Also, Preamble: 'The Union places the individual at the hearth of its activities.'

[8] The right to dignity is also mentioned in Section 10.1 of the Spanish 1978 Constitution but it is only one source of constitutionalism amongst others. Article 23 of the 1994 Belgian Constitution equally protects human dignity but this is tied to certain economic, social and cultural rights.

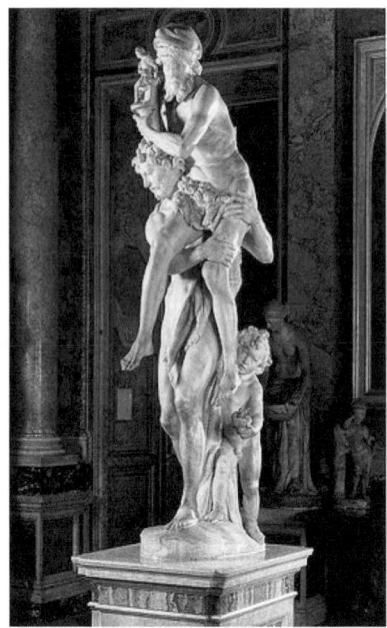

Gian Lorenzo Bernini
Aeneas, Anchises, and Ascanius, 1618–1619

"The group sculpture represents Aeneas fleeing from the burning city of Troy carrying his elderly father Anchises on his shoulders, and his son Ascanius following them. Anchises holds the 'penates' or family household gods." (Web Gallery of Art)

Image reproduced from Wikipedia Creative Commons. Permission: GFDL